MW01383108

A Professional Legacy:

The Eleanor Clarke Slagle Lectures in Occupational Therapy, 1955–1984

Library of Congress Cataloging in Publication Data
Main entry under title:

A Professional Legacy: The Eleanor Clarke Slagle Lectures in Occupational
Therapy

   1. Occupational therapy—Addresses, essays, lectures.
I. American Occupational Therapy Association.
RM735.36.P76   1984   615.8'5152   84-24159

ISBN 0-910317-11-9

Copies may be ordered from:
AOTA Products
The American Occupational Therapy Association
1383 Piccard Drive
Rockville, Maryland 20850

Contents

Foreword

This is a book for practitioners, educators, students—for all occupational therapy personnel. It contains scholarship, philosophy, history, and the wisdom of a distinguished group of individuals, the Eleanor Clarke Slagle Lecturers. Once a year, over a span of 30 years, one of these lecturers has publicly addressed a topic in occupational therapy. Collected here, their lectures form a unique record of the steady progress and increasing sophistication of occupational therapy. They offer a historical perspective and a base for discussion and reflection.

The history of a profession can help its practitioners relate to their field in its broadest context, and can help them define their professional commitment. Learning about the individuals who formed the history can also help practitioners define their commitment. The Slagle Lectures are part of the history of occupational therapy and the lecturers serve as exemplars, role models, or mentors, who by virtue of their character and performance can contribute to learning. The lessons they teach differ from those taught in textbooks; these individuals help to round out a person's education with the more personal lessons of human experience and wisdom.

The Eleanor Clarke Slagle Lectureship was established by AOTA in 1954 as a memorial to Mrs. Slagle, an outstanding pioneer in occupational therapy. The purpose of the lectureship is:

1. to honor a member of the Association who has creatively contributed to the development of the body of knowledge of the profession;
2. to acknowledge the development of improved methods and techniques in the practice of occupational therapy that improve service to clients or the public and that foster public awareness of the profession;
3. to recognize contributions to the profession made by or through research, education, and practice in occupational therapy;
4. to enable members to benefit from new or revised knowledge and developments in the profession; and
5. to give Occupational Therapists, Registered and Certified Occupational Therapy Assistants the opportunity to express and publish the results of their studies and to share their knowledge and experience with the membership.

Lecturers are chosen by the AOTA Recognitions Committee, which receives nominations from the general membership. Candidates qualify by making a significant contribution to the knowledge of the profession of occupational therapy either through the development or refinement of professional theory or techniques, or both, or through involvement in or completion of an outstanding research project. In addition, they have shared knowledge and inspired others through publications, workshops, lectures, seminars, and conference presentations. Each lecture is first presented at the AOTA Conference, and is then published in *The American Journal of Occupational Therapy*.

This volume presents 25 Eleanor Clarke Slagle Lectures, from the first one in 1955, through the 1984 lecture (no awards were made in 1963, 1967, 1969, 1977, and 1982). The first 15 lectures are reproduced from *The Eleanor Clarke Slagle Lectures 1955–1972*, a book published by AOTA in 1973, and no longer available. With one exception to correct an omission, no changes have been made from that volume. The remaining 10 lectures are published in book form for the first time here. The two sets of lectures differ in their appearance because old and new typefaces cannot be matched precisely, and costs prohibited resetting the early material. To make this volume more useful for those who will study the origins and development of leaders in the field, and to add to its historical value, biographies, bibliographies, and photographs of all the lecturers are included.

Eleanor Clarke Slagle was a role model for occupational therapists. She had a stake in shaping occupational therapy, and left a legacy of leadership, achievement, and inspiration. In her memory, this book aims to celebrate individual and collective achievement; to inspire by increasing awareness of the professional environment occupational therapists have created, developed, and improved; and to help readers appreciate the learning that is available beyond the textbook. This legacy is a nostalgic and valuable record of professional endeavor.

Biography of Eleanor Clarke Slagle

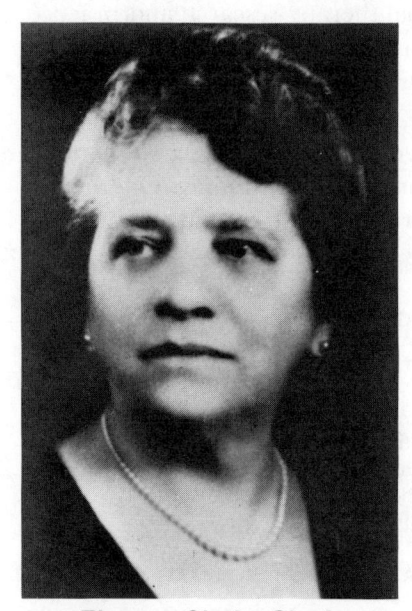

Eleanor Clarke Slagle
1876–1942

Eleanor Clarke Slagle was born in Hobart, New York in 1876, the daughter of the late William and Emmeline Davenport Clarke. She was the sister of John D. Clarke, who was a U.S. Congressman.

First educated by tutors, she then attended Claverack College, a summer school of Columbia University. She was graduated as a social worker from the Chicago School of Civics and Philanthropy, which eventually merged with the University of Chicago.

In 1909, she was a social worker under the direction of Jane Addams and Julia Lathrop who encouraged her interest in the then new field of occupational therapy. Slagle's interest stemmed from a chance visit to the Illinois state hospital at Kankakee. According to an article in the *Chicago American* (1939) at Kankakee she "found treatment and housing of the insane woefully inadequate. Mrs. Slagle saw an unkempt young woman surreptitiously raveling her undershirt from within her waist and with two straightened-out hairpins for needles, trying to knit a crude little shirt for a child. She spoke to the woman, 'That must be for your little girl, isn't it?' she asked. The woman's face lighted. 'I have four children,' she said and went back to her raveling." The article goes on to quote Slagle on the curative values of work and the benefits of activity that restores orientation or community consciousness. "Even if [the ill] were hopeless," she says "I felt that they might have a little happiness. Something of happiness is possible for anyone in any condition."

In 1913 Slagle became director of occupational therapy at Henry Phipps Psychiatric Clinic of the Johns Hopkins Hospital in Baltimore, Maryland. In 1917 she became director of the Henry B. Favill School of Occupation in Chicago where she conducted the first training courses in occupational therapy at Hull House. During the war years she was field supervisor of the reconstruction service, and from 1918 to 1922 she organized and directed occupational therapy research and practice for the State of Illinois. In 1922 she was appointed director of the New York State Department of Mental Hygiene, a position she held until her death in 1942.

An active leader in civic and suffrage movements, Slagle was a friend of Eleanor Roosevelt and the Theodore Roosevelt family. One of the founders of AOTA, she held office as President in 1920 and as Secretary-Treasurer from 1922–1937.

REFERENCES

Brunyate, RW: Powerful levers in little common things. The 1957 Eleanor Clarke Slagle Lecture, page 29, this volume
Cromwell, FS: Eleanor Clarke Slagle, the leader, the woman. *AJOT* 31:10, 645-648, 1977
Chicago American. Eleanor Clarke Slagle, occupational therapy founder, "back home" for convention. May or June 1939, further citation unavailable
New York Times. Mrs. Slagle dead, a therapy pioneer. September 20, 1942, p 41
Dept. of Public Welfare Bulletin 30:5, June 1939

RELATED READINGS

James, E (Editor): *Notable American Women, 1607-1950*, Volume III. Cambridge: Harvard Univ Press, 1971, p 296
Reed, KL, Sanderson SR: *Concepts of Occupational Therapy*, 2nd Edition. Baltimore: Williams and Wilkins, 1983, pp 198-199

The 1955 Eleanor Clarke Slagle Lecture

Equipment Designed for Occupational Therapy

Florence M. Stattel

It is difficult to find words that would adequately express my feeling and appreciation for the honor which you have extended to me in electing me to present the first Eleanor Clarke Slagle lecture. With deep humility and profound professional pride, I thank you for this privilege.

Occupational therapy had its conception in the faith and convictions of our early founders. It developed as a profession because of strong beliefs. Eleanor Clarke Slagle, along with the men and women who shared her convictions, is responsible for our presence here today as the American Occupational Therapy Association. We have been given a wonderful professional heritage of courage and wisdom and as we continue to extend our hand to benefit mankind, may we continue to believe and search for further knowledge.

This knowledge, in our present age, can be secured by correlating and strengthening our beliefs with facts. Empirical methods should be tested when possible, and reasonable doubt should be eliminated. When we consider beliefs we find that they are formations of ideas. Most ideas are really very old. They are rediscovered and formulated and incorporated into one's philosophy and thinking. New ideas are rare, and in a lifetime few individuals are fortunate to accumulate them in even single numbers. In preparing this paper on equipment designed for occupational therapy, it is important to note that the ideas may be old. The newness lies in the formulation of the

Reprinted from *The American Journal of Occupational Therapy*, Vol. X, No. 4, Part II, 1956.

idea into equipment that has a purposeful use in occupational therapy. The keynote to good design of any type is simplicity that will afford real and effectual usefulness. The refinement of design, structure and engineering aspects of the equipment to be discussed were achieved by close cooperation and consultation with the Franklin Hospital Equipment Company and their staff of technical experts. Three pieces of equipment will be discussed in this paper:

1. Tilt table
2. Standing table
3. Bilateral tilt tables

The first two pieces of equipment you are no doubt familiar with. The tilt table and the standing table will be discussed briefly in relation to the design which has afforded broader usefulness in occupational therapy. The major portion of the lecture will be devoted to the thinking behind the design and use of the bilateral tilt tables, which are a new treatment concept.

Tilt Table

In recent years we have been increasingly aware of the emphasis which the medical profession has placed on early weight bearing and ambulation. Man's physiological functions improve when he is in an upright position and his mental attitude is often reflected in improved behavior. The physiological and psychological importance of the vertical position is equally important to all patients ranging from the temporarily disabled to the permanently disabled.

The tilt table is familiar to you. It is a piece of equipment that permits the patient to be gradually elevated to the supported upright position with full weight bearing. Orthopedists have long reported the importance of weight bearing on the long bones of the body to prevent osteoporosis. Neurologists indicate the reinforcement of complex series of reflexes called postural reflexes which control muscle groups so that the upright position can be maintained. Hellebrandt and associates, (1) in 1949, reported on the effects on the cardiovascular respiratory systems and the action of the heart in preventing gravity shock when subjects were gradually brought from a horizontal to a semi-vertical position. As we go through the list of medical specialists, to name a few: the urologist, plastic surgeon, cardiologist, internist, we find further agreement as to the physiological improvement associated with the upright position.

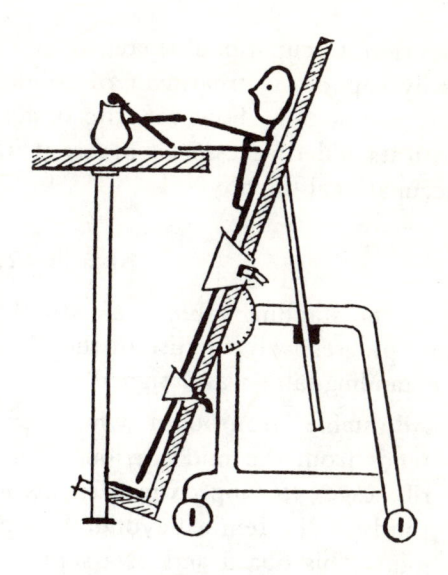

Figure 1. Tilt table—secures correct body positioning, frees upper extremities for treatment activities.

Prescribed degrees of angulation and time are indicated by the physician in the use of the tilt table. The physical therapist reports increased time and angulation tolerance in the severely involved cases. When the patient has been stabilized at a particular angle and can work in that position using his upper extremities, he can be wheeled on the tilt table into occupational therapy. In cases that are routine, without precautionary factors, the patient can be started on the tilt table for the time prescribed by the physician. The *availability of a tilt table with wheels which incorporates a secure lock device,* and the *attachment of suspension slings,* broadens the uses of this piece of equipment and makes it valuable in occupational therapy.

Many patients who normally would not be referred for early treatment in occupational therapy can be started on programs of early specific exercise and self care. The effect upon the patient when he is employed in an activity instead of being a spectator is instantaneous. To name a few diagnoses which can benefit by the use of the tilt table in occupational therapy: quadriplegics, rheumatoid arthritics, muscular dystrophics, multiple sclerotics and cardiacs.

The tilt table permits the exercise of the upper extremities and the skeletal muscle from the waist up. This increases muscular activity, forces the blood through vertical channels, increases heart rate and metabolic processes. For the severely disabled patient, permanent or progressive, it provides psychological as well as physiological benefits in being changed from the supine to the supported upright position. Occupational therapists have long related the use of the full body support in treatment of children in the vertical position. The idea is not new; however, the design and mobility of the tilt table with its added accessories makes it invaluable in broad usefulness in occupational therapy.

Standing Table

The standing table is a natural piece of equipment which follows progressively the use of the tilt table in treatment. This particular standing table was designed to consider the following:

1. Adjustable frontboard which extends from the mid portion of the rib cage to approximately two-thirds of the femur beyond the hip joint. This board acts as a support to the abdominal muscles and diaphragm when the pelvic support is adjusted. In the lower extremities it prevents and corrects flexion contractures due to muscle tightness or spasm;

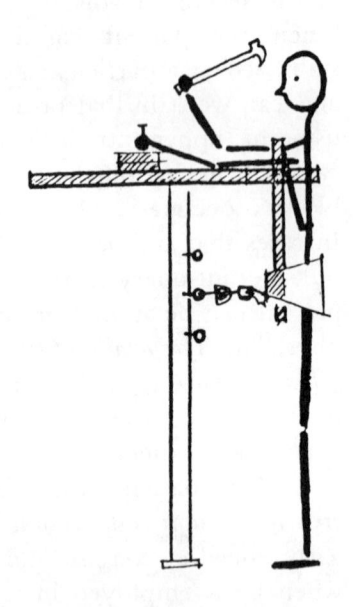

2. Adjustable elbow supports are provided for quadriplegic, ataxic and other patients who need support for anterior, posterior and lateral balance. These elbow supports are not for body weight bearing but for shoulder and shoulder girdle support;

3. The table is firmly bolted to the floor or a planked platform and affords structural security for the patient. A height of 46" from the floor is suggested;

Figure 2. Standing table—frontboard, elbow supports and pelvic band aid in body positioning and stability when standing.

4. The pelvic support is a heavy canvas binder with a leather strap end which snaps, with a double and nautical sail buckle, to one of three eyelets on the metal upright of the table. This support tilts and stabilizes the pelvis against the frontboard. When the feet are

spread to provide a broad base, this stabilization provides correct positioning and enables the patient to use his upper extremities freely.

The table has been used successfully with and without pelvic support. When the support is not used, anterior/posterior balance may be the prime objective. When there is a loss of one or more extremities or where a neuromuscular dysfunction exists, balance must be considered in body compensations. Brunnstrom's (2) article on "The Center of Gravity Line in Relation to the Ankle Joint in Erect Standing" is recommended reading on the subject of posture. Occupational therapists should be aware of the body mechanics involved in maintaining the upright position, as the stability or instability influences the usefulness of the upper extremities in purposeful activities in self care and vocational objectives.

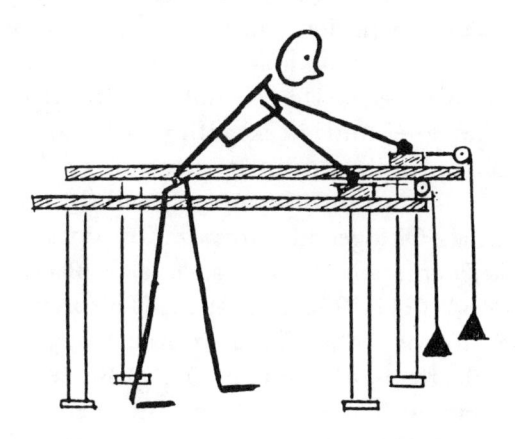

Figure 3. Bilateral tilt tables—alternate bilateral exercise, broad base.

Bilateral Tilt Tables

This piece of equipment is new in design and incorporates the use in exercise of unilateral, bilateral, reciprocal and alternate motions and considers the total body concept in treatment.

For centuries man has postulated on the relationship of mind and body, and sought answers in the study of the physical and psychic development of man. An awareness of the natural process of

physical and mental growth has resulted in consideration of treatment of the total man rather than in single entities. This is further
reflected in the term neuromuscular, which denotes the close integration of neurology and kinesiology. The exercise treatment of the
isolated muscle has been challenged repeatedly as a physiological
impossibility. More and more attention is being devoted to movements and patterns of movements.

In a newborn baby, movements and patterns of movements are
exhibited entirely by reflex. Ford (3) states that a number of these
motor reactions are present in the first few months when they are
not inhibited by cerebral function. When volitional activity develops
the reflex reactions are obscured. These reactions may be elicited
thereafter only in pathological conditions. The neurologists know
that at birth the anatomical development of the nervous system is
not complete. In 1950, Gesell (4) reported on "Tonic-Neck Reflex
and Symmetro-Tonic Behavior." In his comment he states "In spite
of his bilateral construction, man does not face the world on a
frontal plane of symmetry. He generally confronts it on an angle."
He also felt that the tonic-neck reflex behavior reflected three
important principles of development; principle of developmental direction, principle of functional asymmetry and the principle of reciprocal interweaving. Ontogenous organization does not move along
evenly. Periodic fluctuation of dominance takes place.

In the period 1947-1950 and 1951, Hellebrandt and her associates reported on cross education as related to contralateral, homo-
lateral, ipsilateral effects of exercise. (5,6,7) Bilateral, unilateral, alternate and reciporcal exercises were studied to observe the
functional capacity. The vast amount of work covered in these three
papers cannot be condensed and they are references for further
thought. For the purposes of this lecture, selected comments are
brought in to illustrate the influence this work had on the design of
the bilateral tilt tables. The therapeutic use of cross education was
indicated and the validity of the single muscle test was questioned
when considered as a criterion of functional capacity. In the study of
bilateral, unilateral, alternate and reciprocal exercise, the effect of
the exercise on the functional capacity of the weakened limb was
noted. Contractile power and endurance was reportedly increased.
The report of 1951 indicated the lack of justification of limiting
treatment to the affected side. Hellebrandt referred to postural

reflexes as reported by Magnus and Walshe. Reciprocal and alternate exercise and the influence of facilitating mechanisms were considered. In the subjects used for the study it was noted that some gave up because of psychological and not physiological reasons and the reverse was also true. The body will follow the dictates of the mind and the mind will follow the dictates of the body when it is fatigued but the subject controls both and close observation was made to detect differences. In 1952, Levine and Kabat (8) reported on the "Dynamics of Normal Voluntary Motion in Man." The concept that we must think of movement rather than isolated muscle activity was presented. Interdependence of distantly located muscles was stressed. Significant to the bilateral tilt tables was the report that inherent in all movements is the inclusion of the rotation of the trunk and pelvis. Levine and Kabat discussed the purpose of maximum achievement with importance of proprioception, patterns of movement and cocontractions in voluntary movement in man. Eberhard, Inman and Bresler, 1954, (9) in the study on locomotion, report that muscles do not act in the traditional anatomical sense, they fit into the whole pattern of motion. In walking there is rotation of the trunk and pelvis and independent of this, rotation of the femur and tibia.

The premise for the functional design and use of the bilateral tilt tables evolved from the above readings and clinical observation of patients in occupational therapy and are listed as follows:

1. Reflex patterns of movement that are present at birth and are lost when voluntary activity takes over can be elicited in pathological conditions;
2. Functional asymmetric development is found in man and reciprocal correspondence or interweaving of opposite sides takes place;
3. Contractile power and endurance of muscles could be increased by use of bilateral and unilateral alternate and reciprocal exercise, in prescribed rhythmic beat and maximum resistance;
4. Rotation of the trunk and pelvis are inherent in all movements;
5. In locomotion, muscles tend to fit into the whole pattern of motion rather than function in the traditional anatomical sense.

The tables were constructed to permit adequate space for standing or sitting. The tilt is provided by the telescoping mechanism on the forward portion of the tables which permits an angulation of 45°. A series of twenty-one adjustments permit the desired range of motion of the extremities from 0° to over 90° starting from the horizontal position. Surface of the table is a plastic non-friction finish. Full width clamps slide together to wedge and hold project or work of the patient. Small end clamps with pulleys permit the occupational therapist to add resistance or assistance in particular movements. Attachments for a belt support are provided on the stable, upright posts. An audiovisual metronome can be used to establish the rate of speed at which the patient can work and to have a check on the amount of exercise accomplished.

The positions of the feet when standing are:

1. Standing, feet close together—small base;
2. Standing, feet spread—broad base;
3. Standing, one foot ahead of other in pace position.

Exercise patterns of the upper extremities:

1. Unilateral—pertaining to one side;
2. Bilateral—pertaining to both sides;
3. Alternate—complete pattern of movement on one side one or more times; complete pattern of movement on the opposite side, one or more times. Complete pattern of movement on both sides;
4. Reciprocal flow of exercise from one side to another in a continuous pattern of movement. Flow of continuous pattern of movement on one side.

Position of head:

1. Directed toward the involved extremity to reinforce extension pattern;
2. Directed away from the involved extremity to reinforce flexion pattern;
3. Head in mid position.

In occupational therapy many activities are bilateral and unilateral. In the use of these tables, woodworking, weaving and ceramics have been set up in the exercise patterns described above. Finger painting has also worked out successfully. The element of interest which is stimulated by the craft acts as a motivation for the patient to work and achieve and the sometimes inhibiting psychological factor is less apparent.

The audiovisual metronome was mentioned earlier. This instrument provides a sound beat and a simultaneous flash of light. To the patient who has extensive cerebral damage it is advisable to present as many stimuli as possible and this instrument can be used to present this stimulation. The eyes and ears are in this instance reached and the pattern of movement is established along with the stimulus. In all instances it can be used to establish the speed and endurance of a patient to a particular exercise; for example, the patient is set up at the bilateral tilt tables in a selected position, the metronome is set for 40 strokes a minute. If the exercise is unilateral, the 40 strokes would indicate the amount of exercise; if the exercise was bilateral, it

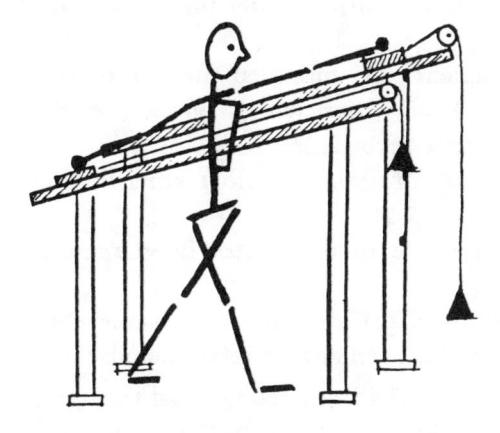

Figure 4. Bilateral tilt tables—reciprocal bilateral exercise, pace position.

would indicate that 20 strokes for each extremity had been accomplished. By setting a timer the occupational therapist could be certain how much the patient had accomplished in exercise at the end of one, five or ten minutes or more. The metronome can often be used to set the exercise pace and through its use it is possible for the patient to maintain the established rhythm.

In preparing this paper, an attempt has been made to cover a vast amount of material which represents condensed thinking. The bilateral tilt tables and the premise on which they were designed are presented. The piece of equipment now needs testing in clinical application to remove reasonable doubt and provide facts in terms of its usefulness. It also needs further exploration as to its functional value in other than the physical disability field.

Some of the thoughts that were postulated when the bilateral tilt tables were completed, were as follows:

1. *Mentally Ill.* Would the physical approach in calling into action the primitive pattern of movement be beneficial to the mentally ill patient?

   Would the audiovisual metronome assist in establishing early rhythmic patterns of movement in craft activities with varied tempo and duration?

2. *Cardiac, Tuberculosis.* Can improved work classifications result in timed, specific work output under supervision of the occupational therapist?

   Could vital capacity be improved through prescribed, closely observed, selected activities which would be closely timed and amount of exercise recorded?

3. *Prevocational Exploration.* Should testing be done in patterns of movements?

   Would it be possible to test motor fatigue and gauge sensory fatigue?

   Would minimum effort and maximum achievement result in analyzing patterns of movements in job demands?

As each selected field of occupational therapy seeks to improve its clinical application, it is earnestly hoped that more questions will be the result. Study of the vast amount of material that is available in the medical field will result in research that will bring answers and improved treatment techniques in occupational therapy. Our educational backgrounds provide us with a basic philosophy along with knowledge and skill to carry it out. Some occupational therapists have selected the psychiatric field, others the tuberculosis field and so on down the list of specialties. Their efforts in selected fields have increased their knowledge and skill in that field. However, it must be remembered that any knowledge or information in any specialty field is related to helping the human being. Our basic philosophy in occupational therapy embraces in treatment the physical and emotional makeup of the total person. With this thought in mind we are all occupational therapists first, reduced from our specialties by the common denominator, the human being who needs our help.

Early in this paper the beliefs of the pioneers in our profession were mentioned. Our profession is a stimulating and deeply satisfying one, which has grown because of our individual and united beliefs. It is sincerely hoped that this lecture will stimulate broad thinking and that indications of individual and group studies of professional importance will develop; that the growth of a national research laboratory in occupational therapy will result as in individual instances and as an organization, we continue to extend our hand to benefit mankind as we search for knowledge.

REFERENCES

1. Hellebrandt, F.A. and Associates, "The Relative Importance of the Muscle Pump in the Prevention of Gravity Shock," *The Physical Therapy Review*, Vol. 29, No. 1, Jan., 1949.
2. Brunnstrom, Signe, "Center of Gravity Line in Relation to the Ankle Joint in Erect Standing," *The Physical Therapy Review*, Vol. 34, No. 3, March, 1954.
3. Ford, Frank R., M.D., *Diseases of the Nervous System in Infancy, Childhood and Adolescence*, Springfield, Ill.; Charles Thomas, 1952.
4. Gesell, Arnold, M.D., Ames, Louise, Ph.D., "Tonic-Neck Reflex and Symmetro Tonic Behavior," *The Journal of Pediatrics*, Vol. 36, No. 2, Feb., 1950.
5. Hellebrandt, F.A., M.D., Parrish, Annie M., Houtz, Sara Jane, "The Influence of Unilateral Exercise on the Contralateral Limb," *Archives of Physical Medicine*, Vol. 28, Feb., 1947.
6. Hellebrandt, F.A., M.D., Houtz, Sara Jane, "Influence of Bimanual Exercise on Unilateral Work Capacity," *Journal of Applied Physiology*, Vol. 2, No. 8, Feb., 1950.
7. Hellebrandt, F.A., M.D., "Ipsilateral and Contralateral Effects of Unimanual Training," *Journal of Applied Physiology*, Vol. 4, No. 2, Aug., 1951.
8. Levine, Milton G., Ph.D., Kabat, Herman, M.D., "Dynamics of Normal Voluntary Motion in Man," *Permante Foundation Medical Bulletin*, Vol. 10, 1-4, Aug., 1952.
9. Klopsteg, Paul E., Ph.D., Wilson, Philip D., M.D., *Human Limbs and Their Substitutes*, New York: McGraw-Hill Company, Inc., 1954, Chapt. 15, p. 437.

BIBLIOGRAPHY

Floyd, W.F., Welford, A.T., *Human Factors in Equipment Design*, London: H.K. Lewis and Co., Ltd., 1953.
———, *Fatigue*, London: H.K. Lewis and Co., Ltd., 1953.
Levens, A.S., Inman, V.T., and Blosser, J.A., "Transverse Rotation of the Segments of the Lower Extremity in Locomotion," *Journal of Bone and Joint Surgery*, 30A:859, 1948.
Magnus, R., *Korperstellung*, Berlin: Julius Springer, 1924 (Sectional translation by Signe Brunnstrom).

Therapist into Administrator
Ten Inspiring Years

June Sokolov

Foreword

To my peers and colleagues: You have seen fit to confer upon me a high award, the symbol of your respect and affection. I have been awed by this honor. I spent many hours deliberating a fitting subject for my discourse with you today and settled finally, not without some misgiving, upon the core of those philosophical beliefs which have been tempered during the past ten rewarding years of practice as a therapist and administrator. I am not an innovator; what I say here is far from new. I would only have you know that what I humbly share with you is representative of the deepest convictions I hold as a therapist, as an administrator, as a human being.

* * * *

Therapist into Administrator
Ten Tempering Years

Some ten years ago the writer sat in a classroom attempting to assimilate and commit to indelible memory an impossible array of facts about the practice of occupational therapy. We were being prepared, in time-honored fashion, for the registration examination. From today's vantage point it is difficult to refrain from comparing that process with those rituals which accompany tribal customs. Certainly we resembled the uninitiated in all respects too closely for the comfort of either teachers or pupils.

Reprinted from *The American Journal of Occupational Therapy,* Vol. XI, No. 1, 1957.

Today, undeniably older if questionably better informed as a result of exposure to practical considerations, it is possible to recognize with some degree of equanimity that the makers of that first registration examination undoubtedly faced its trial run with something of the same apprehension that dogged the students who were soon to provide the test of its validity. However, ten years ago, such reasoning was at least temporarily denied to me. I could sense only considerable foreboding, reproach myself for my lack of faith in teachers and God and return to the fine print of the almighty text books there to search unremittingly for the meanings to puzzles which persisted in eluding me. What accounted for the sudden and bewildering synergistic action of a muscle which, up to a point, had behaved in calculable fashion as a prime mover? What nature of chemical compound was known to remove printer's ink from some spot where it had no official business? (And, wouldn't it be more efficacious in this instance to remove one's offending self from the premises as rapidly as possible?) What precautions did one observe with a sixty-five-year-old hemiplegic complicated by total aphasia, cardiac insufficiency and diabetes mellitus? Or, more to the point, what kind of occupational therapy program did one offer because, of course, there had to be one. This major faith, at least, in the unlimited scope and authority of one's chosen profession was unshakable.

So we pondered the technicalities of our profession, secure only in the one, irrefutable fact that all this was worthwhile and even possible because it would eventually permit us to realize our common aim of helping people to help themselves. What a rude surprise then, as we sat in that relatively peaceful classroom, to be singled out for the prediction that within three years' time I should have left the practice of occupational therapy for the province of administration. Impossible! Cold, forbidding word and world of topside decision and responsibility, devoid of all patient—nay, all human contact. How could one help but react with immediate rejection of such a fate. This could not happen to me. I wanted nothing to do with boards and committees, community action, finances, services and all the rigamarole of executive responsibility. I wanted to work with people. (Heaven forgive me and ascribe to the naivete of youth my repudiation of communities and their citizenry as something other than people. For among these were later to be found the generous affirmation of a personal faith.)

I have wondered since how many young people draw the same faulty inference. And, if they do, may our incorrect assumptions be traced to certain common administrative practices we meet as we move toward maturity and responsibility, as well as to our human way of prejudicing a situation by seeing it in the narrow framework of imperfect knowledge rather than against the unlimited horizon we can flush with a little vision.

The predictions of our teacher were painfully accurate. Were I not so well acquainted with her discerning and judicious approach to life, I might well have suspected her of consulting a crystal ball or dabbling in extra-sensory perception. Almost three years to the day after taking up my duties as an occupational therapist, I found myself involved in administrative functions and by the time five additional years had elapsed, this had become the provocative and rewarding substance of my working existence.

I have no inclination here to propound the role of the administrator in scholarly or detailed fashion. The accepted texts devoted to this subject are adequate if not overwhelming. It shall be my pleasure (and yours, I hope) to dwell for a while on the art of administration which is essentially an art of working with people to encourage and assure those personal and group satisfactions which tend to result in affirmative, effective performance.

The great American myth of the push-button executive to the contrary, executives in social agencies, at any rate, must work chiefly with and through people. Some measure of their success may be noted in the degree to which this capacity for working through the medium of people bears fruit in the improved and even inspired performance of staff and the consequent greater good that accrues to those served. Obviously, we subscribe to a definition of success which pivots upon the quality of our human relationships. We are not primarily concerned with the size and scope of endeavors, the number and variety of personnel, the roster of services, the soaring annual budget, indicative as these may be of growth and development. Such attributes seem to be all too easily come by in an era of prosperity when rehabilitation of the ill and injured receives almost as much daily attention from the press as the political scene receives in an election year. The trick becomes how to avoid a mushrooming growth and hold to a realistic operation, a qualitative service, to moderate change that suits the circumstances and is not dictated by the artificial stimulus of a current trend.

What, then, are some of the values one perceives, infers and confirms in the process of working with and through people to achieve group goals.

If one tends to be inherently a "doer," a prime but difficult lesson to master and practice is the restraint and rechanneling of energies. The goal changes from personal performance to eliciting increased assumption of responsibility from others. For many people (therapists not excepted) doing comes easier than talking about it. In consequence, we may resort to showing or performing rather than sketching in a backdrop or opening a door, as it were. As has been said, a good teacher is one who leads the pupil to the threshold of his own mind and bids him enter. While more difficult to achieve, this is the procedure of choice and tends to insure more lasting satisfactions and greater gains in personal stature.

In any case, the pangs of relinquishing proof of personal competence are lessened at the earliest observation of staff satisfactions. And these staff satisfactions are the natural corollary of expanded horizons and the chance to come to grips with new and more challenging responsibilities. The first time one is suffused in a glow of pure pleasure because a staff member has ventured into new and untried territory to emerge either bruised and questioning or victorious and wiser, becomes the memorable date of a new romance with the art of administration. This is the moment when one feels the bite of conviction and knows where the greatest rewards will henceforth lie.

We hear frequently that young people of today do not crave responsibility—that they seek freedom from the burden of responsible choice and decision. As always, one does well to be chary of such generalizations. In those rare cases where the glove fits, we should perhaps be quicker to recognize true personality disturbances instead of chalking the response up as yet another "sign of the times." In our admittedly limited experience, an atmosphere in which the premium is placed on achieving personal satisfaction through exploring, investigating, making mistakes, finding out why, pooling group thinking and reaching out constantly to new accomplishment in the name of commonly cherished ideals, exerts the irresistible tug of a strong current and carries the worker with it magnetically. There is no substitute for the exercise of reason and self-trust and the reward thereof is constant. Given the basic aim of wanting to help people help themselves, human beings tend to gravitate toward those ways of life which promise to transform their intangible aims into realities. The administrator is on the scene to provide this opportunity, to set the stage for personal growth and to allow the accomplishment of group and agency objectives. How does he go about his role of catalyst?

One significant contribution he can make is to free the work atmosphere of irritating fears and tensions. We readily acknowledge that no one works successfully or happily in an atmosphere charged with constant anxiety or apprehension. Yet the evidences of such circumstances are legion. The writer has frequently been called on to define and analyze the reasons for ineffectual performance and poor standards of work, only to find that something akin to staff demoralization exists which freezes into immobility every healthy human and professional impulse. A change of leadership is contemplated, staff cutbacks are being considered, financial problems loom, a new order is in the making but no one has thought it necessary or fitting to discuss these crucial problems with the people intimately concerned. An undertow of panic results.

Let us illustrate the administrative function in such a situation. A new worker has been added to a well-integrated and functioning staff. This worker has left a secure position in the highly organized and orthodox field of education to seek new opportunities and horizons in the field of rehabilitation. He represents an unexplored aspect of service in the agency and brings with him a host of techniques, talents, beliefs, practices and prejudices which are new to the staff. He brings with him, also, a natural concern about the merits of his decision which was perhaps arrived at somewhat rapidly. It seemed like a good idea at the time. After a few days in a totally new environment and some encounters with unfamiliar practices, he's not so sure. During the orientation to the agency's services and the people behind them, it becomes fairly obvious that he is unable to listen, absorb, assimilate. He appears preoccupied, concerned with other things. He catches at details and misses concepts—sees the grain of sand but not the world mirrored therein. These symptoms readily communicate themselves to other staff members. Mental images are stored, calculations and reservations are made. It is time for administration to intervene in an attempt to rectify the situation before the staff begins to reflect an established group attitude which is apt to anchor these early responses. Informal conferences with the worker are aimed at clearing the air. These are not effective. The administrator takes another avenue. He consults with supervisory staff (department heads) about the problem. The possible and probable causes of the worker's reactions are weighed and considered and a potentially influential group attitude is forged. The staff concludes that the new worker deserves all the help they can muster to convert his energies and will to the job at hand. They agree that his unease is, undoubtedly, temporary. To a man, they go forth determined to offer extra assistance, encouragement and support to help channel responses and criticisms to appropriate sources for consideration. Within a very brief period results may be measured in the new staff member's relaxed manner, receptiveness to suggestion and participation in group thinking and planning. After a month or two, he is working with obvious satisfaction and making a substantial contribution to the agency's objectives in terms of his personal endowment. A group of people who have worked toward and achieved a common set of goals have succeeded in communicating their good-will, enthusiasm and positive experience to another human being. The link is forged into the chain. Administration has helped to refocus group energies on meeting client needs. Similar examples abound. Every department, every agency is the scene of innumerable tensions, group and personal. They are a part of the fabric of existence and no more to be frowned upon than the rind we discard with the eating of an orange. But they must be recognized and evaluated for potential damage. Sensitivity to impressions, recognition of a disturbed environment, proper timing, analysis of the problem and bringing to bear upon it the powerful antidote of group acceptance are implicit in the administrative function.

The cultivation of impressions or intuitions is worth a moment's digression. While we may not rely indiscriminately upon a single impression, many such perceptions constitute the genesis of all ideas, the basis for achievement. Henry James has summed this up exquisitely in *The Art of Fiction and Other Essays*. (1) He discusses the business of writing from experience and says, "Experience is never complete; it is an immense sensibility, a kind of huge spiderweb of the finest silken threads suspended in the chamber of consciousness and catching every air-borne particle in its tissue. It is the very atmosphere of the mind; and when the mind is imaginative—much more when it happens to be that of a man of genius—it takes to itself the faintest hints of life, it converts the very pulses of the air into revelations. The power to guess the unseen from the seen, to trace the implications of things, to judge the whole piece by the pattern, the condition of feeling life in general so completely that you are well on your way to knowing any particular corner of it—this cluster of gifts may almost be said to constitute experience . . . If experience consists of impressions, it may be said that impressions are experience, just as they are the very air we breathe . . ." And he goes on to admonish "Try to be one of the people on whom nothing is lost." (2)

One of the major fears which confront occupational therapists as administrators is an expressed or implied fear about the value of occupational therapy itself. Like most fears, this one if suspected must be taken out and viewed in that strong daylight which does so much to dispel shadows and reduce problems to size. Conversely, when it has been examined and analyzed for the benefit of all concerned, doubt and distrust should be dispersed by the active, intensive and changing practice of our profession. The Overstreets speak convincingly of learning to call an episode finished when it is over with, and label this "the art of rescuing the present and the future from the tyranny of the past." (2) If occupational therapists persist in some of the breastbeating and loud self-recrimination which have attended us too regularly in the past eight to ten years, we cannot expect the world to look upon us with either respect or trust. No one denies that we must examine the reasons which invest our practices. We might, however, do well to remember that T.V. Smith, the eminent philosopher, upon his retirement thanked God publicly for the right of old age to "withstand all easy commitment." "All my life," says Mr. Smith, "I have been abashed at having to decide things in the name of reason for which there were no adequate reasons. I know there were not, because equally reasonable men are always deciding such things differently. And the more important the issues, the more differently they get decided. . . . Indeed, I myself incline to the view . . . that there are never adequate reasons for doing anything." (3)

All of us have heard and perhaps uttered the cry of frailty:

occupational therapy will not live to see another decade if it is not perfected as a science; if we do not recruit more therapists; if we do not settle the problem of unregistered personnel. All these qualifications are dependent on which crisis looms largest in the group addressing itself to the problem of our future. These are problems we must deal with, yes, but they do not constitute a final threat to the life and vitality of occupational therapy any more than the rising cancer rate threatens the life or continuous practice of medicine or the hazards of the road threaten the use of the automobile. The seriously debilitating factor is our own lack of faith and conviction about what occupational therapy has to offer the patient. Nothing will erase this basic fault except the cultivation and practice of a genuine belief and its substantiation in the daily revelation of efficacy.

A good deal of our discomfort and uneasiness may stem from the fact that we, along with other disciplines, are living through an attempt at conversion to a more exact science. This is a painful process at best and can be devastating to a profession burdened with amorphous beginnings which lend themselves all too easily, in the hands of the unselective, to branding occupational therapists with currently unacceptable labels, such as "do-gooders."

Daily we are impressed with the revival of interest in religion, the revanescence of handcrafts, the renewed emphasis on a liberal arts education. All about us are signs of the swing of the pendulum from crass materialism to a renewed acknowledgment of man's continuing need for human kindness and compassion, for individual creative effort. What could be more reassuring to people engaged in the practice of healing through doing?

With an apology to our psychiatric colleagues who, I suspect, have always known and held to this conviction, it behooves us to emphasize and underscore the significance of effective human relationships implicit in the practice of occupational therapy whether we are talking to a physiatrist or a psychiatrist. Regardless of our tools, it is primarily by virtue of our interest, enthusiasm and concern that we shall bridge the chasm of illness to draw the patient back into the mainstream of active participation which signifies the return to life and hope.

This is in no sense a repudiation of the effort to improve our practices, sharpen our professional tools, better our methods of work. It is dictated by a deep-seated belief that the medium we use is always secondary to the motives and drives which direct our actions.

The administrator becomes an important avenue for the unequivocal voicing of such sentiments since his attitudes and beliefs will unfailingly be sensed and transmitted to the staff. His is the job, then, of conditioning the atmosphere so that unspoken fears may be voiced, group attitudes reshaped and fused, healing action taken to correct the profound debilitation caused by irritating doubt.

Patient evaluation sessions, used as a teaching device, may provide a useful vehicle for crystallizing group attitudes about occupational therapy. It is more than a passing impression that, given the opportunity to comment on the function of occupational therapy, the therapist too often remains passive and silent only to fester later under an impossible assignment doled out by the attending physician. Administration has a responsibility for overcoming such deadlocks. A leading question directed to the physician, the therapist or both, may instigate the conversational give and take that is essential to the forging of individual ideas, the art of selling them to others, the grace of retreating with good countenance and heart when fairly defeated and the satisfaction of having actively contributed to decisions about the purpose and function of one's own metier. The old, if somewhat impertinent, remark about "put up or shut up" has its merits applied to this situation. Staff members must learn to charge, parry, thrust, defend or retreat in the intellectual arena much as they have previously learned the rules of the game in the sports arena.

Clearing the air of basic fears about the value of occupational therapy is an on-going process. Self-recrimination should give way to the more purposeful activity of meeting problems as they arise for these are the stuff of life and ours the incomparable privilege of rising to their eternal challenge.

The art of administration supposes, also, acknowledgment and cultivation of an atmosphere in which a premium is placed on the making of courageous errors. We do well to recall often the sense of peace and freedom to be found in reviewing our identification with the family of man, that curious groper after knowledge, that colossal maker of mistakes. How comforting to know that one is entitled to try and fail, that it is upon this shifting foundation that all human advances are achieved. From "The Mind Goes Forth," we take heart in the following quotation: "The deeply civil person knows life as imperfect, flawed, limited, self-contradictory; as unfinished; often immature, raw on the edges, unfulfilled; but as remarkable in fact and possibility and as structured for growth. With all these aspects the truly civil person feels at home." (2)

Administration generally has responsibility for inaugurating teaching programs. The example set by first-class hospitals leaves little doubt that clinical teaching enriches and improves services rendered to the client. The new knowledge, the fresh perspective, the spirit of inquiry the student brings with him illuminate the scene and stimulate the staff to their best creative effort. To the degree that all experience is grist to the human mill, we may assume the student also profits. In attempting to qualify the returns to the student over a period of years, certain basic ingredients of a teaching program parade before us for review.

Young people often come to us hemmed in by the safe margins of the knowledge they have assimilated well. They will not readily push these margins out unless we commend the pioneering spirit and, indeed, breast the frontiers ourselves. This should not be promptly equated in the listener's mind with study and research, applicable though they be. It is much more an attitude, a state of mind which invests our every action, from shifting a schedule to tossing out a traditional method for some new system. It is, we believe, a refreshing jolt for the new student who arrives on the scene primed for performance (with the mental image of the rating scale never far away) to be assured that he will be rewarded for imagination and invention, that his supervisor will cherish trial and error rather than past performance according to textbook specifications.

Gradually, we have had the temerity to question the fine line drawn between the status and responsibility accorded the student and the therapist. It seems to us that this is a chimera which cannot be perpetuated if we hope to give to student and patient that sense of security and authority which are prerequisite to a positive relationship. In seeking to create for the student a level somewhat below that of staff prestige, yet to demand from him those things expected of a staff member (with the possible exception of ultimate responsibility to administration), we seem to be pursuing an unrealistic, if not unattainable objective. In good government we underwrite responsibility with authority. The student in training is anywhere from one to nine months short of his first job. Overnight, he will be expected to drop the pose of subservience and assume the mantle of adulthood. Since few of us are quick-change artists when it comes to personal development, the outcome of such a system will generally be an additional year of growing into responsible performance. Yet the current situation demands prompt assumption of leadership and mature judgment from the new therapist. This is often deplored but I suspect it is something we might cease to deprecate. In many of the established giant businesses of today this golden option for personal responsibility has been severely curtailed. Thousands of young clerks and typists seem never to move beyond the immediate assigned task, be it filing the card meticulously under "C" or typing the letter neatly and accurately. The card may bear information of keen signif-icance to the boss and the letter may read like gibberish but there will too seldom be an attempt to check on the information or to read the letter for sense. This is not necessarily the sign of a dull mind but rather of a dependent one which has been denied the God-given opportunity of thinking for itself, of questioning, of investigating even at the risk of appearing foolish.

To a degree our schools perpetuate this state of dependency. We still persist in spoon-feeding substance to students, examining them regularly and all but lifting them through the business of learning with methods and devices as adroit as they are stultifying. We forget or overlook the fact that education in its deepest sense is "life-long discipline of the individual by himself." (4) We assume self-discipline will set in, like grey hair, after the student is on the job.

If the therapist-administrator seeks to engender a dynamic and rewarding teaching program he will do well to examine this dichot-omy and establish the student as a full-grown person of whom is expected the creative effort, natural error, renewed curiosity and growing capacity for responsibility which we associate, whether rightly or wrongly, with the finished therapist. In place of the smothering pat of authoritative approval, we may substitute the lis-tening ear—the sounding board against which the student may try the "ping" of his ideas. While this may play some havoc with established efficiency, it will assuredly contribute to personal and professional growth.

We are reminded of an episode which may illumine these ab-stractions. A student was treating an emotionally labile hemiplegic woman of middle age. The physician in charge was carried away with the importance of self-care for this patient and somewhat arbitrarily emphasized this in his prescription to the exclusion of other activities. In the manner of many busy doctors, he had found little time to examine the background of the case which indicated a long career of drudgery interrupted for the first time in many years by the respite of illness. The student was vaguely aware of this implicit contradiction but failed (in traditional fashion) to verbalize it to the doctor. Instead, she proceeded to carry out the orders to the letter. The patient broke down and sobbed uncontrollably on the day she was first able to master her shoelaces alone. The student, shocked, discussed the situation with a therapist who, neither condemning nor approving, helped the student to voice her desire to try a less orthodox approach. Utilizing a spark of interest the patient had revealed for drawing and painting as a stimulus to other activities, the student encountered some success. She was asked to present the results to the physician, who, in the face of the evidence and the student's newfound assurance was moved to adjust his recommendations. Much was learned; a small world was conquered. Had the therapist, at the outset, issued warnings about deviating from the prescription, we might have succeeded solely in perpetuating a blind and mulish adherence to rule.

Physicians who enjoy the practice of medicine as art and science, rather than the artificial prerogatives bestowed by overawed humanity, tell us that they are neither qualified nor interested in planning discrete occupational therapy programs. They alone can and will set the guidelines for us, indicating the pitfalls and dangers inherent in treatment. We must heed this advice and also the ring of inner conviction which tells us that we alone can create, devise and adjust the program of therapeutic work which is our contribution to the healing process.

The cult of objectivity in human relationships has occasioned a good deal of fanfare in our teaching and clinical training settings. Random observations in our own field and allied situations moved us to examine this precept and to cast our vote with those who believe it is neither possible nor desirable to establish antiseptic relationships with people, to divest our relationships of some degree of emotionality. Undoubtedly some of the existing confusion we experience here rests upon problems of semantics. The word "emotional" is often viewed in the narrow sense of uncontained feeling. It appears to the writer that what we bring to patient or staff relationships rests largely upon our ability to manifest a warm interest in individuals as people. An axiom of our profession is the importance of our approach to people. Just what do we mean by this? Is it a kind of come-on that we hold out as bait until the fish is hooked, then to withdraw rapidly into our shell of cool aloofness? Or does it mean that we are able to convey to people at all moments of our relationship that they are important and valuable to us, that we have an investment in their future, that we care considerably what happens to them. If we accept the evidence that what we do and say often influences even momentary or fleeting relationships, how much more obvious is this potential in daily association? As members of the genus homo sapiens we all move in a constant search for understanding. As human beings we are not constituted to live together without involvement. We have learned that events across the span of oceans and continents affect us, that we are in more than an abstract sense our brothers' keepers. This is no less true of our more intimate associations with patients and colleagues. To the degree that these feelings are neither unrecognized nor unmanageable, they are, we submit, the most powerful tool we have for evoking response and encouraging movement forward. And, if we should err, let us remember that we were not meant to be omnipotent. People will forgive us the errors made in the name of earnest belief more readily than the achievements which result from calculated planning. We should differentiate this kind of response to others from the casual benevolence that rests upon familiarity with the size and fortunes of Joe Doake's family as the base of association. The kind of interest we propose as a part of the administrative armamentarium is an enlightened concern with personal growth and achievement.

In this role of helping people to achieve commonly held objectives, nothing is more rewarding than our deepending awareness of human strength and frailty. One learns to hold aloft the ideal, to expect from people the most and the best of which they are capable yet to respect human frailty and hence to treasure the least of the offerings. As the staff family grows from a few people who have learned to harmonize "exceeding sweet" to a whole chorus which is more apt to give out with a sour note from time to time, there is, for the administrator, the endless fascination of reading an increasingly complex score. The bass are the conservative element, holding the line, providing the foundation; the tenors are the mercurial element, given to temperamental sallies and sudden bursts of melody; the contraltos are the mediators creating a blending of voices; the sopranos carry the design ever onward. All have their inalienable place and the whole is the less for any loss or absence.

The importance of expecting the best from people is illustrated by the remarks of a famous dancer who, as she exhorted young and very green converts to attempt greater feats, pointed out that few of us know even the inside limits of our endurance, nor do we take the time or trouble to find this out except when life itself calls the turn. I remember that we students had been complaining that we could not run any longer. The artist dared us to test this statement. She suggested that we run until we dropped of breathlessness or a stitch-in-the-side. Some of us took the dare and learned, in the process, an illuminating lesson about the depth of our endurance and physical powers. This can be translated into mental efforts. People may gripe and complain about being stimulated and provoked to new and greater efforts but, in our humble opinion, they respond to challenge as the hound to the hare. This is no more nor less than a reflection of man's eternal striving after perfection. Attainment may, indeed must, in many instances fall far short of the goal. This is secondary. It is the reaching that counts; not the thing we grasp. The sense of joy and accomplishment, of participation, are to be found on the march. The goal, achieved, has already altered and is elusively beyond us again.

Another lesson to be mastered in this complex and provocative business of working with people is the sharpening and refinement of the sense of timing. How easily one loses the golden opportunity to communicate an idea or advance a plan when the time is either too soon or too late. We might speculate lengthily that timing is the essence of success in all things great and small. Certainly it has a place in successful administration. The atmosphere of a staff or board meeting, the readiness of people for a concept or plan, the degree of skepticism, the point at which this turns to argument, the introduction of personal motives and consequent loss of focus on the objective, all these are as significant to the development of the administrative sense as the scent of smoke on the air is to a present danger for animals of the forest. Reactions like these are not to be overlooked in the ardor of one's own beliefs. Personal conviction and zeal spice an offering but they must be preserved within the framework of group readiness much as a treble phrase plays a counterpoint against a holding base.

While the sense of timing can be enhanced with experience, it has in common with all true things an intuitive basis. We say of the gifted politician that he can sense the mood or will of the people, and uses this to introduce advanced ideas and doctrines. This is equally applicable to the administrator who, seeking to inaugurate a new policy with staff or board, must consider group structure, mood and will. Long ago Shakespeare immortalized this idea when he said, "There is a tide in the affairs of men which, taken at flood, leads on to fortune . . ."

By way of example, a staff may resist the introduction of a timesaving procedure for the exchange of routine information. They are unmoved by the suggestion that such measures will reduce the burden of frustration upon individuals. The matter is discussed and, wisely, tabled for the present. Soon the moment for which our administrator has been waiting arrives. Several staff members register complaints about the lag in communication. While this irritation is prominent the staff is convened to hear an expression of the problem by its own members. Together the group seeks an answer and happens, magically, upon the plan originally proposed by administration. The time is right; the goal is realized. Astute members of the group recognize some semblance of coincidence, to others this is not yet revealed. This is unimportant. With faithful practice, everyone is eventually in on the secret and common obstacles may be hurdled with the speed and coordination that endow the polished athlete.

The tempering years have sustained our conviction that the goal of harmonious group performance, per se, is a false idol. One insurgent and gifted human being is worth twenty robots who have been chastened into the uncomplaining performance of assigned tasks. New ideas, new people, new projects may threaten to disrupt equilibrium, upset patterns, create temporary dissensions. Do we decide for or against their injection into our midst?

Some of our social scientists have been preaching that "the whole is greater than its parts, that the system has a wisdom beyond the reach of ordinary mortals." William H. Whyte, Jr., writes tellingly of this quandary in *Is Anybody Listening?* (5) Says Mr. Whyte, "The individual can be greater than the group and his lone imagination worth a thousand graphs and studies. He is not often a creator, but even as spectator, as the common man, he can rise in ways his past performance would not predict. To aim at his common denominators in the name of ultimate democracy is to despise him, to perpetuate his mediocrities and to conceive him incapable of responding to anything better than the echo of his prejudices. . . . It is not in the nature of social engineering to be creative; it must necessarily be based on what is already existent. It can measure what is or what was . . . It cannot dream or conjure; it cannot find out from people whether they would like something new, something untried, because people cannot judge what they do not know. And they will not know until someone is damn fool enough to stick his neck out and have faith in his intuition, his perception and his hunches."

There is room for rugged individualism within the staff framework; room for these insurgents, these uncommon men and women to make their contribution to the patient and the agency and to claim in return the honest respect of other personnel. To the administrator falls the challenging job of placing such people in optimum positions to insure their productiveness, of providing the environment which will foster their creative effort.

The incomparable privilege of working with people, lay and professional, leads inevitably to a reaffirmation of principles expounded by great men in every era. Man hungers after beauty, goodness and truth. He seeks to experience life first-hand and in so doing develops a personal independence and esteem which sustain him through trial and tribulation. He seeks also to identify with mankind, to give and receive warmth, affection and love. He is a problem-solver and so dispels, inch by painstaking inch, the fears which beset his way. He responds to the challenge of perfection yet craves acceptance of his frailty. Although actually he may present a less than admirable figure, he is potentially superb. The practice of administration, like the practice of occupational therapy, is another way of recognizing these truths.

REFERENCES

1. James, Henry. *The Art of Fiction and Other Essays*. Oxford Press.
2. Overstreet, Harry and Bonaro. *The Mind Goes Forth*. New York: W.W. Norton and Company, Inc., 1956.
3. Smith, T.V. "The Leisure of the Theory Class," *The Saturday Review*, August 25, 1956.
4. Barzun, Jacques. *Teacher in America*. Garden City, New York: Doubleday Publishers, 1954.
5. Whyte, William H., Jr. *Is Anybody Listening?* New York: Simon and Schuster, Inc., 1952.

The 1957 Eleanor Clarke Slagle Lecture

Powerful Levers
In Little Common Things

Ruth W. Brunyate

Preface

Madam president, occupational therapists and guests. It is with great pride, an overwhelming sense of inadequacy and profound humility that I accept the award you have conferred upon me. It is strange how small one feels in perhaps his biggest hour.

Worthiness for such an honor is never singly earned. An occupational therapist is, after all, merely a tool through which the doctor treats his patient. The value of the therapist can be judged only on the soundness of his contribution to treatment—for this is the culmination of his professional training. The therapist who participates in the administrative phases of a treatment program is again a tool through which the patient receives his treatment. The value of an administrative therapist can be judged only by the extent to which he is able to mold professional knowledge with sound business practice in such a way as to hold the patient in true perspective—for this is the culmination of his nonprofessional training.

These values are learned through formal education and experience but above all through the inspiration of others. I would, therefore, acknowledge the three people beyond my own family who have most affected the development of my abilities: Miss Helen S. Willard, Doctor Winthrop M. Phelps and Mr. Christopher H. Wiemer. Under Miss Willard's guidance I developed my philosophy of occupational therapy and my faith in my profession. Under Dr. Phelps' leadership I have developed my philosophy and techniques of treatment of the

Reprinted from *The American Journal of Occupational Therapy*, Vol. XII, No. 4, Part II, 1958.

cerebral palsied and a concept of education as a continuing process based on simplicity, honesty, patience and diligence in the approach to complex problems. Under Mr. Wiemer's counsel I am beginning to learn the value of the individual in the ordered structure of the treatment unit, and a faith in oneself to see that value, to nurture it and direct it.

You have given me a very beautiful gift which I shall always treasure. I thank you each individually and pray that the hours of deliberation and the final thoughts presented here may be worthy of your trust.

Foreword

Forty years ago, on September 3, 1917, the first annual meeting of the National Society for the Promotion of Occupational Therapy was held in New York City. The meeting was called to order by the vice-president, Mrs. Eleanor Clarke Slagle. Who was this woman leading a pioneer group dedicated to a new profession? Occupational therapists who were active prior to 1942 had the privilege of knowing her. Some had met her, others knew her intimately. But for those who knew her not at all we would like to review her life, that each may understand why an award has been established to perpetuate her memory and why we value our Slagle heritage. (1)

Eleanor Clarke Slagle was born just eighty-one years ago this October 13th in Hobart, New York. (2) Her brother was one day to become a prominent United States Senator from their native state. Mrs. Slagle was educated by tutors, then attended Claverack College, summer school of Columbia University and graduated from the Chicago School of Civics and Philanthropy. Here, as early as 1908, and largely through the inspiration of Julia Lathrop and Rabbi Harris, a course in invalid occupation was offered to attendants and nurses from hospitals for the insane. Dr. Adolf Meyer, professor of psychiatry at Johns Hopkins Hospital, gave continued advice and encouragement to the course.

In 1913, when the Henry Phipps Psychiatric Clinic of the Johns Hopkins Hospital was opened, Mrs. Slagle became the director of occupational therapy. This position she continued to hold until 1917 when she became director of the Henry B. Favill Memorial School in Chicago. She returned to New York in 1922 to become director of occupational therapy of the New York State Hospital Service to which she devoted her energies until her death.

In March of 1917 at Consolation House, Clifton Springs, New York, the National Society for the Promotion of Occupational Therapy, forerunner of the American Occupational Therapy Association was founded. Incorporation papers were drawn and later signed by five people, two of whom, Dr. Dunton and Mrs. Slagle, are familiar to even the youngest of our present members. Mrs. Slagle became vice-president in 1919, president in 1920 and was secretary-treasurer from 1922 to 1937.

When she resigned in 1937 she retired to Tarrytown, New York, but continued her work in the state program where she established the practice of holding annual institutes for chief therapists to discuss problems and review new methods. She, in a sense, pioneered the very type of conference that we have only this year perfected. The last ten years of her life were complicated by a heart problem which was greatly taxed by a fall and back injury in 1940. Her insistence on continuing to practice her profession undoubtedly contributed to her death on September 18, 1942.

Reports of the early meetings of our Association tell us much of Mrs. Slagle and of the spirit which fostered our early development. (3) Forty years ago at our first annual conference the treasurer noted receipts of $109, expenses of $72.36 and an indebtedness of $150 to the lawyer for the cost of incorporation. The Society numbered 39 members of whom 26 attended this first meeting to enjoy a program including papers entitled, "Comparative Methods of Hospital Teaching," "Arts and Crafts in Medicine," and "The Teacher in Occupational Therapy." A review of patients followed and is notable, for it presented a depressed patient and an apparent case of paralysis, thus contradicting the now popular belief that early interests were devoted only to psychiatry. Finally a banquet was announced with great enthusiasm and later reported with equal interest, though Dr. Dunton tells us that it was a very sad occasion, for only three people appeared at Keen's Chop House to bolster their spirits and show their faith in a future profession. One of the three, of course, was Mrs. Slagle.

At the second annual meeting of the National Society for the Promotion of Occupational Therapy, September 2-4, 1918, in New York, Mrs. Slagle again played a prominent role and, again as vice-president, she presided. The treasurer reported a balance of $38.73 and noted that with the aid of a loan of $30 the costs of incorporation had been paid, for the lawyer was growing impatient. He also noted there was owing this Society $64 in unpaid dues. (4) (Perhaps we have inherited some early weaknesses?) Twenty-five members attended this meeting and heard papers on "The Problems of the Invalid Occupations in War Hospitals," "The Principles of Occupational Therapy," and "The Remuneration of the Teacher." The word "teacher" in the early literature refers to the one who teaches the patient, thus the therapist. The speaker here suggested that his topic was untimely "since more than half the world is giving its all in sacrifice," (5) but continues that we are assured a "laborer is worthy of his hire." The topic initiated much discussion and the consensus was that the average salary for the occupation teacher seemed to be from forty to fifty dollars a month with maintenance. The salaries offered for reconstruction aides averaged $1350 for home service, $1500 for head aide with ten assistants, and $1800 for supervisors. Postdepression graduates will note how this compared with their initial salaries of $1300 with maintenance.

Another note of interest is Mrs. Slagle's comment on training for occupational therapy. She stated that after considerable experience the speaker felt that two months of crafts training and three months of practice teaching in hospitals made an ideal arrangement for a short course. The candidate should have college education or its equivalent in other experience. (6)

The third annual meeting was held September 8-11, 1919, in Chicago at the Favill School, probably the first of all occupational therapy schools. The Favill School had for three years been housed by Hull House and the renowned Jane Addams greeted the convention and congratulated the Society "because you are really the vanguard on the line of philanthropic effort and you are beginning at the bottom as all great social experiments have always done." (7)

At this meeting Mrs. Slagle was elected president and so formally began her many years of leadership in our profession. As time goes by fewer therapists will be able to recall her personality, for fewer will have known her. Future therapists will instead have to do as we have done, turn to her letters, the minutes of meetings in which she participated and the memories of her friends to learn of the heritage she left to them. They must read of her dominant personality, her sense of humor, her abiding interest in children, her ability to be outstanding in any situation, her dignity and handsome manner of dress and carriage, her astute mind, and her ability to rise above adversity. These traits of character were forceful factors in her influence on the growth of our profession as she moved from office to office and helped determine the framework of our present American Occupational Therapy Association.

But Mrs. Slagle's greatest contribution was to the practice of occupational therapy, not to its organization. This phase of her work is less known perhaps because it is a more personal thing or because it is less tangible and more difficult to study. She was tremendously interested in students, in their education and growth and in the direction of their work that they might share her enthusiasm in patient treatment. To perpetuate her memory we will now turn to this her greatest heritage and, using her own writings as a point of departure, will incorporate some of our own thoughts on student training and its meaning to the individual student, to the director of his course and to the members of this Association.

As we begin this third Slagle lecture we would use her own words from the presidential address of 1920, "this happens to be my turn and, like the measles and mumps or various and numerous other labelled states of mind or body, you wish me well, and hope it will be over soon." (8)

"Powerful Levers—in Little Common Things"

Clinical training is an outmoded phrase. We now speak of student affiliation and indeed date ourselves when we fail to do so, yet the original phrase has meaning for us as a review of definitions will show. The dictionary defines "clinic" as "medical instruction at the bedside of the patient," and defines the world "train" as "to bring to a required standard of knowledge or skill to give education by instruction and discipline." Since education is "the systematic development or cultivation of natural powers by inculcation or example," the concept of clinical training immediately implies apprenticeship. In clinical training one is assigned to a clinic to apprentice or "serve in order to learn." Initially then our choice of the phrase "clinical training" was to describe that period of the professional education devoted to serving another that through instruction and discipline one would cultivate his own natural abilities.

More recently we have adopted the phrase student affiliation. A student is "a person engaged in a course of study especially an advanced scholar—one who closely examines or investigates." To affiliate is "to receive on friendly terms, associate with—to adopt as a child." And here we would better cease to quote for the dictionary goes on to say "to associate with, usually reflexively or passively," (9) and we know of few training experiences which could be called passive. Our new phrase "affiliate" has, we believe, a meaning too often overlooked, namely, to receive on friendly terms—to adopt. Our traditional concept of clinical practice is usually in terms of an assigned period spent in each of four or five clinics in which the student bridges the gap from the classroom to the job, a period of trial under supervision, a period in which to practice all that has previously been theory, thus the climax of academic experience.

We would think of student affiliation in a far broader sense for we believe that it is a period of transition to a whole new way of life. In an early paper Mrs. Slagle said, "A study of the greatest teaching personalities is a revelation of the powerful levers they found in little common things to lift their pupils up and out into a fuller life, and it is to the study of such methods that the most successful teacher will look for help." (10) Mrs. Slagle was using this thought to describe a therapist's work with a patient for she again used the word "teacher" as we now use the word "therapist." We feel, however, that this same key to success in treatment is the real key to success in teaching and indeed even the key to success in the performance of all of our daily tasks.

The nine month period of clinical affiliation must be a period of time in which the student gains far more than the opportunity to put his new knowledge into practice. It must be above all else a period of time in which those who teach "lift the student up and out and into a fuller life." Those who direct the student do not perform their roles successfully until they place the development of the individual in true perspective—above the importance of interpreting the theory and practice of occupational therapy in a particular disability area. The student who enters the affiliation period just to become proficient in applying his professional skills fails miserably if he does not first develop the personality and character through which the professional skills receive their most potent meaning.

Too often we forget that the majority of occupational therapy students are gaining their college education and professional training at one and the same time. We try to graduate a professional tool for the doctor and lose sight of the basic need of all college students to find time to grow as they learn.

The period of affiliation is, we feel, the most important of all educational experiences for it is true education lifted beyond the framework of what is purely academic. It is a practical experience and a period of transition in which the student must gain the ability to live as an independent person—which is to say he must begin to jell his own philosophy of life, of work and of his profession.

Sometimes those who teach are so preoccupied in following the essentials set down by the American Medical Association that they fail to see that a student is also trying to live with himself and others. Each affiliation must have a "well-defined program to interpret the function of occupational therapy in its own area or type of service," (11) but of more permanent value is the atmosphere and personalities through which this program is introduced. People are more important than things. Personalities are remembered long after course content is forgotten. In the clinical field even more than in the formal setting of the professional school, the character of the teacher makes a lasting impression, for here there is daily contact under all sorts of conditions, here there is a sharing of responsibilities, here there is an apprenticeship. The importance of the individual therapist in training a student in any one affiliation will be notable to you if you will but for a moment recall your own affiliations. It is not true that even those of you who have been out of school for "generations" can recall to this day the individual personalities of those who counselled you in each affiliation while you may have forgotten some once favored classroom professor. We remember the things we do rather than the things we hear about. We remember the things we see rather than the things about which we are told. We remember the things we feel rather than those we experience only through others.

For these reasons therapists involved in student affiliation programs must evaluate themselves as well as their staffs and programs with utmost care. We should have a very sound philosophy of student training if we are to accept the challenge and privilege of student education. This philosophy must enable us to give to the student through our own example an opportunity to develop a wisdom, an acceptable law by which he will live his adult life. It must give him, too, an appreciation for and thus the desire to share our own way of living, of working, of practicing our profession. If we teach these things we are successful in student training. As a guide to teaching them we would now suggest some factors so common and so little that they have a tremendous effect upon us all. Let us enumerate a few as an index for individual thinking.

The ability to make one's way alone. College is the time when a young person makes the transition to independence—independence of action and of thought. It is the time when personality is developed and character molded, the time when he must realize that he becomes an adult and must make his way alone. This transition is a difficult one and yet must occur while the student is under the stress of study. All such experiences are learned under stress, for this is when one uses the ultimate of his own discipline, and discipline is innate to the process of education. If a student learns to habituate himself to his environment he will have matured tremendously, for his environment is only temporary and will always change as long as he shall live. If he learns to adjust himself to living with his own kind and with those who differ in every way he will achieve some measure of both success and happiness.

The acceptance of things you do not condone or choose. Along with growth in independence must come the realization that things cannot always go according to one's own choosing. This is perhaps the most difficult of all experiences which occur when youth accepts adulthood, and many individuals of senior years bring unhappiness to themselves or others through never having understood the lesson. Students have so recently acquired freedom from the dictums of others that they have a false security in the justifiability of their own ideas and wishes, and so resent having to accept again a control even in this new form—self-discipline and tolerance. Sir William Osler, the famous physician, once said "Things cannot always go your own way. Learn to accept in silence the minor aggravations, cultivate the gift of taciturnity and consume your own smoke with an extra draught of hard work, so that those about you may not be annoyed with the dust and soot of your complaints." (12) This attitude once acquired becomes ingrained and is the fountain from which we gain our ability to understand others and so to be comfortable in our work with them. It must become part of an individual before he is able to follow direction and share departmental responsibility and it must be so inherent in his personality that it is no longer a conscious thing if he is to be successful in the direction of others.

A willingness to listen. This is another trait which must develop in college years and crystallize at the time of student affiliation. Too often freedom from the classroom, assigned reading and prearranged group participation gives an exaggerated feeling of importance and fosters an eagerness to express oneself and a restlessness which leaves no time for reflection. New-found information is assumed to be seasoned knowledge which the owner is impatient to share—or at least reiterate. Quietness or meditation and attentiveness are scorned as the shy attributes of the inexperienced and are accepted only with embarrassment unless the student is given the opportunity to practice them and encouraged to realize their value. Today's students are being groomed for a world geared to the pace of group dynamics and the workshop exchange of ideas. They will lose half the value of participating if they have not first learned to listen. Sometimes it would appear we are all afraid of a moment of silence.

A willingness to seek advice. Perhaps this is felt to be a feminine trait yet some of the biggest men in history personify it. It begins again in little things, the recognition that we cannot know everything, that we are human and therefore even forget part of what knowledge we have acquired. One must learn to turn to others when the need arises but to turn cautiously and select our source wisely, then meld the counsel with our own experience and thus accept it as advice, not as a directive or decision. Mrs. Slagle once wrote to a friend, "I seek advice—I also seek to please." (13) Some would say this is a contradiction and that she was in a sense just trying to see-saw by herself and was thus running from the seat at one end to that at the other. Others would feel she was straddling an issue, thus standing over the fulcrum and so successful in see-sawing alone. We feel that the two thoughts frequently go hand in hand, for seeking the thoughts of others often results in giving pleasure to both of the individuals involved. At any rate there seldom, if ever, comes the time when we arrive at the point of never needing the help of others.

An ability to appreciate the commonplace. An occupational therapist will always work with people from all walks of life. Frequently he is pulled far from his own native environment and thrown into the problems of varied standards of living. Sometimes the sordid, the filthy, the crude come hand-in-hand with illness and disability and overwhelm the inexperienced. The ability to appreciate the commonplace, to note a touch of beauty in the midst of squalor or be aware of tenderness even in frugal living, this is the trait that refreshes and strengthens the individual as he is introduced to the ways of others. Osler once said, "Nothing will sustain you more potently than the power to recognize in your own humdrum routine as perhaps it may be thought, the true poetry of life—the poetry of the commonplace, of the ordinary man, of the plain, toilworn woman, with their loves and their joys, their sorrows and their griefs." (14)

The ability to retain the buoyance of youth. The young have a wonderful zest for living which carries them through many a difficult hour. Unfortunately, as we take our place in the working world we gradually lose that enthusiasm, that eagerness and spontaneity. The student who learns to modify it yet retain it will be well repaid. True, the exuberance and clumsiness of the puppy, particularly the big puppy, is humorous but not continuously desirable nor is it compatible with the dignity of maturity. However, who will deny the strength derived from the ability to rebound after rebuff, or the desire to adventure after mishap—and are these qualities not rooted in buoyance and vivacity?

An understanding of the value of time. Our modern world is time conscious and we are keyed to schedules and to a rapid pace, that we may accomplish the utmost immediately. We know a doctor who mourns that people no longer have time to be sick, nor to get well. He says that we used to crawl into bed and suffer our colds for four or five days but now must have a shot of this or a dose of that to stay on our feet. This trend is infectious and our students soon catch the disease. We must, through our own example, give them a truer concept of the value of time. Each day is a very real and integral part of one's life, for each individual is but the sum total of each day's experience. The student, busy with each affiliation, is keenly aware of blocks of time—four weeks here, eight weeks there— and prone to work through those blocks. If he will pause to realize that that which he adds to each day becomes the sum total of all his days, he will build a far better life. This is particularly true if he thinks he does not like the area to which he is currently assigned and is anxious to get on to another disability area. Someone has said,

"Time is not always something to beat, it is also something to linger through and enjoy." (15) If we check off the days, we lose time, if instead we take each in turn and add to the day, we profit.

A realization that privilege is bound in duty. Traditionally as one moves up in status to more responsible positions he is granted more privileges. Those who are just learning the structure of an institution and the relative rank of services and positions frequently see the privileges that go with increased rank and perhaps even envy those who have found them. It is again at the student level that we must begin to realize that privilege and duty are closely interrelated. The apparent freedom of hours, of expression, of entrance and exit, carry a duty which should outweigh the privilege. One of the early members of the Dupont dynasty taught his sons that "no privilege exists that is not inseparably bound to a duty." (16) Privilege must be recognized by the one who receives it, must be guarded, never flaunted, must be doubly repaid through the sense of obligation that others in turn may respect it.

An equanimity of mental and moral outlook. Each student has lived through years of counsel from his elders, his family, his minister, his professors, but there comes a time when he must realize that the problems of the great moral issues of his time are now his own to solve. Many of our occupational therapy students attended college in areas close to their own homes, even perhaps commuting from their family residences. For them the affiliation period is the first real break, particularly if they are not receiving maintenance, for now they find themselves in a strange city completely independent. Those of us who are busy with such a student in duty hours frequently forget that he may be experiencing for the first time the pressure of living the moral code that he has inherited. We must somehow help him to see that while mores change, fundamentals do not. This is the time in which an innate sense of the fitness of things becomes his own possession rather than a hand-me-down. If he gains an appreciation of the good which is inherent in every fellow being whatever his station in life, and a commiseration for the evil again in every human being whatever his claim to godliness, (17) then he will be able to secure his own personal code of behavior upon which he will operate for the rest of his days. This phase of a student's adjustment to life is a very personal one and does not routinely come under the scrutiny of his director, for a student lives this in his own privacy as he justly should. Let us then just be aware that it is going on and that the atmosphere which we create in our own living can aid and abet it.

A desire to represent the best in manhood and womanhood. This is perhaps the summation of all the factors we have named. In this period of transition a student may easily struggle against that which his seniors expect of him. Now he is preoccupied with trying to become a good therapist, he is bombarded with tangible things, patients, techniques of treatment, records, supplies, and we must not so emphasize them that he fails to realize that becoming a good therapist is dependent upon first becoming a good person.

These are but a few of the common little things which the director of student affiliation and his junior staff members must hold in their consciousness if they are to give the student the best of any training experience. These are the little things which should be part of our own lives given through example that a student may develop his own philosophy of living—an acceptable law by which he will live each day of his life.

The student affiliation must also create an atmosphere in which the student may evolve his own philosophy of work and of his profession. This again is not a tangible thing taught in lecture or through supervised patient treatment but it is a very real factor in graduating successful therapists. There are many elements in our working lives which go to make up our philosophy of work and of our profession. Most of these are common to all paramedical or ancillary services. Some are peculiar to occupational therapy alone and are so taught in our theory classes on ethics and etiquette. We feel, however, that there are certain basic concepts which the affiliation centers exemplify and would again enumerate a few in random order, for they too are the common little things which collectively make the big person if he will encompass them in his philosophy of work.

A dedication to the patient. The patient is the reason we exist. This maxim is so true and common that frequently it is forgotten. In our big clinics, particularly in our teaching clinics, the patient is frequently outnumbered twenty to one. He is surrounded by doctors, nurses, technicians, social workers and therapists and though he is always the focus of the group, he is not always given his rightful place. In our eagerness to teach we frequently categorize patients, lump them into groups and label with symptoms to tag for specific modalities. Here the student comes to prominence and the patient recedes. In our anxiety to give full treatment we surround the patient with a mass of records, tests, reports and schedules even to the point of eclipsing the human element. We tell ourselves too frequently that patient welfare has priority over all else and then we busy ourselves with the myriad of mechanical details related to his care. Mrs. Slagle was acutely aware of this and always directed her attention to the patient first. Even as she became more and more involved with the administrative phases of her department she kept her patient in proper perspective. This is a trait seen in all great physicians even as their work calls them into teaching and research fields. The ability to understand the patient and his human problems as well as his physical or mental handicap is always the clue to successful treatment.

An appreciation of where the textbook ends. In many fields we have accumulated a vast amount of knowledge and so have devised given treatment routines. In arts and crafts we have inherited through the ages acceptable techniques and methods. These have been formalized and expounded in textbooks. Usually it is true that a subject is not taught until texts are available and we are accustomed to this type of learning; it is comfortable and gives us security as we practice the knowledge so gained. Yet there comes the time when textbooks do not validate what is practiced, where techniques cannot be defined in print, and it is here that experience has the advantage over mere education. It has been said that the successful person is not always the one who envisions an idea, but rather the one who is able to sell that idea to others. Freedom from established fact or directive is gained through the years but respect for it should start in college. In helping her students understand the approach to patients Mrs. Slagle said, "There can be no set of rules or theories applied; simple tact, patience and common sense assist more than anything else." (18)

Here again is one of the reasons we support the apprentice type of learning experience. Let us encourage students to examine and observe the staff in its performance of duty, and foster a respect for things that are successful through experience, not alone through the textbook. A staff member should not be embarrassed if he cannot always produce a fact to support his premise or his act, if execution of that idea is successful in its end effect on the patient.

An avoidance of overconfidence in our methods. In her report as president in 1920, Mrs. Slagle said, "Much valuable time, no doubt, was lost in the beginning by an over-agitation of standards—nothing is more stultifying to progress than standardization in a comparatively new field of service—keep your program flexible—let us have ideals always, fine, strong and true to the proper development of the individual patient but let us not be overconfident of our methods yet. A great many of us have opinions concerning the proper way of administering occupational therapy, all, no doubt, perfectly good opinions, but the chief point for us to remember is that we are still representing only a small part of the treatment given . . ." (19) Continuous reevaluation is a must.

A willingness to get in step with each institution. Preconceived ideas seldom helped anyone or any situation. Each clinic has its own problems, its own idiosyncrasies, its own weakness and strength. As we move from one to another we must be slow to criticize and quick to analyze. We must be willing to learn and to understand before we venture to change. Again Mrs. Slagle said that "we must carefully get in step and in line with the individual problems presented by each situation in which we serve, that the emotion toward our particular branch of work does not determine its force." (20)

A knowledge of how to support as well as to lead. Some say that leaders are born, others that they are developed, yet whatever you hold to be true you must grant that leaders follow before they lead. A supporting role is inglorious yet can be the most satisfying of experiences. We cannot graduate a profession of leaders for immediately we have nothing to lead. We must instead give proper respect and recognition to those who follow. In a treatment situation the individual who contributes the most is the one who quietly goes his way treating his patients with sincerity and compassion without an overlay of wishing to do otherwise. The being of the clinic lies with the patient, the greatest contribution to its functioning lies immediately with those who work closest to the patient, for as they are successful the clinic justifies its very reason for existence. The routine treating therapist is the backbone of the whole program as is the duty nurse. Such a therapist contributes in other ways too—through his enthusiasm for his job, his optimism in difficult times, his flexibility in accepting assignments, his willingness to do the menial if needed, his "acknowledgment of the dignity of the cure of disease," (21) his assumption that he must give beyond what he receives.

A recognition of the average, not just the superior. We cannot create a profession peopled only with the outstanding, the superior, the talented, but instead must remember that the majority of us will have average ability. We must respect this average and recognize it as our balance wheel for frequently it will prevent us from wandering at a tangent. We must develop a respect for the average and not give it a stigma by apparent oversight in our eagerness to acknowledge those who have unusual capabilities. We must appreciate it and encourage those who have this status, that they too may have the security of knowing that they contribute to our profession.

An acceptance of learning on the job. We cannot graduate experienced therapists. A new staff member cannot be proficient in all disability areas nor is he qualified to meet every situation presented in daily treatment. We are vocative in complaining that our young therapists do not know this or that fact or technique so vital to our own job or disability area. We fret because schools and training centers do not supply this needed skill. We should instead expect a new graduate to continue to learn—always, if he is wise. We must provide that opportunity and consider his first few years of employment as a continuation of professional training. We are each morally obligated to give this training whether or not our department has an active teaching program.

An awareness that facts need no embellishing. Again we quote Mrs. Slagle whose comments on record writing are pertinent. "From the beginning of hospital practice students are taught the value of accurate notes, that a fact needs no embellishing in the way of narrative." (22) This art is almost impossible to teach without benefit of practical experience and is one that we continue to learn for many years. We would interpret Mrs. Slagle's words another way, too, and apply them to the problem of argument versus the expression of opinion. A student must learn that a staff member must always supply facts to support his position or ideas but must never embellish them by narration which then turns the situation into an argument. This is true when any staff member is asked to inform his seniors of a given problem. If that staff member does not like the situation he is justified in reporting the fact of his dislike and may support that fact with comments to prove its logic. He may, however, never go beyond that point to argue or harangue for in so doing he only weakens his own position. Facts accurately presented stand alone and are well interpreted whether they apply to treatment progress or to a working situation.

An enthusiasm for small job benefits. As jobs become more plentiful in our profession and therapists continue to be short in supply, we frequently find ourselves trying to sell our vacancies. This is done through formal job analysis, or an advertisement or a letter. Let us never forget the value of the unsolicited selling which is done in the daily performance of the job. Our own enthusiasm for fringe benefits, our loyalty to the institution, or interest in our chosen field, these frequently form a more impressive bit of information than does the listing of hours, pay scale, increments and the like.

A recognition of the value of extra-professional interests. Not every therapist is a so-called career therapist. Some practice their profession with less enthusiasm than others. Those who devote added hours to their profession and exhibit an extensive interest in its organization become mechanical participants unless they have learned to add other outside interests. There are only so many hours per day and the therapist who works and then participates in extra-curricular professional activities must be particularly alert to other interests. Again we turn to Osler who said, "No man is really happy or safe without a hobby, and it makes precious little difference what the outside interest may be—botany, beetles or butterflies, roses, tulips or irises, mountaineering or antiquities—anything will do so long as he straddles a hobby and rides it hard." (23)

These are but a few of the common little things that we must cherish in our philosophy of our profession. There are many more but these will serve to indicate why we feel that the concept of student affiliation must be in the broadest sense an apprenticeship. These things are learned by example, by experience, they become part of an individual as he sees what they have meant to others and so accepts them himself. This then is why we must today adopt a student for we must inculcate by example that through us a student will increase his own self-discipline and thus multiply his chances of enjoying his profession.

Many occupational therapists are concerned directly with the problems of student training and develop an amazing enthusiasm for this phase of our work which tends to overwhelm those therapists not so involved. This is understandable for it is a dynamic problem and a tremendous responsibility. Most of us are so absorbed with the vastness of it all that we tend to get it out of all proportion to the total practice of our profession. We would do well to think on the implications of this for a moment. There has developed, we fear, an aura which surrounds that occupational therapy department which trains students as compared to one enjoying a similar program but without students. As we educate more and more students and particularly as we see them go through the same clinical centers, we build up a whole wedge of our profession intimately familiar with a limited number of departments and their staffs. If a student has enjoyed his affiliation he carries with him a deep and genuine respect for those who taught him. As he attends his initial conferences he feels strange and young and unrecognized. It is natural then for him to welcome the familiarity of those with whom he trained.

We feel that the total membership of the American Occupational Therapy Association should carefully evaluate several current trends which we believe are directly related to this perhaps inordinate attention on the training departments. We have the greatest respect for our schools and their personnel and for the student affiliation directors and their staffs. We would, however, sound a word of caution that we of AOTA must not put undue emphasis on them in conducting our national affairs. The 1957 Yearbook lists 1257 agencies which have occupational therapy departments. Of these, 250 are recognized student affiliation centers used by the accredited schools. These departments employ 973 OTR's and the school staffs number approximately 86 OTR's, hence a total of 1,059 OTR's associated with students. The Yearbook lists 4,762 registered therapists of whom 3,138 are known to be working. Only one fifth of our departments and one third of the OTR's are participating in student education. A review of our Association shows that twelve out of thirteen standing committee chairmen, twenty-three of thirty-seven members of the House of Delegates, fourteen of the seventeen Board members and all of the officers are now, or were at the time of election or rise to national prominence, involved in student training.

We apparently choose our leaders from the schools and student affiliation groups and probably do so because they are familiar as well as capable people. Whether or not this is healthy is not for discussion here, but we would suggest that it should prompt those who are in training units to direct the attention of our students to the nontraining departments. You of these departments can help.

You can do so by your very active participation in local associations so that your names and abilities may become familiar to the students we bring to these meetings. Your expression of opinion on local and national matters is a vital factor in maintaining the proper balance. It is your key to gearing the policies of the Association to the particular needs of your departments. Your willingness to express yourselves clearly at local meetings will enable the student to understand the problems of the nontraining departments in which they will more than likely find their initial employment.

A quick review of a recent issue of AJOT shows that seven out of ten of the papers written by OTR's were written by training personnel. So, too, were seven out of ten of the letters to the editor. Does this reflect the day-to-day practice of our profession? Where is the lone therapist who works without other registered occupational therapy staff members and without students? The common thought is that student affiliation staff members have more time, more freedom to write, more secretaries at their disposal. We suggest that they are simply prompted by their habit of teaching and by the very students who take up their time. A well-directed affiliation is never a labor-saving device for it takes hours of staff time and energy if it is properly guided. The nontraining therapist has just as much time if he will but seek it. We urge that every practicing therapist consider it his duty to evaluate his work and to contribute some portion of it to professional literature. The expression of an idea or an opinion will do if there is neither time nor material for a full paper.

The nontraining therapist can help offset the prominence of the affiliation center in many ways just as can the center itself. The combined efforts of both, and of the schools, must arouse a greater respect for the lone therapist and a greater opportunity for him to participate, perhaps through attendance at student affiliation council meetings or at institutes. Whatever the method may be it must develop in an atmosphere which encourages the value of nonacademic learning and this atmosphere can be created by all training and school personnel. Let us not formalize everything to the point of overlooking the value of the individual. What we need most of all is a contributing membership to the American Occupational Therapy Association, not in the financial sense of a paid membership, but rather as an inherent part of each registered therapist's practice of his profession.

We have endeavored to present here our thoughts on student affiliation and its meaning to the individual student, to his director and to the members of this Association. In summary we would say that education belongs to the individual who receives it and, as we were once told, it is not to bank, to hoard, nor to squander, but is to ease the rigors of one's existence. If we would share our education we would do well to look to the little common things to lift one up and out and into a fuller life. As we earn our own education or guide others as they attain it, let us, however, always hold it secondary to a far greater thing—service—for service is the real meaning of our lives and of our careers. To it we must be dedicated or we do not live our profession. And with this thought we would give you one closing quotation from Mrs. Slagle, for we feel it is the true theme of all our lives, both personal and professional. "If we look to service, not to reward, we shall see in our own day, OUR work ministering to the highest needs of man." (24)

REFERENCES

1. Slagle, Eleanor Clarke. "Development of Occupations for the Insane," *Maryland Psychiatric Quarterly*, IV:1 (July), p. 19, 1914.
2. ———. Editorial, *Occupational Therapy and Rehabilitation*, 21:6 (December), 373, 1942.
3. Proceedings of the first annual meeting of the Nat. Soc. for the Promotion of OT. Spring Grove Hospital Press, Sheppard Hospital Press, 1918.
4. Proceedings of the second annual meeting of the Nat. Soc. for the Promotion of OT. Sheppard and Enoch Pratt Hospital Press, 1918.
5. *Ibid.*
6. *Ibid.*
7. Addams, Jane. Proceedings of the third annual meeting of the Nat. Soc. for the Promotion of OT. Sheppard and Enoch Pratt Hospital Press, p. 41, 1919.
8. Slagle, Eleanor Clarke. Proceedings of the fourth annual meeting of the Nat. Soc. for the Promotion of OT. Spring Grove State Hospital and Sheppard Pratt Hospital, p. 1, 1920.
9. Funk and Wagnall's. *Desk Standard Dictionary*. New York, 1946.
10. Slagle, Eleanor Clarke. "Development of Occupations for the Insane." *Maryland Psychiatric Quarterly*, IV:1 (July), p. 19, 1914.
11. "Essentials of an Acceptable School of Occupational Therapy." *The Yearbook*. New York: American Occupational Therapy Assoc., 1957.
12. Cushing, Harvey. *Life of Sir William Osler*, Vol. I, Ch. 22. Oxford Univ. Press, 1940.
13. Slagle, Eleanor Clarke. Letter to William Rush Dunton, Jr., M.D.
14. Osler, *op. cit.*, Vol. II, Ch. 26.
15. Etting, Gloria Braggiotti. "Go by Sea." *Town and Country*, August, p. 96, 1957.

16. Dupont (Irene Dupont's father, 1784). "The Duponts of Wilmington," *Life*,
    42:8, p. 101.
17. Brunyate, William L. Letter to daughter, 1935.
18. Slagle, Eleanor Clarke. "Development of Occupations for the Insane." *Mary-*
    land Psychiatric Quarterly, IV:1 (July), p. 19, 1914.
19. ———. Proceedings of the fourth annual meeting of the Nat. Soc. for the
    Promotion of OT. Spring Grove State Hospital and Sheppard Pratt Hospital,
    p. 1, 1920.
20. *Ibid.*
21. Pledge and creed for occupational therapists.
22. Slagle, Eleanor Clarke. "Training Aids for Mental Patients," *Archives of*
    Occupational Therapy, 1:1 (February), p. 17, 1922.
23. Osler, *op. cit.*, Ch. 29.
24. Slagle, Eleanor Clarke. Report of president, proceedings of the fourth annual
    meeting of the Nat. Soc. for the Promotion of OT. Spring Grove State
    Hospital and Sheppard Pratt Hospital, p. 1, 1920.

Every One Counts

Margaret S. Rood

Introduction

As the activation of every reflex is necessary in the proper sequence toward coordinated effortless muscular control, so the activation and learned control of basic reflexes in developmental order are necessary for the highest level of emotional maturity. Intellectual maturity, independent thinking, can never be achieved by stuffing the mind with rote learning or facts without progressing onward to individual comprehension and application to original contributions based on the work of others.

If emotional and intellectual maturity are developing dynamically, then professional maturity can be attached happily and wisely for the warmest interaction of all, to secure the best treatment for the patient. And if we are truly maturing then the needs of others will be our guide in the considerate give and take of professional life.

And as we come to the full realization of the need for stress for growth so we must realize that the attitude toward stress will make it a challenge toward increased development or a block to our progress. Unlike the school situation where a grade remains static on the record, in living one has a chance to try again. Having achieved, that record counts as does the strength gained from trying.

The course was charted for us a long time ago. Each individual is a product of his heritage, his experiences. We benefit by the drive and vision of those who have gone before and we in turn have a responsibility to add our particular share whatever it may be. And as

Reprinted from *The American Journal of Occupational Therapy*, Vol. XII, No. 6, 1958.

Eleanor Clarke Slagle had the vision and selfless devotion in the initiation and development of our professional organization, we must build on that foundation to pass on an improved heritage to those to come.

In turn may I discuss briefly the physical, emotional, intellectual and professional aspects in relation to selected principles of muscle reaction.

Physical Development

Activation of muscles proceeds from reflex or involuntary stimulation to voluntary control. In the loss of voluntary control of muscles from many causes it may be possible to reactivate muscles if the cause is physiological discontinuity and not anatomical destruction. But it is necessary to stimulate the first reflex pattern. Therefore, the sequence is important and the total pattern within the sequence. If balanced development does not occur early the problem of treatment will always be more difficult because there will be parts of many reflexes acting in an imbalanced pattern.

For efficiency of a part, interaction with an antagonist is necessary for (primary) shortening and (secondary) lengthening before cocontraction of both at the same time is possible. If one of a pair of muscles does not function in reciprocal innervation, eventually the normal one will be seriously affected. Gravity or stress is essential for the stimulation of the heavier work muscles and for bone growth. Cocontraction or static support positions are essential before heavy work movement is effective. As in cocontraction for support— whether on elbows, all fours or standing—the distal segment is stable, so too the heaviest work a muscle does in movement in its biological purpose is with the distal segment stable. One of the most difficult muscle problems is the lengthening reaction of heavy work one-joint muscles such as the soleus, vasti and anconeus. Slow knee bends with heels flat will get both lengthening and shortening reaction of the vasti and soleus. This is different work from the lighter guiding (lengthening) reaction of the longer muscle passing more joints. Lengthening reactions are important to flexibility as well.

As an example of this approach to muscle action, we might contrast the Delorme heavy resistance at ankle for knee extension versus squatting, which is the normal functional use of the muscle.

The quadriceps loom or kick wheel which embodies this same principle is excellent for the rectus femoris but not for the vasti which is our major problem usually.

In squatting the feet are on the floor or, in other words, the distal segment is stable and the muscles must pull the rest of the body into alignment, a heavier job than just moving the distal end of the extremity.

In life, the rectus femoris comes into play in walking which is a lighter work demand. Therefore in actuality, occupational therapy procedure involving squatting is more effective than kicking if it is the vasti which needs strengthening.

In learning patterns or movement to reproduce at will, the individual must do his own learning. As therapists we must give sufficient stimulus but prevent ourselves from helping too much. Passive action is not the answer. Light work patterns of skill require cortical or voluntary attention. The shoulder rotator cuff muscles of a patient with subluxation of the humerus may be activated by heavy work grip of the hand but not by light work.

Postural cocontraction for erect position can be gained by dental dam rubber resistance to top of head or over each shoulder following appropriate stimulation. Therefore, rather than asking for voluntary correction of posture or traction, resistance is used to cause postural cocontraction without conscious thought. During passive activity such as TV viewing, no attention need be paid because there are more reflex feedbacks below the level of consciousness for heavy work. Stimulus from the muscle spindles found in heavy work muscles pass only as high as the cerebellum for integration. Also repetitive, rhythmical patterns will release top level control after patterns have once been learned. Therefore rhythmical music is the most effective tool; not the metronome with its interrupted tone which requires a more cortical response.

The last two examples would give some indication that fatigue is involved not in the muscle but the cortical control of the pattern. These same points might well serve to illustrate developmental reactions in emotional, intellectual and professional growth.

Emotional Development

As the give and take of shortening and lengthening reactions of muscles is necessary for the health of both, so the giving and receiving of love and of stress is necessary for healthy emotional reactions, and these must be in the sequence of normal development. The baby receives care, love and protection. From this early selfish taking he should progress to wise receiving and giving. That which an individual desires and that which is most ego satisfying to the giver may create or prolong dependence. There will be many, many steps in human relations with definite sequences and experiences necessary for full maturity. Accepting one's parents as interesting individuals on their own merit is one of the higher steps.

The facing of stress is essential to full emotional maturity. Sympathetic nervous system arousal needs repetition so that it can be assessed as non-critical, and therefore may result in a controlled learning experience rather than an uncontrolled emotional reaction. Some withdraw from hurt, others become aggressive. The former is more serious since the damage is to self while the exterior signs do not bring forth the social disapproval attendant to aggression. Aggression, or any pressure of ideas, begets resistance, so care should be used in pushing ideas. Attitude on the part of the recipient toward stress will determine whether it be a healthy challenge to growth or a stimulus for withdrawal in an unhealthy pattern. Comprehension of the fact that insecurity breeds resistance will allow for more intelligent handling of such problems. Holding firm under stress is important also for the individual to learn.

Muscles need light and heavy work patterns in movement and holding to keep in the best equilibrium. Making a point of having friends of all ages is one of the surest ways to prevent atrophy or contractures of the spirit.

Careful selection of most important things will prevent the hyperkinesia of too great superficial stimulation. Heavy work stimuli lead to relaxation and renewal of the body. The physical and emotional are interdependent. It is important that there be a balance of gross physical activity when the mind creates tensions. Likewise the joys of simple as well as the more complex, pleasures should be kept and fostered.

Dependence on outward approval may be too strong. There is a need for developing one's own goals and these may be higher than those set by others. Insecurity requires constant repetition of approval. A secure person realizes that if a decision is thoughtful and right insofar as one knows, one must try to face without bitterness the criticisms which will inevitably come. There is adaptation of the sensory receptors only if the situation is too static or repetitive, however there is some slight adaptation of the sensory receptors to the criticism; nevertheless the criticism should be listened to carefully and the soundness of it judged in the light of what one knows. The interference of emotional reflex reaction will not allow sound judgment, as reflex emotion and intellect are at variance.

Intellectual or Educational

Thinking too must have the reciprocal innervation of give and take to be of the greatest value. Light and heavy work will give an appropriate balance.

Rote learning or easy receiving is supposed to be at its peak up to fourteen years of age. Are we continuing it beyond this age unnecessarily? One knows how hard it is to set students free to think. It is easier in the beginning of professional life, but if set patterns have been established, insecurity and emotional reactions will delay the establishment of new habit patterns. The new student can more easily relate principles to the basic sciences since he does not have old techniques to uproot.

In professional life, are we properly stimulating our therapists in give and take at small unit meetings as part of our association activities? Individual study assignments to key free-for-all discussions would stimulate greater effort than the more standard passive reception of lectures, worthwhile though they be. Efforts on this line have been more notable on the national than the state level.

Although study and reading with a specific goal is difficult initially, repeated exposure provides its own self-ignition because of the interest created, and if done in relation to a patient's problems, solutions are easier. Answers to the theoretical questions which might take months to secure can be found far more quickly if they relate to a specific patient's problem. Not as much cortical driving is necessary since many of the clues are there at hand and certainly the motivation. Comprehension gained this way is more rounded and better remembered since it need not be translated learning.

In the majority of occupational therapy schools, the scientific preparation in physical disabilities is less than in physical therapy schools when functional activities would seem to require as great a knowledge of structure and function if not more.

Professional

As supervisors are we preventing growth by too much supervision? Are we allowing others to help set their own goals? Dependence does not develop strength in staff, students or patients. By setting sights, we risk setting lower goals than they might set for themselves. The safety and security of well-defined boundaries such as specific 'assignments, authority over ideas as well as work, prevents individual development. Once exposed to the headiness of individual projects rather than merely satisfying someone else, the exposure usually takes.

All occupational therapists should add to our store of knowledge and general growth, not suffer technique and equipment contractures. We have a tendency to be dependent when there is need to exercise our muscles of initiative. Each must contribute at his own level so that the whole may be more complete, since each with different background and interest will see different facets of the same problem. The richness of research material and its application to treatment techniques has been slow to seep to the therapy level. Our responsibility is to read widely and observe, to think and bring to the doctor's attention those things which might affect the patient. Therapy will be only as good as the therapist.

The establishment of an advanced study treatment center should be contemplated, not in conjunction with any school of therapy but of and for the Association and its members. This would provide for dynamic interaction of minds under medical guidance. Some of the points to be considered in relation to such a center would be:

1. Inclusion of small groups of occupational therapists and allied professional groups. In the physical disabilities area, the physical and occupational therapist would be the basic interacting unit.
2. A nucleus of top therapists each with special abilities that all might learn from one another.
3. Therapists selected should have five or more years experience.
4. Theory and its application and practice must be integrated with enough time for studying, thinking and thoughtful application.
5. Individual courses for special weaknesses (such as written and oral communication) could be secured in other facilities.
6. This might be a central bureau for the proper consideration of new

developments in the field, including testing of new treatment procedures and equipment ideas as well as evaluating existing procedures.

7. Preparation of abstracts and papers for professional publications should be a requirement.

Support could come from grants from numerous foundations and quarters are secondary to personnel and ideas.

Summary

It is important in development and growth that there be stimulation from without and from within so that autogenetic or self-igniting facilitation and inhibition be developed. There are many steps along the road but heavy work patterns of effort and stress must be faced and overcome before the finer, higher level patterns are possible. Both movement and holding are necessary. In the past we have performed reciprocal innervation patterns for movement only, without the cocontraction patterns against stress. We have been assisting weak muscles and giving them the lightest work when a heavier work pattern given first would make the skilled pattern possible or easier. To change to the thought of heavy work patterns will be difficult, but by knowing all of the sensory stimuli for the appropriate sensory receptors it is possible to aid the desired pattern through the nervous system. Thought is necessary in order to put patterns of muscle work through the proper sequential order of normal development. Any omission or transposition of order will prolong the process or make the results imperfect.

The most important points in all of our developmental patterns are sequential order, activitation for primary and secondary action in movement, and the resistance to stress. These apply to emotional, intellectual and professional development as well as physical growth. With mastery of these points will come the auto-inhibition and facilitation so necessary for functioning alone as a human being within the total group. We will then add our share to the heritage which has been given to us by others and which will be carried on in the future by many more. May our journey as explorers in life be fruitful and satisfying, and increasingly stimulating mentally. Our physical age of maturity has definite limits but our mental and spiritual age need not.

The 1959 Eleanor Clarke Slagle Lecture

The Essentials of
Work Evaluation

Lilian S. Wegg

Preface

The principles of occupational therapy established by our pioneer occupational therapists, and most particularly Eleanor Clarke Slagle, have given us the foundation upon which to build advanced techniques and approaches.

Although prevocational occupational therapy is a recognized part of our work, it seems apparent that there is still a need for a discussion of the basic principles and practices essential to such a program.

The essentials which will be considered today are the expression not only of myself, but also of the members of the work evaluation team of the May T. Morrison Center for Rehabilitation. The recognition you have given to me must, in truth, go to this team as a whole.

Introduction

In the consideration of vocationally oriented occupational therapy, it is essential to provide an effective means of determining needs, measuring abilities and predicting capacities of an individual. One of the most effective means is through the use of tests. Experience in helping to develop a work evaluation service has taught me that tests are basic to such a service and that the work tests developed in occupational therapy are the very essence of such a program.

Reprinted from *The American Journal of Occupational Therapy*, Vol. XIV, No. 2, 1960.

It is, therefore, this subject of tests which will be our primary consideration today; what a test is, what a test should do and the role of the occupational therapist as a tester.

In the field of physical disabilities, certain tests have become standard to good treatment. Some of these are range of motion tests, muscle examinations and functional activity tests. Initially, we use these various evaluations as a way of establishing tentative goals. Throughout the course of treatment, we use them as a means of measuring progress or abilities.

The work evaluation team, in an examination of the vocational needs of the patient, realized that these tests did not reveal, to any practical extent, the person's ability and capacity for work. The need for a more thorough appraisal and accurate prediction of vocational capacities was evident. It was appropriate that an approach be developed which would attempt to deal with this need and which would be suitable for all diagnostic areas.

In work evaluation, tests using the reality situation or work sample method have proven to be such an approach.

Statement

If we recognize that tests play a part in determining needs and act as a guide to the attainment of goals, then we can assume that the purposes of a work evaluation program are the testing and evaluation of work abilities, including skills; the testing and predicting of work capacities, including the level of employment expected; and the testing and exploration of interest and work aptitudes.

More specifically, the objectives of the tests, are:

1. To evaluate ability as related directly to recommended and specific job tasks. The evaluation of the person's learning ability, retention of skill through tests and recall of skills on retests should be considered.
2. To determine capacity to perform job tasks. Such factors as production and proficiency in terms of the specific samples should be carefully evaluated.
3. To evaluate such physical and psychological factors as work tolerance and work habits.
   a. To evaluate work tolerance, such factors as ability to work in the required physical position for the required length of time;

tolerance to job demands, such as noise, dust, people and tools; tolerance to routine, repetitive work or skilled work should be considered.

b. To evaluate work habits, such factors as responsibility, cooperation, attention span, response to authority and criticism, method and manner of performance, mood and relationship to others, should be examined.

4. To devise and evaluate work simplification methods as indicated.

5. To provide the patient with an opportunity to participate in a realistic work program.

In order to meet these testing objectives based on vocational needs, it is necessary to have media closely related to job demands. Work sampling and evaluation is job-oriented, not disability-oriented. We are evaluating the ability of a person to work. Because the individual is vocationally in need, our media and our roles must have a vocational orientation. The fact that a medical diagnosis rendered the person in need of vocational rehabilitation means that we must be aware of the diagnosis in the work program. We are dealing, then, with a medical and a vocational program, with consideration of the former but emphasis on the latter. This change of emphasis influences the role of the occupational therapist.

To understand this clearly, we first need to know what a test is and what a test should do. A test is defined as "a means of measuring the skill, knowledge, intelligence, capacities or aptitudes of an individual." In preceding remarks, it was mentioned that a work testing program should provide a reality situation, an accurate measurement of abilities, and an accurate prediction of capacities.

Let us keep the definition of a test and these essentials of testing in mind and determine how work tests should be organized to accomplish the objectives.

Many of you will be familiar with the *Dictionary of Occupational Titles.* This publication has been prepared by the Division of Occupational Analysis, of the United States Employment Service. It has provided a suitable framework upon which to organize the structure of work tests. This structure allows for division and selection of appropriate work samples according to the major job families: such as, technical work, clerical and sales work, service work, mechanical work and manual work.

The test should measure as nearly as possible the movements required on the job. In addition, such intensity factors as the distance walked, directions reached, and weights lifted and carried should be evaluated. It should be of sufficient length to evaluate both ability and endurance. This means that the test should involve normal units of work rather than single units which would evaluate only the momentary capacity. If, under normal working conditions, the individual would be required to work with 500 or 1,000 parts for a given period of time, then the work sample should be set up accordingly.

The tests should be provided in a special atmosphere which is tailored to fit the demands of the various job families and which is in keeping with the demands of a testing situation. Unless group testing has been specifically recommended, the tests should be administered in a room separate from the occupational therapy department or workshop area.

The test should provide both an objective and a subjective analysis and standardization in all tests is a recognized goal. Standardization does not relieve the occupational therapist of interest, ingenuity or initiative. On the contrary, as each client varies so greatly from the next, the tester's entire thought and time will be directed to the evaluation of that particular person's performance in terms of the test objectives established for him. Without standardization of the testing procedures, there would be no reference point or base line for the tester, there would be no opportunity to accumulate reliable data and, indeed, the entire process would lose the scientific concept.

The test should be easily administered. Each test should have a test kit indexed according to the occupational classification and titled with the test name itself. For example: handwriting is classified under the major heading of "Clerical Work, General Recording," with the numerical classification of 1-X2-0. Assembly, packaging and sorting of miscellaneous items is classified under the major heading of "Manual Bench Work" with the numerical classification of 6-X4-3.

Each test kit should contain a test outline composed of a description of the test in industrial terminology, the purpose of the test, the physical demands of the task, the psychological factors to be considered, a list of the equipment and supplies required, a detailed explanation of how to prepare the work place, an explanation of the exact information to be given the client, and full instructions as to what should be included in the timings and what items should be recorded as errors. The equipment, tools and supplies should be assembled in a portable kit if possible.

The test results should be readily evaluated. This requires a standard and quick method of scoring and checking for accuracy. Several systems for the latter can be used, such as: special marks, numerical codes, or answer sheets. When evaluating craftsmanship, models for comparison should be used. When evaluating work samples classified as repair work, the tester should be sure that the finished project works. Discussion of scoring will come later in the paper.

The test should be acceptable to the individual taking it. This is not a problem if there is rigid adherence to the reality situation. There is some danger when devising a work sample to make something do for the sake of economy in time and money. This is false economy. It results in the test appearing silly to the client and thus losing its predictive value.

The test should be available to facilities and occupational therapists at a moderate initial outlay. Replacement or maintenance should not be costly.

The use of work evaluation tests means that the occupational therapist must be a work tester and, as such, is assuming a function of more vocational emphasis than medical. This change in emphasis, however, does not change our functions radically. The following outline of the essential functions of the tester will indicate that these are basically the same as the defined and accepted functions of the occupational therapist. The items with which we work, the factors which we consider, the terminology which we use, the goals which we set, may be adapted to fit the need. The basic or fundamental things that we do, however, have not changed.

Essential Functions of the Tester

Referral. Included in the referral for work evaluation should be as many known factors as possible, such as; the work history, the medical, social and educational histories and the results of psychological evaluations. There should be a recent physical examination or medical approval of the program. In our facility, it has been the occupational therapist and the rehabilitation counselor who have procured and assembled this data.

Acceptance. Once this information is obtained, the referral should be followed by a staff review for determination of acceptance and choice of work samples. At the May T. Morrison Center, we have termed this review the work sample prescription conference. The occupational therapist, the physiatrist and the rehabilitation counselor select the appropriate tests. If the referral comes from the Vocational Rehabilitation Services, the counselor active in the case attends the conference. The selection of tests is based on the client's physical capacities, personality appraisal, social history, vocational interests and aptitudes and the tentative vocational objective.

The occupational therapist should assist in recommending the actual tests to be used. He should suggest whether or not retests or equivalent tests seem indicated and at what stage these should occur in the program. Retests refer to the same tests done more than once and can be administered within the first tryout period or scheduled for a later date. Retests given within the initial period will evaluate the individual's ability to recall skills. If given at a later date, retests will not only evaluate recall but also will serve as a measurement of progress in abilities. Equivalent tests refer to tests which are similar to others in that they can evaluate similar factors but will differ in such things as the test outline, the instructions or the tools. These are generally done within the initial tryout period. Such tests are useful when evaluating the client's tolerance to working with a variety of materials, such as wood as opposed to metal or vice versa.

Preparation. In the planning stage, preparation refers to the scheduling of the client. Various social, psychological or physical factors enter into the choice of time and days. The time of the day, the day of the week, the time of the month, the attitude of the family can, and will, influence the client's participation in the testing program.

Pretesting

Preparation. The equipment should be kept in working order, the supplies should be adequate for each testing period and the work room should be properly arranged for the client and the job.

Presentation. In the explanation of the testing program, it is important to orient the client to the purpose of the testing and of the tests. Terminology should be used which is in keeping with the job and suited to the client's needs, such as in the case of the deaf, blind or the brain injured. Initial contact will structure the total testing atmosphere.

Instructions will be oral, written or schematic depending on the nature of the job. Instructions should be kept to the test outline as they have been carefully worked out according to normal job conditions.

Demonstrations of the movements required and the various methods needed to complete the work sample will be necessary. This is particularly true in jobs requiring a high rate of production. Our test outlines are written for the nonhandicapped person and adapted as necessary for each client. This adaptation would be required in the case of a functionally one-handed individual performing a task normally requiring the use of two hands.

Tryout phase. The client should be allowed to try out part of the test to learn the procedures and to allow the tester to observe his capacities. The learning time should be recorded for comparison with the average learning time. The need for accuracy should be stressed during this phase and all errors should be corrected and discussed with the client as they occur.

Test

Administration. An accurate administration is essential otherwise the scores cannot be validated. Strict adherence to the work samples as prescribed, however, should be up to the discretion of the tester—a judgment which is used constantly in the treatment of patients.

Instructions and comments should be confined to the testing situation. The performance must be by the client's own efforts in this phase. Unnecessary words or actions will disturb the worker.

Observation. Both direct and indirect methods of observation should be used. An example of the direct method would be the close observation essential to note the number and types of errors which the client makes. Very often an individual will make consistent errors. These could be due to an oversight during the instruction period, or something that the client has failed to comprehend or something that he is prone to do. Without close attention to this detail, the wrong conclusion could be made. An example of the indirect method would be the subtle observation of manifestations of behavior.

Recording and evaluation. When making observations, it is easy to overlook certain factors, forget certain details or emphasize unimportant events. Therefore, for recording and evaluating, it is recommended that the tester use a work test sheet, check list (work sample prescription) and stopwatch. A slide rule is optional.

The work test sheet is an ideal place for recording the client's name, diagnosis, date, numerical classification and title of test. It also allows space for a description of the client's performance and his production, proficiency and final ratings. If this sheet is carefully written, it can serve as a part of the final report. Only the most significant material should be recorded. This places additional importance on the work sample prescription as the testing objectives will then serve as a guide.

To evaluate performance, it is necessary that some method of scoring be established. The Morrison Center has a norm for each work sample test. This norm was established by methods used by our industrial engineer, Mr. Paton B. Crouse. The norm is set up so that 100% represents the normal good performance of nonhandicapped workers familiar with the job and working at a tempo that would be required in competitive employment.

These norms, written in decimal figures, are recorded in each test kit. If the test involves several parts, each part will have a norm. A decimal stopwatch is used to record the client's time. At the conclusion of the test, the norm is divided by the time achieved by the work. This establishes a percentage and is known as the production rating. To obtain a proficiency rating, a certain percentage is then deducted for errors. This percentage is based on the degree of skill needed and the quality required by the job. All final ratings are based not only on the production and proficiency ratings, but also on the subjective analysis of the client's coordination, attention and interest for that particular job. These ratings are expressed in terms of "good," fair," or "poor" depending on where they fall in the numerical scale of 100-0. For example 0-30 represents poor or questionable performance and means that the client is capable of selective work in the sheltered shop area or noncompetitive employment. A score of 30-50 represents a fair performance and means that the client is capable of sheltered shop work at that time with the potentiality for competitive employment with training or adjustment. A 50-75 score represents good and means that the client is an adequate worker for competitive employment. A 75-100 score represents superior and means that the client is a good to exceptional worker and capable of competitive employment.

The final evaluation must also be based on the atmosphere and deviations which have been allowed by the tester. These deviations may or may not be acceptable from the vocational viewpoint. It is imperative that this be determined before the tester ventures too far from the standard procedure. This again is one reason why a discreet choice or prescription of samples is so essential. If the elements of a test have to be varied to such a degree that the test loses its identity, then an appropriate work sample was not selected.

Reporting

Quite detailed and structured reports should be prepared. Adoption of standard terminology by the team is essential. To avoid unnecessary repetition when preparing the report, our evaluation service has adopted a standard organization of the report and standard phrases for certain parts. For example, the opening paragraph always states:

> The following work samples were selected on the basis of the client's education and employment history, psychological test results and physical (or psychiatric) information in order to evaluate his physical ability and capacity, his emotional tolerance and capacity, his interest and aptitude to engage in the following work.

The prescribed or selected work samples are then listed, after which is a description and evaluation of the client's performance on each test. A summary of the overall performance relating directly to the testing objectives with recommendations for future course of action or possible areas of placement concludes the report. Whatever the organization of the report, however, the tester must strive to be objective in his remarks. The tester must not be influenced by previous evaluations. His opinions must be based solely on the observations during the testing period.

The preceding essentials form the scientific basis of a work evaluation program. The success of such a program depends on the most important essential of all—that is, the tester. It is obvious that there are certain traits that a tester should possess. First, the tester should be one who can perform concise analyses, both of a qualitative and quantitative nature. As he will be confronted with varying abilities, diagnoses and degrees of intelligence, he must be one who can react consistently and objectively. He must be sensitive to the needs of the client during the testing—needs which could result in a shift in the task or the atmosphere. The tester should be one who can adopt and maintain a scientific concept. He should be one who is willing to work in harmony with a team. He must be one who is interested in learning new concepts, in developing new programs and in the broadening of his education.

The opinion of the work evaluation team at the Morrison Center is that the occupational therapist is the natural choice for the work tester. An occupational therapist's training and work experience is geared to dealing directly with human beings—not just for a few brief moments, or in an hour's interview, but hour after hour throughout a day. An occupational therapist's thoughts and techniques provide him with a unique approach. This approach is ideal for, and essential to, a testing situation.

Before concluding, there are certain other practical considerations which should be noted at this time. First of all, one should not assume that a vast number of tests are required for a work evaluation service. There are four major job classifications which are most commonly requested. These are: clerical and sales work, service work, skilled mechanical work, semi-skilled to unskilled manual work. Of these four classifications, the first and the last are the most used and the most practical from the standpoint of placement areas for handicapped individuals.

Although our tests number 83, only 25 of these are most commonly used. These 25 are:

Clerical and sales work

   1. Computing work using the calculator machine
   2. Handwriting
   3. Simple bookkeeping
   4. Typing
   5. Checking of equipment, invoices
   6. Routine recording work, using adding machines

7. Classifying work
8. Filing
9. Clerical machine operation
10. Collating
11. Telephone and switchboard work
12. Cashiering and vending machine

Service work

1. Kitchen helper
2. Domestic worker

Skilled mechanical work

1. Electrical equipment repairing
2. Radio repairing

Semi-skilled to unskilled manual work

1. Inspection
2. Electrical unit assembling
3. Wood unit assembling and woodworking machine operation
4. Miscellaneous bench work
5. Metal bench work
6. Miscellaneous metal working
7. Miscellaneous paper work: assembling, cutting, sorting
8. Light elemental work: simple routine, repetitive jobs
9. Elemental service work: janitorial or dishwashing jobs
10. Miscellaneous physical work. This is work requiring simple, routine tasks such as might be found on construction projects or in maintenance areas and which would range from light to medium to heavy in degree.

A second major consideration is the number of days suitable for testing. We have found that a period of three days is quite adequate. This is a concentrated period, lasting all day, with one occupational therapist handling one client at a time. Such an arrangement is ideal, but this period must be solely confined to testing and not include training or adjustment. It is my feeling that there is a time and a place for testing, and a time and a place for adjustment or training. An attempt, on the part of one occupational therapist, to do both of these simultaneously loses the scientific approach. This is not to say that adjustment and training cannot be scientific, but in the combination of the two, the true purposes become obscured. The purpose of the testing is to diagnose and evaluate the client's ability and capacity for work but not to condition him for employment. Testing is required to determine the area of training, the level of training and, indeed, if training should be considered. The purpose of a work adjustment program, on the other hand, is to adjust and condition the client to the demands of work by providing opportunities for him to develop work habits or improve such work assets as were noted in the testing situation. The opportunity to participate in a testing program, with close relation to an adjustment program, has made me realize that similar but not identical evaluations can be gained. It would seem apparent, therefore, that both a work testing and a work adjustment program is needed to provide a thorough vocational appraisal. These programs must be coordinated in a team approach. As the work training or adjustment program should occur in a variety of places depending on the results of the work tests, a coordinated team approach implies the integration of an in-center and an out-center team.

There is one last consideration. This is the implication of a testing and evaluation program to our patients, our media and our selves. It means that we are able to offer a more thorough program to our patients by determining their vocational needs and assisting in their fulfillment. It means that occupational therapy can offer a scientific approach. It means that the occupational therapist has a new and stimulating concept. All of these factors have a far-reaching implication as they extend to the potential occupational therapist, our students, a challenge to enter our profession.

In conclusion, certain basic essentials must be considered and adopted in order to provide an effective work evaluation program. It is apparent that such a program must be composed of several phases. The phase which has been discussed today, namely work sample testing, is just one step towards the determination of the patient's ultimate vocational objective. This paper has been an attempt to outline work evaluation essentials and to show the effectiveness of occupational therapy when planned with a group of experts and executed with a goal in mind.

Devices:
Development and Direction

Muriel E. Zimmerman

Preface

As the sixth occupational therapist to receive the Eleanor Clarke Slagle award, I find myself not without a feeling of great humility as well as one of pride. I am respectful of the achievements and high standards of my predecessors and also of the many other occupational therapists who have made and are making a fine contribution to our profession. Thus I am most honored by this confidence you bestow upon me and hope I shall be worthy of it.

I should be remiss if I did not say that whatever I have learned has not been due solely to my own efforts nor to my own inspiration nor to what I am. For I have been fortunate in knowing and working with so many very wonderful people, each of whom has played a significant role in my growth and understanding. To all of them I am deeply indebted for their faith, encouragement, counseling and guidance which have directed my path. My only regret is that it is not possible to name them here; the list is long and I could not be happy with any omitted. To both professional and personal friends, and to my own understanding family who have suffered growing pains with me, I wish to express my deepest gratitude.

Foreword

We need no temple gong, village bell, television commercial or other fanfare to quicken the pulse and the pace or to get attention for a discussion of the use of mechanical devices or aids which have

Reprinted from 1960 *The American Occupational Therapy Conference.*

become by now an integral part of the rehabilitation procedure. We are no longer skeptical as to whether this ought to be the concern of the occupational therapist. We know only too well what has been and can be accomplished for the physically disabled patient by the application of mechanical inventions. And we are fortified in our enthusiasm by rapid technical advances.

Just why we should have waited so long to consider the fact that man has always made use of such skills to help himself is perplexing. It might in part have come when it was recognized that we did not necessarily do the patient a service by doing things for him and that we aided only when we helped him to help himself. Perhaps it could simply have been the result of man's inventiveness coming to his rescue out of necessity, in this area of his life as well as in others. By whatever circumstances it evolved, we can only be delighted that it happened and comforted that from mankind's tragedy came also his means of escape.

Yet not every therapist may have as much time at his disposal as he would like for participation in such helpful procedures. He may also still be meeting some frustration in the form of lack of cooperation from staff in other services and lack of referral. And there may be others who seek more and better ways for advancing the knowledge and skill already available.

It is then at this time my pleasure to present a discussion of this exciting aspect of treatment.

During these past ten years of investigation and search into practical and satisfactory devices to help achieve independence for the physically disabled, a basic philosophy and a technical approach to selection of the proper devices have been a natural development. Trial and error methods, if carefully observed and studied, must lend direction to further pursuits. In 1956 I presented to this same body, at the annual conference in Minneapolis, some of my first organized findings. The analysis discussed at that time consisted of the following approach: (1) evaluation of the patient's physical needs; (2) evaluation of the psychological factors involved in use of special devices; and (3) selection and design of suitable materials and methods of fabrication in relation to the first two factors.

It is not my intent to repeat what I have said before, but to present any additional findings that have refined and improved former methods and which still leave a challenge for future growth.

The study of physical needs by analysis of motions used in the performance of various activities has pinpointed for us the specific losses to be compensated for, either wholly or in part. Through observation, the process of eating has been described and charted. This has shown us which motions are used and for what purpose. We have had some indications also as to relative importance of each of the motions, the extent used and whether it is an "active" motion or a "holding" or "stabilizing" motion.

Such studies are naturally based first on motions as observed in a "normally" functioning arm. As such, our analysis seems relatively simple—especially as we all have very similar habits and patterns, due to our common anatomical structure and the fact that we have all been taught a similar way of accomplishing various activities.

We must realize, however, that even normal functioning varies, and since the upper extremity is fitted to perform many activities, the motions that we use for one activity do not necessarily require ALL the movements available. Thus, if we are minus some of the usual motions in eating, for example, we may still easily be able to manage quite satisfactorily. This we can observe frequently in many of our patients. Often the substitutions or variations are hardly discernible or are performed with such efficiency and ease that we are not quick enough to detect them immediately. This is apt to be true when the loss is minimal or when it is confined to only one location or joint. Here, substitution of either another body motion or use of a device is relatively easy to achieve.

But let us take the patient who may have multiple weaknesses or losses, the one who may be classified as having so much and yet so little. Here the dynamics of motion become much more complex. Let me illustrate with the problem as presented by a rather typical disability limitation such as is often found in the patient with quadriplegia as the result of a spinal cord injury. Upon examination it is found that elbow flexion tests **good**, extension is **zero**, shoulder flexion is **poor** or **trace**, but abduction is **fair plus** to **good minus**, supination and pronation are **fair**, wrist extension is **poor plus** to **fair minus** and grasp is **zero**. There are no range of motion limitations. This patient, if left to his own resources, might be able but for lack of grasp to feed himself, if he were so motivated. But you would probably observe a rather bizarre pattern of motion. The arm would be raised outward by shoulder abduction to shoulder height, then the hand brought in toward the mouth. (One must also remember that in such patients trunk balance is apt to be very poor, so that they cannot bend forward to meet the hand; and wearing a neck collar will further lessen their ability to compensate in this direction.) Another reason why you will find such patients using more shoulder motion than elbow flexion, even though the shoulder is weaker, is that by so doing they eliminate the problem of hitting themselves in the face. This situation is due to lack of triceps muscle, which comes into play after the forearm is raised to a vertical position and then drops toward the face.

According to this report, it would seem that only a substitute for grasp and some assist for shoulder flexion would provide the needed aid and the preferred eating motions. A simple device such as a leather utensil holder or a built-up handle will provide a substitute for grasp. Either an overhead sling with one support under the elbow or a ball-bearing arm support with "flying saucer" used as elbow rest (both standard devices) may be used for providing shoulder flexion positioning.

Such devices, however, have been found to enable only partially satisfactory performance. Too often I have found that the shoulder assist as described above did not accomplish what was expected of it; rather, the patient was frustrated and hampered. Instead of using the support, he is apt to revert to his own substitution; and this bizarre pattern may put undue strain on the shoulder, often bringing on early fatigue and sometimes pain. Why is not the flexion assist as described helpful? We have observed two principles of dynamics which seem to contribute to this happening. One is the result of the type of device used to substitute for grasp. In equipping a patient with a holding device, we must remember that the most frequently used devices position the utensil as though held with a hook grasp rather than pinch grasp. This is not the usual grasp of adults. Also, hook grasp positions the forearm in pronation rather than the mid-supination used in pinch grasp. As a result, when picking up the food, because further rotation of the forearm is impossible, some rotation and abduction of the shoulder is usually necessary. This automatically lifts the elbow from any support provided. Once lifted, the natural tendency is not to lower the elbow to the support and use elbow flexion to bring the hand to the mouth, but to continue shoulder abduction and, as described before, bring the hand to shoulder height and then toward the mouth.

What then should be done? A holding device utilizing pinch grasp may be provided, although thus far any device made for this purpose is far more complicated than those designed for the hook type of grasp. If a fork is used, the tines can be turned down rather than up. Or the fork end can be bent downward. This works very well unless the food is too soft or slippery, in which case it may be lost before the fork is partially raised. Some wrist flexion and ulnar deviation may be used as a substitute, and the normal individual would employ these other motions. But when some weakness of the wrist is present, wrist strength is apt to be utilized mainly for a stabilizing force, which is also one of its purposes. The presence of a wrist splint may impose further limitations.

Of the two shoulder flexion positioning assists, I have found the overhead sling with elbow supports the most helpful. The sling ought to be equipped either with a spring of the correct length and tension or with a device to provide similar action. Then, as the elbow is raised up and away from the body, the sling shortens, thus keeping the elbow-piece under the elbow, ready to support it and encourage its use by lowering the elbow before raising the hand to the mouth. This sling support is simple, but it is also conspicuous. Moreover, there must be some conscious effort and cooperation on the part of the patient to make use of the support as intended.

It is rather obvious from the above-presented description of dynamic functioning that we are still in need of better assisting devices. It should remind us that we are dealing with a part of the body in which more than fifty muscles, wonderfully constructed, are working together for an integrated performance. When the loss of function is minimal and confined to one joint or motion only, the problems arising are relatively uncomplicated. Also, when total function is lost, a fairly satisfactory substitute performance can be achieved through a contrived mechanism. Yet, to aid satisfactorily when there is a multiple combination of varying degrees of loss of function, and to keep pace with adjustments needed as function improves, meanwhile making certain that undesirable motion patterns or substitutions are avoided, requires careful evaluation and proper selection of equipment.

Let us further examine this human tool, the upper extremity. To assist mechanically the functioning of all the components of hand and arm requires as varied an approach as mathematical law dictates for possible combinations of the many units involved and the varying degree of participation of each.

An early study made by the engineering department of the University of California was entitled "Studies to Determine the Functional Requirements for Hand and Arm Prostheses." Because of the need to sort out of all of these movements those that would be most useful, the kinematic analysis of the motions of the activities of daily living was one of the main aspects of the study. Those conducting the study scientifically determined, through many engineering processes, the most useful types of hand grasp. Of the two needs, (1) to pick up an object and (2) to hold objects, it was found that the pick-up motion most frequently used a lateral grasp (58 to 34) with the thumb against the lateral aspect of the index finger. The hold-for-use motion most frequently employed a palmar prehension grasp (64.5 to 34) with the pads of the thumb tip and first two finger tips together. It was found that both grasps were about equally employed. However, it was also found that palmar grasp could be used to substitute for picking up many objects normally using lateral grasp. It was not so with substituting lateral grasp for palmar. Therefore the hand prosthesis was designed to provide a palmar prehension as the most useful motion for the hand. (1)

These hand activity requirements would be the same whether a prosthesis or a splint is desired. Hand splints are also designed to provide a palmar prehension type of grasp. This is true of both the Warm Springs type of opponens hand splint and the flexor hinge tenodesis hand splint.

So far, this last analysis has considered only the hand or terminal device. While it can be studied separately, it is also dependent upon arm function for placing it in a position of use. Let us consider each of the arm parts and its contribution to the total hand-arm functioning.

The wrist as a positioning device is well known. Most persons agree that either a neutral or a slight cock-up position, if there need be any limits set, is the most useful. This is perhaps true. However, depending upon the type of object grasped and at what height it is in relation to the body, other factors must be considered in any analysis, such as whether other accommodations are possible, as supination and pronation, internal and external rotation of the shoulder or trunk, or body bending. Again, citing the study by Boetler, Keller, Taylor and Zahn as an example, it takes 42 degrees of supination of forearm for picking up a plate. The action can be accomplished if only 30 degrees of supination are present; however, there must be additional compensations, such as depressing the arm or bending the body to the right. (1) Nevertheless, while this compensation may be anticipated as a possible and satisfactory accommodation in the average amputee, it generally is not possible to expect many persons with flail upper extremities resulting from poliomyelitis or a spinal cord injury to do this.

Elbow flexion and extension are obviously important in most activities and are provided for fairly easily. The motions or various positionings of the shoulder are complex and again, as in the hand, realistic replacement of all of them is almost impossible, at least today. Stabilization against the force of gravity, some flexion and abduction and some internal and external rotation are probably the most useful.

Let us go back for a moment to the selection of a suitable design for a functional splint for the hand. The pinch type of grasp has seemed to prove the most useful, yet the design as now used does not seem to be totally adequate. In various patients we have tested with this device we have found that many objects are still difficult to pick up. The difficulty seems due, largely, to lack of ability to position the hand. And if we observe an amputee using a hook we will find that even with his many arm and body accommodations he may have to pre-position the article. If these accommodations or the ability to position the hand are impossible, then we must often accept limited performance. Just recently a patient whom we were fitting with a splint was experiencing some of these difficulties, and he offeréd us a suggestion for possible improvement in the present flexor-hinge hand splint, which was designed to position and stabilize the thumb in abduction and hold the interphalangeal joints of the first two fingers in slight flexion. Motion (of a hinge type) is provided at the metacarpal—phalangeal joints. When the wrist is in a cock-up position, picking up objects is difficult. If, however, pinch grasp were provided by stabilization of just the interphalangeal joints of fingers and thumb, while motion (opening and closing of grasp) occurred in both fingers and thumb, then pick up might be easier. This means another moving part and usually that complicates any device. However, the suggestion as mentioned to us is being tried experimentally and a sample splint has been constructed with very good mechanical results at the time of this writing.

We have not had time to use this splint on a patient. Therefore, it is only a first-test model and cannot be classified as good, poor or bad. Rather, it is being shown as an illustration of how, when a specific problem is defined, an attempt may be made to solve it (Figures 1, 2, 3, 4). The only results we can state at this moment are that less wrist motion is used and more opening of grasp is obtained. Wrist motion required in the original model was approximately 70 degrees. In the new design, it is 25-30 degrees, or less than half. Opening of grasp was increased from 2 3/8 to 2 1/2 inches. It is possible, however, that the new design may call for greater strength for operation, which could negate the advantages.

Again, we have presented another functional problem to illustrate the extent to which our present knowledge and efforts are still limited, in terms of our needs. A helpful procedure to follow would be (1) to evaluate for loss of necessary motions for a specific activity; (2) to select devices to compensate or substitute for lost motion; (3) to note whether devices provide for a normal functioning of the specific part or whether they impose abnormal patterns; and, (4) to note substitute motions imposed because of abnormal patterns and adjust the equipment accordingly.

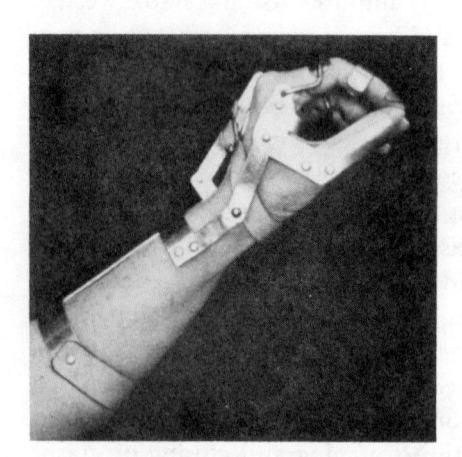

Figure 1. Hand splint (old design) with wrist extended and fingers closed.

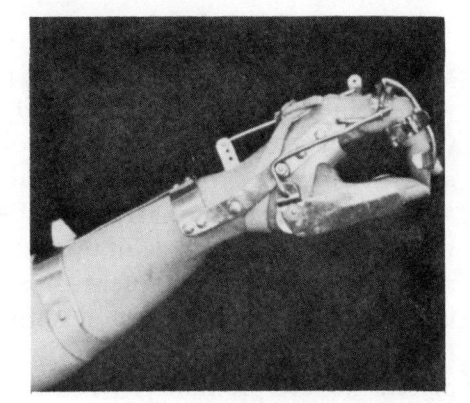

Figure 2. Hand splint (new design) with wrist extended and fingers closed.

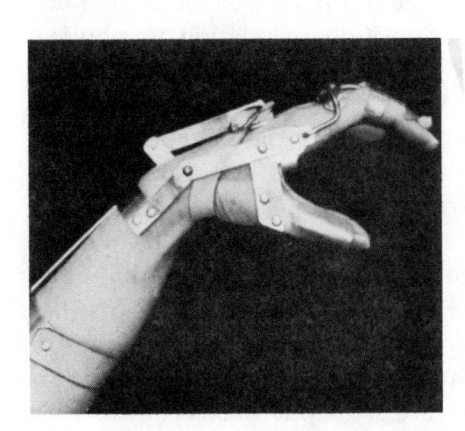

Figure 3. Hand splint (old design) with wrist flexed and fingers open.

Figure 4. Hand splint (new design) with wrist flexed and fingers open.

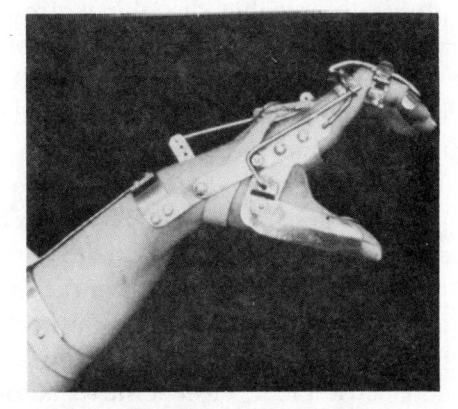

Such studies as are currently being undertaken by the University of Michigan in their research program on orthotics should be most helpful to all of us concerned with this field of rehabilitation. One in particular (2) is the study of total arm function for specific activities in relation to space, a study being made on a much broader scale than ever before attempted. A parallel might be drawn here with motion studies made in the field of homemaking in which it was shown that the most frequent trips made in the kitchen are between the sink and the stove. The resulting energy-saving principle arising from this situation is that these two pieces of equipment should be placed in close proximity. When this is not done, ways and means of compensating must be provided.

Thus far I have discussed only additional problems of one factor, namely, that of the study of motion in relation to physical needs. The second factor is that of the psychological implication of devices to the patient.

Many of the responses of the patient are the same as those he exhibits toward the disability itself and are, of course, the psychologist's concern to evaluate, not ours. But we can recognize also some attitudes directly related to the devices and we ought to be aware of why they make an additional emotional impact. I believe the sociological attitudes of our society are greatly at fault for much of what occurs. The term independence to most of us, for example, is apt to mean sheer physical strength. And in today's world this is not so strange, as often the nondisabled are hard put to keep pace with work and leisure activities of a busy and highly competitive culture. Here, however, is a paradox. Although man thinks of himself as physically capable of taking care of himself, he at the same time strives to help himself more and more with mechanical inventions.

Let us look for a moment at the busy executive. He gathers information, communicates it, and directs much of his business via the telephone, intercommunications system, dictaphone and possibly TV or radar viewing screens. Most of the time while doing this he sits behind a desk in a chair. Physical energy used is at a minimum. This same person, as a good many other citizens of today, probably whisked himself out of bed in the morning, got ready for the day and traveled to work using many other mechanical devices such as modern plumbing, which provides instant hot water at the turn of a tap; an electric razor, electric stove, automatic coffee maker; packaged or frozen foods; a bus, taxi, automobile or subway; and an elevator to lift him from the ground floor to wherever his office is located. Whenever I am in our workshop and glance out for a moment to the towering structure of the Empire State Building, I am reminded of the fact that without elevators this building would be only an empty structure, except for a few rugged individuals; and they would undoubtedly be found on the first ten floors, with just possibly an isolationist above, rejoicing in his ivory tower.

Man has continually striven to extend his power beyond his own physical ability. Could we learn of the heavens beyond our reach without our great telescopes? And now we are designing rockets to take us to these great outer spaces. From the beginning of the discovery of flint and the invention of the wheel, man has steadily reached forth for new and better ways to help himself.

This being so, why should any person resist using devices just at the very time they can mean so much to him? Let us look at the other side of the picture. The ideal of the anatomically perfect person is shouted at us from the pictures and slogans of advertising, from road signs, magazines, radio and television. So the need for outside assistance is like adding insult to injury. If any of us has any doubt of the real importance of this trauma to the ego of the individual, I can ask you to reflect on how so many of us react to the more or less accepted use of eyeglasses, hearing aids and even certain easily recognized styles of clothing. Spectacles are given all sorts of added glamor in the form of color, shape and decoration; or contact lenses deny the presence of glasses altogether. Hearing aids are mounted behind the ear, some on the ends of spectacle bows to make them less conspicuous. I have come across an advertisement by a hairdresser in which he showed hair styles designed to hide a hearing aid. And certainly the manufacturers of our nationally advertised commodities make use of a real or fictitious person who represents the American ideal to enhance selling appeal. Have you ever noticed how often this person is a handsome Adonis or a rugged outdoor sportsman or both? Why do we cling to such ideals? Probably because physical perfection represents strength and beauty. We still need reminding that there are other types of strength and beauty besides that which we see—goodness, truth, achievement and thoughtfulness.

It is all too infrequently that we see an advertisement representing these other qualities. But we do have them occasionally. One that

I clipped showed the "egghead" modeling a new style boy's shirt. A well-known magazine, which is famous for typifying the American public, showed on its cover the college campus with the girls clustering around the top science student while the football hero passed by unattended. And some of my colleagues may have heard me comment on one of the cigarette ads which purports to appeal to the "thinking man." (Even so, the "thinking man" shown usually has a spectacular hobby.)

We must remember that ages ago, when many of these concepts had their origin, brute strength was important. Survival often depended upon it. And we must admit that in those days it was man's greatest attribute. The person who survived by his wits was rare. Because of these occasions brains were given a high regard even then. But there was little opportunity to use them and physical labor was paramount. Today we live in a different age, a highly mechanized one. We employ all our ingenuity and skill to improve our lot. Is there really much difference between the robot arm which aids the man in the atomic laboratory to handle radio-active material and the artificial muscle and CO_2 which enable a powerless hand to pick up and hold the objects necessary to his daily activities? There is nothing really unique in the dependence of the physically disabled upon equipment except in the degree and type of design for operation. And it would be helpful to all of us if we could remember the philosophy of Antoine de Saint Exupery that just as man has created these many tools that he uses, he is also master of them and slave only when ignorance and prejudice keep him from trying to help himself. (3)

It may seem that I have been talking rather at length concerning man's use of mechanical aids. However, if we are going to be working with patients who need such equipment, then we cannot lightly ignore such influences but must deal with them. We do our patient no service by stating merely, "He is uncooperative" or "He does not wish to help himself," and by feeling that he must automatically consider us the angel of deliverance from his problems.

What can we do then to make these devices acceptable to the disabled? I believe there are several definite courses of action to take. One method of making equipment more palatable is to introduce it into the treatment program as early as possible. This takes away from that stigma of being "the last resort," which is inevitable if devices are sought only after all other measures have failed. It is easier to accept help in the beginning with the hope that it may be discarded later—as well it may be, for recovery comes for some—and it has been found that devices can have some part in enhancing the possibility of recovery of skills. Also, familiarity with equipment can lessen the threat of its continued use, if such is the need. Let me give one example to illustrate the early use of devices.

Sometime last spring I was confronted with a challenging situation which called for definite action. A patient in his early twenties, a first-year medical student and a victim of Guillain-Barre syndrome, was referred to the service for evaluation in terms of supports and other self-help equipment for the upper extremities, both of which had very little muscle power in shoulders or elbows. The wrists and hands were fairly good, although not completely normal.

I first introduced myself and explained the function of our service. Whereupon the patient turned to me and stated very positively, "Of course, you realize I shall have no need of your services because by September I shall be completely well and back in medical school!"

Before I could make any comment he continued, "And I may as well tell you that in the other hospital, where I was before coming here, the occupational therapist tried to rig me up in all sorts of contraptions, treating me like a hopeless cripple."

I gulped inwardly, thought fast, and then replied, "Well, you are quite right in that devices are designed to help the person who is or may be permanently disabled to become independent; but they are used in other ways as well. They can be set up as therapeutic agents to provide independence while one is working on a treatment program. Can you, for instance, feed yourself now?"

The reply was, "No." So I explained that I could provide him with a device with which he could do this. The device, if properly set up, would do nothing for him that he could do for himself. It would only substitute for those motions that he could not make now. And as soon as any progress was made, adjustment would be made in the device accordingly, to gradually lessen the assistance as he became able to take over. He was then asked whether he would like to see the equipment. He agreed and was willing to give it a test. He was fortunately so impressed that we were able to set up the equipment for his use. For several days he was visited regularly to check whether everything was satisfactory. He was then left to continue its use. Later, at an opportune time, I visited him again to see whether any changes were needed. When I remarked that possibly we might consider some lessening of the assistance, the reply was, "Oh, let's not do it yet!" The patient continued to use the equipment and gradually less and less assistance was needed. Today, fortunately, the patient does not need any aid for the upper extremities. It is not to be inferred that the apparatus provided was solely responsible for return of strength and function. Many other treatment measures were being provided simultaneously. But the patient was able to start performing many activities very early, and it can be assumed that the devices were contributory and did enhance other programs by providing early coordinate use of the arms and build-up of tolerance and skill.

In addition to the early use of devices, there are other measures that can be taken to insure their success and value. We can and should make the best devices possible. We must first be certain they will really serve the purpose for which they are intended; the study of motion, as described, helps to determine this. Then we must ask ourselves whether the device is performing as efficiently as possible. Is its operation simple? Free from breakdown or need of frequent adjustment? Within the understanding and grasp of the operator after a minimal amount of practice and supervision? Or is it inconspicuous, so as not to attract undue attention? Is it as near to the accepted mode as possible without being freakish? Is it cosmetic and attractive? In regard to the improvement made in eyeglasses, for instance, it should be recognized that not all the recent advances are a result of our need for ego-building or just to keep up with the Joneses, although we cannot deny this aspect of the picture. The use of color is pleasing and satisfying, and that, as well as the shape, can either add to or detract from one's appearance. And perhaps most important is design for function. Contact lenses certainly were originated with that purpose in mind. They are much more simplified than glasses and reduce the breakage hazard. They eliminate possible discomfort from pressure irritation on the nose or ear as well as interference of vision from the frames.

Modern designers are more and more alert to function and efficiency. While they do not yet advertise many of their products as designed for the person with a physical limitation, they do promote the fact that they require only one hand to operate and thus will take less effort to do the job. The development of improvements in kitchen and household equipment has been a real boon to any homemaker whether physically impaired or not. The major reason we have been so happy about our new Functional Home for Easier Living is that its selection and adjustment of features do provide easier living for anyone.

If you wish to remind yourself some time of these various requirements of equipment, let me suggest a simple method. Just ask yourself what you would demand. Let us look at clothes. Function and versatility: as few pieces as possible to serve as many needs as possible; easy and quick to put on and take off; design or style in keeping with today's fashion trends; becoming to you; wearability and ease of care; "travel-a-bility;" and, of course, a price within your budget.

These are high goals and to provide all of these answers is not yet totally within our scope. But if we try to do our best, so may the patients be more willing to try also.

There are two other brief thoughts that I cannot exclude. One is that although we must do everything possible to provide equipment to aid our patients, if this is the answer to their problems, we should never try to impose anything upon anyone just because it is one way of giving assistance. All equipment has its limitations and must be judged according to its usefulness and the need for it as against the disadvantages. Socioeconomic factors also must be considered. A favorite story of ours at the Institute is that of the patient referred to ADL for dressing activities who finally said, "But do I have to learn to dress myself now when I've always had and will have a valet to do it for me?" Electric wheel chairs, as helpful as they are, are not the answer for persons going home to remote areas or underdeveloped countries where as yet no facilities for repairs or adjustments are available.

The last factor is that of patient participation. Full explanation from us of what is to be accomplished, leading to understanding by the patients, is the easier road to acceptance. In these busy days we often let lack of time rob us of this responsibility. Also needed is the willingness to listen to the patient, to his ideas or complaints. The patient not only feels that you are interested in him, but you may discover many interesting facts and learn better ways of doing things.

For after all, it is the patient who is experiencing the satisfactions or difficulties of devices made for his help.

The third and last factor in selection and provision of equipment is the fabrication or construction of the device itself. Again, this is an area that I have already covered previously and therefore I shall not make more than a brief resume.

It is important to know something about materials and principles of construction design and to evaluate this information in terms of the tools, the time, and the personnel and skill at our disposal. While devices are becoming more and more available as more people enter the field professionally, the occupational therapist, I believe, still has a role to play, if not in construction, then in understanding so as to improve his ability to work with the team in evaluating, testing and training.

The engineer does not select or choose at random the various materials he uses, nor create a design out of idle fancy. He uses fundamental principles regarding properties of materials and laws of mathematics and physics. Even the clothing designer relies on more than just the need for a new fashion. As it was expressed to me by a well-known dress designer, a sure sense of such things as the very "feel" of a material, which suggests the "hang" and "hinge" of the weave—the pull and tension of the threads themselves—is basic to good design.

And we can make another contribution. This is to seek and find the different types of devices that will meet the needs of many different disabilities and many activities and will satisfy the various other demands of a majority of the disabled, their therapists, doctors and families. Upon such a basis, and by means of the production line, manufacturers will eliminate some of the higher costs of today's individual construction. At present, because some production is limited and prices therefore high, we have a tendency to complain that this goal is not being achieved. But we must remember that their inability to provide us with lower costs is in large part directly related to our own inability to accomplish the above and thereby come into some accord on what we want.

To appreciate fully the manufacturer's problem, let me give you a simple illustration. I asked our staff to tell me how long it would take them to make an ordinary spring-clip clothespin. Estimated time was from one-and-a-quarter to six hours. Obviously, various levels of skill are represented here and must affect the cost of labor which, if figured accordingly, would run from $1.75 to $6.00 for this one simple, dime-a-dozen clothespin. Manufacturing costs also are high for a single clothespin, for making the necessary jigs may take longer than to make a whole clothespin. The only answer to this lies in quantity production.

This can only be desirable, for it is also an answer to helping more patients. We must recognize and accept with standardization, however, the fact that there will always be the extreme deviations from the average or norm, which will leave us with some unanswered problems requiring special solutions. And, as with all standardization, we must never fall into the trap of believing we have found our final goal. There must remain the challenge of further improvement.

It is within this last framework of thought that I would like to call attention, before I close, to the contributions of research and special studies and the place of the occupational therapist in these endeavors. When I, as an occupational therapist, entered the field of self-help devices, there were no specific boundaries or limitations as to who should be doing this work or how it was to be done. With time, we are lending direction to how it should be done and, to a certain extent, by whom. The role of the occupational therapist is being defined. It seems necessary, as we shift from the unique to the standard, to fit into the pattern and scheme of organization and teamwork.

Nevertheless, when one problem or set of problems has been solved, automatically new goals are set, new needs discovered. I like to recall the words of Robert Browning. (4)

> "Ah, but a man's reach should exceed his grasp,
> Or what's a heaven for?"

For occupational therapists looking for new worlds to conquer, there is always one waiting at our finger tips. And while we may not recognize at first where the path lies, if we seek we shall find it.

At a time when there came a deeper recognition of the need for stepped-up development and use of self-help or assistive devices, occupational therapists along with others made available their talents and skill to help find the answers. And out of all these efforts there has been achieved a beginning science of this new field. We recognize that we have certain techniques at our disposal: (1) the study of motion requirements for specific activities and how these relate to the possibilities of the total functioning of an individual and to limited function; (2) the understanding of the patient's psychological needs and ways of meeting them and (3) the understanding of mechanical requirements through study of materials and fabrication processes. And, finally, we can come to determine how and where our contributions as occupational therapists will serve most potently in the total process. Most probably it will be in testing for selection of devices, check out for use, and training. Sometimes, depending upon need and suitability, occupational therapists' skill may be used in fabrication.

In conclusion, we have met our responsibility to the patient who needs devices by lending our resources to this field. We must continue to meet these responsibilities so long as there remains a need for our skills. And finally, we must remain eager to participate in any way where the vision of others or our own vision can create a better world for the disabled.

REFERENCES

1. Boetler, Keller, Taylor & Zahn, *Studies to Determine the Functional Requirements for Hand and Arm Prostheses.* Los Angeles 24, Calif.: Department of Engineering, University of California, July 25, 1947.
2. University of Michigan, Ann Arbor, Michigan. Orthotics Research Project.
3. Saint-Exupery, Antoine de, *Wind, Sand and Stars.*
4. Browning, Robert, "Andrea del Sarto."

The 1961 Eleanor Clarke Slagle Lecture

Occupational Therapy Can Be One of the Great Ideas of 20th Century Medicine

Mary Reilly

Specifying the Theme

As an occupational therapist honored by her peers, I join my Eleanor Clarke Slagle predecessors in feeling the awesome responsibility of the award. The occasion, it seems to me, makes it obligatory for an awardee to objectify a lifetime experience and then speak of an issue of concern to all. With this in mind, I have elected to present an issue which impinges upon the very root meaning of our existence. In developing the idea I have sought to reflect it against the changing background of the world in which we live. My hope is that its exploration will add to an understanding of the profession which we practice.

The question I would like to speak to is one which each one of us has asked at some time or other in our professional lives. Some of us have asked it many times. It has been raised in different ways and expressed in different words, both within and outside our field. In all probability, it will continue to be asked by those who follow us. I am referring to an anxiety about our value as a service to sick people. This theme I have identified by the question: *Is occupational therapy a sufficiently vital and unique service for medicine to support and society to reward?*

The anxiety begins in a primitive form when we stand before our first patient and sense the enormous demands that a treatment

Reprinted from *The American Journal of Occupational Therapy*, Vol. XVI, No. 1, 1962.

problem makes upon the occupational therapy brush, hammer or needle. The wide and gaping chasm which exists between the complexity of illness and the commonplaceness of our treatment tools is, and always will be, both the pride and anguish of our profession. Anxiety accumulates as we become increasingly involved in treatment, teaching and research, and even more sophisticated questions tend to arise from that same source to plague us.

The theme of today's presentation is focused, therefore, on the critical appraisal of the essential worth of occupational therapy. I say critical because the technique of criticism will be the method by which the issue will be explored. The subject was selected because I found from my experience that the value of occupational therapy exists in a controversial state. Among any group of my colleagues who have practiced long and well, I found that this question of value constituted a continuous and almost lifelong dialogue.

The Theme Converted to an Hypothesis Test

Where and how does one begin to make dependable and hence usable judgments about value? Taking full advantage of the freedom inherent in the Slagle lectureship, I reasoned that the idea most basic to our practice ought to be searched out and then converted into a kind of a question which might be answerable to some degree. This search, I further reasoned, should begin in the time of our earliest days. I began there and found that there was a single root idea embedded deep in our foundation and this deeply imbedded belief is what we call occupational therapy. In the stormy years between then and now, I found that there were few opportunities given to examine the roots of our foundation and to consider the growth which sprang from it.

My reexamination of our early history revealed that our profession emerged from a common belief held by a small group of people. This common belief is the hypothesis upon which our profession was founded. It was, and indeed still is, one of the truly great and even magnificent hypothesis of medicine today. I have dared to state this hypothesis: *That man, through the use of his hands as they are energized by mind and will, can influence the state of his own health.* This is the inherited occupational therapy hypothesis passed on for proof by the early founders.

The splendor of its vision goes far beyond rating it as an idea conceived once in a lifetime or even once in a century. Rather, it falls in the class of one of those great beliefs which has advanced civilization. Its magnificence lies in the optimistic vote of confidence it gives to human nature. It implies that there is a reservoir of sensitivity and skill in the hands of man which can be tapped for his health. It implies the rich adaptability and durability of the central nervous system which can be influenced by experiences. And more than all this, it implies that man, through the use of his hands, can creatively deploy his thinking, feelings and purposes to make himself at home in the world and to make the world his home.

For a profession organized around this hypothesis it sets few limits to its growth. It merely endows a group with the obligation to acquire reliable knowledge leading to a competency to serve the belief. Because this is an hypothesis about health, it requires that this knowledge be made available for the guidance of physicians and that it be made applicable to a wide range of medical problems.

The Role of Criticism

Before preparing a brief for its validation I would like to make a detour into a description of the method whereby the issue will be explored. The method is in harmony with my temperament because, by choice, I am neither a conservative nor am I a conformist. I am a devout and practicing, card-carrying critic. Since criticism as a technique of public discussion has yet to emerge in our association affairs, I feel a need to define and describe it. Its philosophy, techniques and tactics will constitute the point of view from which I will speak.

The public use of criticism by a profession has been spelled out best by Merton (1) who sees it as a prevailing spirit within a group necessary to maintain a group's progress. Its greatest usefulness is that it acts to repudiate a smugness which assumes that everything possible has already been attained. Its presence commits an association to keeping its members from resting easily on their oars when they are so inclined. In general, Merton finds that criticism stings a profession into a new and more demanding formulation of purpose and maintains a policy position of divine discontent with the state of affairs as they are.

A disciplined person in either the sciences or the professions uses critical thinking as a personal tool of reality testing and problem solving. When a professional organization as a whole accepts criticism as the dominating mode of thought, then indeed, theorizing flourishes and the intellectual atmosphere of their gatherings is characterized by sweeping controversies. In this atmosphere of controversy, progress becomes somewhat assured.

But a card-carrying critic must do more than merely engage in critical thinking. Judgments made by a critic must emerge from a discreet use of techniques which are difficult to master and dangerous to apply. Basically, the skill is dependent upon an ability to analyze, interpret and synthesize. A critic must have a sharply developed capacity to see deficiencies in data and fallacies in interpretation. The best stock in trade that any critic has is a discerning eye for trends and an ability to pattern and verbalize them. Whether a critic is worth listening to is usually decided by an ability to use language well, by a creativeness in synthesizing new relations and by courage to propose provocative hypotheses. Ultimately, however, a good critic rests his case upon how well he has been able to restructure the issue so that the necessary powers for its resolution can be freed. These idealistic but difficult standards are the ones I hope to follow in restructuring the issue of how valuable is occupational therapy.

Design of the Presentation

Having discussed the point of view from which I will speak, it is now necessary to describe the plan of attack which will be made on this global theme. For the sake of this presentation let us suppose that the hypothesis I have proposed is the wellspring of our profession and that it is worth proving. It would not follow necessarily from this that it is provable. A large part of the power to act on the hypothesis, of course, resides with us, the members of the American Occupational Therapy Association. But the society in which our profession lives holds power too and can rule on its growth. Even before we begin the validation, we must look at the probability that this idea may not be capable of proof in this century. I plan to ask first whether the American culture can tolerate such an hypothesis. Next I shall question whether the 20th Century is the right time for the test. The most crucial aspect of the presentation will be an attempt to identify the point at which the process of proof ought to begin. This will be followed by an attempt to identify the basic pattern of our service by which the hypothesis will be proven. Finally, I shall comment on some ongoing crises which the hypothesis is undergoing and then leave for history its continuing proof.

Is America the Place to Test the Hypothesis?

Let us first consider the tolerance in America for the occupational therapy idea. In his social history, Max Lerner (2) identified certain dynamic forces which impelled the greatness of this country. He cited in the American mind two crucial images present since the beginning. One was the self-reliant craftsman, whether pioneer, farmer or mechanic. He was the man who could make something of the American resources, apply his strength and skill to nature's abundance, fashion new tools and machines, imagine and carry through new constructions. Without taking himself overseriously, Max Lerner's American has generally regarded the great engineering, business, government and medical tasks as jobs to be done. Progress in technology was seen simply as agenda for the craftsman.

The second image Lerner drew was from the American environment. It was that of a vast continent on earth, as in space, waiting to be discovered, explored, cleared, built-up, populated and energized. Lerner contends that our culture is dominated by an American spirit which hates to be confined. A drive toward action, he postulated, is a part of the American character.

This drive towards action seems to me to make reasonable the American idea of a patient. Our cultural concept of the man of action suffers little change when an American moves into a hospital community. It has been supported by a series of principles which merged and fused into what we now call rehabilitation. Early in this century, there emerged the principle in medical management that patients were easier to handle when they were occupied with mild tasks. Later when it was found that an active patient tended to recover faster, early ambulation became an acceptable principle of physiology and blended well with the principal of patient occupation. Concern for the psychological nature of patients brought forth the widespread acceptance of craft, recreation and work programs in hospitals. The need to train patients in self-care became almost a crusade to insure the rights of patients to be independent. Within the community, laymen cooperated in ventures to assure the handicapped's right to return to work. Now we are implementing in full swing the socioeconomic principle that it is good business for society to support such programs with public monies.

There are some obvious things which can be concluded about America's tolerance for the occupational therapy hypothesis. It would seem almost axiomatic that the American society in general, and medicine in particular, has need of a profession which has as its unique concern the nurturing of the spirit in man for action. In every way it knows how, America has said that this spirit must be served and served in a special kind of way when it has been blocked by physical or emotional ills. That this need will be persistent in American culture seems fairly certain. That occupational therapy will persist is not quite so certain. It is true, however, that if we fail to serve society's need for action, we will most assuredly die out as a health profession. It is also most assuredly true that if we did dissolve from the scene, in a decade or so, another group similarly purposed and similarly organized and prepared would have to be invented. I believe, therefore, that the occupational therapy hypothesis is a natural one to be advanced in America.

Is the 20th Century the Time?

The timeliness of the hypothesis is the next question I should like to raise. Are we the people and these the times for the test? We are all deeply entangled in the forces and events of the century in which we live. But if this entanglement commits our energies to the endless treadmill of survival, then the hypothesis cannot get off the ground. The social scientists tell us that the world we live in is in a state of indigestion from too much change. We have yet to absorb the disorganizations brought on by a depression, two wars and an ongoing massive technological revolution. This change is being reflected by society into all its component institutions. It follows naturally that we feel its reflection in our professional lives.

But our state of turmoil was not always so, because occupational therapy was born in the quieter times of this century. In the first several decades of our existence, medicine offered us a tranquil and supportive setting. Our literature reveals that physicians tended to nurture the development of our schools and clinics. In these earlier times we were helped to meet the challenges of contributing to the ongoing medical scene. The last several decades, however, have put excessive stress for expansion upon a profession whose role had been barely defined. We have seen our practice organized into specialty fields by the demands of World War II. Our clinicians have only recently been systematized into team behavior by the pressures of rehabilitation. Now in the sixties we are confessing to a mounting sense of confusion and voicing a need for direction. We are keenly aware of the conflicting demands being made upon our practice. The problems that our schools face in digesting the accumulating technical knowledge which practice demands, is a matter of growing distress. Caught up in these forces how free can we be to control our growth?

If we are anxious today, the social scientist offers the explanation that it is because we are now aware that the hopes we had cultivated in gentler times of the past are being threatened by the pace of the world around us. Historians, however, are quick to counter that when times of great change appear, they are forecasting a death to the old and a birth to a new way of life. It is inconceivable that we or any other group with organized intelligence would stand idly by and permit the random destruction of the old and encourage blind birth to the new. Fortunately, most institutions have centralized their action for controlling change through planning groups variously called the Task Force, Master Plan Committee or the Role Definition Study. Our national association has not remained aloof from such efforts and is currently involved in three change controlling studies. As many of us know well, the studies involve professional curriculum and clinical practice, the functions of the organization and the future development of the profession.

We may conclude that we have shown by our action that we have felt the buffeting of great change and are attempting to control it. But how can we know whether the efforts we are making are sufficient and are of the right kind? This difficult question has some partial answers. One common sense answer is that we must recognize the fact that we have grown and have changed as we grew. In our forty years of existence our sense of purpose, our anchorage points have shifted. It is only logical to reason that we will not rediscover a sense of purpose by merely reflecting within our professions the problems of the larger society in which we exist. Few rewards are granted to those who are content to reflect problems. Society demands that its problems be answered. Therefore, to any group which aspires to be a profession, there is placed before it a clear-cut mandate. This mandate says that if we wish to exist as a profession we must identify the vital need of man which we serve and the manner in which we serve it.

I contend that this is the point at which the proof of the occupational therapy hypothesis begins. The reality of our profession depends upon an identification of the vital need of mankind that we serve. How free we are in these troubled times to reconstruct our thinking at this basic level I do not know. But I do know that the crucial nature of our service cannot be spelled out in the loosely constructed way that it is today. I personally have little trust that we can continue to exist as an arts and crafts group which serves muscle dysfunction or as an activity group which serves the emotionally disabled. Society requires of us a much sharper focus on its needs. As the next step in the development of the theme it becomes necessary to make a critical examination of what, if any, vital need we serve.

What Vital Need Is Served?

As the first order of the business at hand we ought to have it clearly in mind what constitutes a vital need. Of all the descriptions of the need states of man which I have heard I like Eric Fromm's (3) the best. He says that needs are an indispensable part of human nature and imperatively demand satisfaction. The need we serve must fall within this category. He says further that they are rooted in the physiological organization of man and consist of hunger, thirst and sleep and that in general they all belong to self-preservation. He proposes a simple, forthright formula of self-preservation which is directly applicable to occupational therapy. According to Fromm, when man is born the stage is set for him. He has to eat, drink, sleep and protect himself from his enemies. Therefore, for his self-preservation he must work and produce. Work, in the Eric Fromm sense, is a physiologically conditioned need and therefore a need to work is postulated as an imperative part of man's nature.

In our forty years of practice we have accumulated some fascinating odds and ends of understanding about the need to work. For example, early in my training I was taught that work was good for people. All people needed to work and sick people even more so. This kind of justification of service reminds me of the old story about the man who died and woke up surrounded by all kinds of delights which were his for the mere bend of the finger. After he had satiated himself well, he called for the headman, expressed his appreciation for the manner in which he was treated and then said, "Now that I have pleasured myself well, it is my wish to do something. My good man, what is there for me to do in this paradise?" The answer given to him was, "You are doing it now." "But," replied our man, "I must do something or else my stay in heaven will be intolerable." "Who" replied the headman firmly, "said that you were in heaven?" In the past I have been guilty of believing and having my patients persuaded that work was good and heaven would prove me right. The rationale that man works because it is good for him, regardless of its comfort to us, makes little contribution to our understanding of work as a basic need.

During the thirties, the economic depression gave us an unparalleled opportunity to learn that when able people could not find work, certain psychological disorganization occurred. These changes were deemed to be over and above the changes which could reasonably result from economic loss. We are able to generalize from the depression that human nature does not thrive in idleness. In the last several decades we have accumulated a few more broad generalizations. One is that the stress of work produces psychosomatic conditions in modern businessmen. Another generalization which is now being formulated is that when people retire from their work, they retire from life itself.

A vital need to be occupied however, is not to be inferred from such global generalizations. It is being left to the more rigorously controlled experimentations to do this. Now under laboratory conditions man's need-state for action is being rigorously investigated. In the United States and Canada basic research is going on in an area called sensory deprivation. The work began in reaction to the Russian brainwashing attempts. The research was designed on the principle of restricting man's interaction with the ongoing world of reality. Under controlled conditions of isolation man was found to suffer profound disturbances of his thought processes. In isolation men regressed to unrealistic and prelogical modes of behavior. The sensoy deprivation findings suggest strongly that the concepts of man's response to his environment must be sharply revised. The behavioral aberrations which were observed in the idleness of depression and retirement, and the stress of overwork, appear to have been confirmed by the laboratory induced sensory deprivations. The data were checked out by neurologists, psychiatrists, biochemists, pharmacologists, mathematicians and engineers.

The final sensory deprivation report sums up to a concept that the mind cannot continue to function efficiently without constant stimuli from the external world. The central nervous system is now seen as a complex guessing machine oriented outward for the testing of ideas. The experimenters postulate that each individual constructs a different development pattern with respect to strategies for dealing with reality. Jerome Brauner, (4) as one of the researchers, concluded that early sensory deprivation prevents the formation of adequate models and strategies for dealing with the environment. Later sensory deprivation in normal adults, he suggests, disrupts the vital evaluation process by which one constantly monitors and corrects the strategies one has learned to employ in dealing with the environment.

To summarize at this point, it seems to me that the American drive toward action as identified by Max Lerner and the human drive toward work as identified by Fromm have been verified in the laboratories. I believe that we are on safe ground right now to say that man has a vital need for occupation and that his central nervous system demands the rich and varied stimuli that solving life problems provides him that this is the basic need that occupational therapy ought to be serving.

What Is the Unique Service?

A profession, however, must do more than identify the need it serves. There is a twin obligation to spell out its unique pattern of service. The next gigantic task which this presentation faces and with some trepidation, because of the limitation of time, is an attempt to identify the basic pattern of our service by which the hypothesis may be proven. The charge is gigantic because it makes it obligatory to define the occupational therapy body of knowledge, its treatment process and techniques.

A search for valid content, process and methods has been my preoccupation in the past ten years of reading, study and practice. If I had the ability to do all this with any degree of clarity, I would not be here talking about it. I would be in a clinic doing it. However, I am now admitting to a rising sense of satisfaction in the project and a receding sense of frustration. At no time in technological history have the behavioral scientists been producing so much knowledge directly applicable to our field as they are now. The material is emerging from sources as divergent as neurological theory, animal psychology, developmental and personality theory and from psychologists as diverse as Allport, Murphy, Harlow, Hebb, Goldstein, Piaget and Schlachtel.

In order to plunge directly into this material I am going to have to make use of a device in logic known as a First Principle. For if we were to have a First Principle in occupational therapy it would provide us with a way to specify our knowledge. To those who may not be familiar with the meaning of First Principle, it is a device in reasoning to account for all that follows. For instance, the idea of God is a First Principle which accounts for the Universe. There has been a First Principle postulated to explain the nature of man. We are told that the first duty of an organism is to be alive. Medical science derives its premise from this first law of life. If it were not desirable to cure disease and prolong life, the rules of science and the skills and practice of medicine would be irrelevant. The second duty of an organism is to grow and be productive. Occupational therapy ought to derive its premise from the second law of life. If it were not desirable to be productive, the skills and practices of occupational therapy would be irrelevant.

These two laws merge into a concept of function which asserts that both the existence and the unfolding of the specific powers of an organism are one and the same thing. This concept of function is expressed as: the power to act creates a need to use the power, and the failure to use power results in dysfunction and unhappiness. The validity of the First Principle is easily recognizable in the physiological functions of man. Man has the power to talk and move, therefore, if he were prevented from using the power, severe physical discomfort would result. Freud utilized this First Principle to build a powerful theoretical position from which emotional illness was so successfully attacked. He accepted man's biological necessity to produce and generalized that when sexual energy was blocked, neurotic disturbances resulted. He endowed sexual satisfaction with all-encompassing significance. He developed his theory of sexual satisfaction into a profound symbolic expression of the fact that man's failure to use and spend what he has is the cause of sickness and unhappiness. The Freudian theory that human action is primarily sexually based has thrown a strong but restrictive shadow over other behavioral fields. It has been only lately that attention has been given to human productivity in nonsexual areas. Occupational therapy's focus, it is asserted here, lies in the nonsexual area of human productivity and creativity.

In Gardner Murphy's (5) brilliant defense of human productivity he makes us aware that there is a distinct path which leads to becoming human. This path is not seen as being sexually directed. The direction lies largely in the enrichment and elaboration of the sensory and motor experience and the life of symbolism which depends upon them. He maintains that the sheer fact that we have a nervous system, the sheer fact that we can learn, means that we can prolong and complicate sensory and motor satisfactions, can make them richer, can give them more connections, can avoid boredom, can recombine them, can feed upon them, can become immersed in them and make them a part of ourselves. In all these respects, Murphy says man is most completely human. His primary thesis is that man achieves satisfaction in using what he has, in using the equipment that makes him human; and this entails not only the sensory and motor equipment but that central nervous system upon which the learning and thinking processes depend.

Murphy's spirited description of the conditions necessary for being human can provide the basis for an occupational therapy First Principle. This logic constitutes our mandate to discover and organize our body of knowledge; to develop a treatment process; and to devise techniques for its application to the health of man. The logic of occupational therapy rests upon the principle that man has a need to master his environment, to alter and improve it. When this need is blocked by disease or injury, severe dysfunction and unhappiness results. Man must develop and exercise the powers of his central nervous system through open encounter with life around him. Failure to spend and to use what he has in the performance of the tasks that belong to his role in life makes him less human than he could be. With this principle in mind I would like to summarize my thoughts of the last several years of work on our body of knowledge, our treatment process and techniques.

Regarding the body of knowledge. Because our profession is focused on influencing the health of people there will always be a need to include in our body of knowledge the fundamental material of anatomy, neurophysiology, personality theory, social processes and the pathological states to which these functional areas are subject. However, I do not feel this is our unique content. We should have as a special contribution a profound understanding of the nature of work.

Knowledge of work capacity lies scattered over many behavioral fields. We do know, for instance, that man's ability to work has been developed in the long evolutionary process. It began when man hunted and fished for his food and continued as he grew his food and fabricated objects for his comfort. The lot of man was considerably improved when he freed himself from arduous labor through tools and machinery. His comfort was immeasurably assured by the social institutions he built and operated with increasing skill over the centuries. It is my contention that this evolutionary process, plus a bit more, is present, symbolically expressed in today's culture. The concept of work capacity as being an outgrowth of an evolutionary process I call the phylogenesis of work. I believe that cultural history of work ought to be deeply embedded in the occupational therapy body of knowledge and its phylogenetic nature considered particularly in program building.

We know that as a child grows, he recapitulates the history of his race in the stages through which he himself must pass en route to maturity. The need to pass through phylogenetic experiences in work is necessary for mature work capacity to be developed. There is historical evidence that a child's ability to play, to explore his environment, to exercise his motor skills are the foundation for his later school experiences. The problem-solving processes and the creativity exercised in school work, craft and hobby experiences are the necessary preparations for the later demands of the work world. Because we know that the random movements of the infant progress in developmental sequence toward the job competencies of the mature adult,

I postulate an ontogenesis of work. I believe that the ontogenetic nature of work ought to be considered in the case study approach to each treatment problem.

The occupational therapy body of knowledge should include therefore, an understanding of the developmental nature of the sensory-motor systems, the patterning of aptitudes, abilities and interests, the nature of the learning process involved in the acquisition of skills. It should include also an understanding of the developmental nature of the problem-solving process and process of creativity. My epistemological conclusion is that the biological, psychological or social knowledge we select as part of our thinking content must be intermeshed deliberately with the knowledge of work-phylogenesis and work-ontogenesis.

Regarding the treatment process. The capacity to work develops in the long socialization process through which a child becomes an adult. It proceeds along the path of growth as man learns to intermesh his motor with his intellectual functions and adapt this integration to the tasks of his life which satisfy his need to control his environment. Work capacity, in this sense, can be said to develop out of the struggle with gravity for motor control, the struggle with learning for manual and mental skills and the struggle with people and people purpose for economic and social control. When the struggle is great, the personal involvement is high; although conflict and frustration are high, so, too, is work satisfaction high. It follows, too, that when involvement is low, work satisfaction is low. The occupational therapy process becomes primarily concerned with that special aspect of the socialization process called work satisfaction. Its approach in treatment is biographical because work satisfaction is, by its nature, the result of past experiences expressed in the present ability to cope with the environment. Its focus is on the meaningful involvement in problem-solving tasks or creative performances. The parameters of its concern are the ability to experience pleasure in achievement, to tolerate the frustrations of struggle, to sustain the burden of routine tasks and to maintain the level of aspiration within the reality level of work skills. The goal of the process is to encourage active, open encounter with the tasks which would reasonably belong to his role in life. The process is paced and guided by the supervision of the prescribing physician.

Regarding treatment techniques. Techniques which would

emerge from the body of knowledge and the professional process as just described would be concerned with program and treatment execution. Methods would include all those administrative techniques of program building which would provide a laboratory setting for human productivity. The treatment technique would be all those procedures associated with modifying sensory-motor dysfunctions, perceptual difficulties and the difficulties inherent in coping with the world of play, work and school. It is suggested in terms of today's thesis that in the merging of our content, process and methods, the unique pattern of our function will be spelled out. If this pattern is focused strongly on man's need to be occupied productively and creatively, the hypothesis will grow stronger.

Major Tests of the Hypothesis

Of all the ongoing tests of the occupational therapy hypotheses, I have selected a few major ones upon which to comment. The first and obvious one is whether a need to accumulate substantial knowledge about human productivity and creativity will be recognized and acted upon in our schools and clinics. The problem of balancing our knowledge has been with us for some time. Until now our attention has been preoccupied with the medical science which supports the application of our craft knowledge to medical conditions. But medical science knowledge is a means for the application of our service and not an end in itself. A profound knowledge of human dynamics of productivity and creativity is the end to which our knowledge ought to be designed. As far as our practice today is concerned, we have more medical science knowledge than we know how to apply and we are applying more knowledge about human productivity than we actually have on hand.

The second, and not so obvious test, is the delimiting effect that psychoanalytical practice has on the promotion of a nonsexual concept of human productivity. The fundamental doctrine of the Freudian pleasure principle is that the essential movement of a living organism is to return to a state of quiescence and that primary pleasure is sought in sensual gratification. A fundamental principal of work is that primary pleasure can be sought through efficient use of the central nervous system for the performance of those ego integrating tasks which enables man to alter and control his environment. In this sense psychoanalytical theory is seen to focus on subjective reality while work theory becomes largely concerned with objective problem-solving reality. It is not that these points of view run counter to each other. They simply do not meet or interact except under very special conditions of intimate supervision by a psychoanalyst.

In 1943 Hendrick (6) raised this issue in the *Psychoanalytic Quarterly*. He argued that the psychosocial activities of the total organism are not adequately accounted for by the pleasure and reality principles when these are defined, in accordance with Freudian tradition, as immediate or delayed response, respectively, to the need for sensual gratification. He suggests that work is not primarily motivated by sexual need or associated aggressions, but by the need for efficient use of the muscular and intellectual tools, regardless of what secondary needs (self-preservation, aggressive or sexual) a work performance may also satisfy. Hendrick postulated a need for a work principle which asserts that primary pleasure is sought by efficient use of the central nervous system for the performance of well integrated ego functions which enable the individual to control or alter his environment.

In psychoanalytic practice today sexual satisfaction is seen as being influenced by ontogenetic, phylogenetic and biographical considerations while no such considerations are seen needed for work satisfaction. Although many analysts have agreed that sexual capacity correlates highly with work capacity, the idea has not been developed much beyond the statement. Work is seen as a kind of experience a patient ought to have and whatever satisfaction he derives from it will be dependent upon his subjective state. As a result, extensive activity programs have grown up around psychiatric treatment which have been designed for participation, but not specifically for ego involvement. These programs are now being called activity programs and those implementing them are called activity therapists.

Such activity programs encourage the participation of large groups and usually appeal to the automatic, learned patterns of behavior. However, activity programs so designed, deny the dignity of a human being to struggle, to control his environment as witness the fact that they tend to make man quiescent within the hospital community. They tend to depersonalize, institutionalize and, in general, debase human nature. The occupational therapy hypothesis makes the assumption that the mind and will of man are occupied through central nervous system action and that man can and should be involved consciously in problem solving and creative activity. It is believed that psychoanalytical theory and the occupational therapy hypothesis can profitably coexist if a work principle is postulated and executed. This will be even more true if occupational therapy deepens its understanding of the phylogenetic and ontogenetic nature of work and makes a case study approach to ego involvement of patients. It is not so possible, however, that activity therapy and occupational therapy can coexist. It is believed that the major crisis in the proof of our hypothesis will not be how to coexist with psychoanalytical theory but to know the difference between activity and occupation and to act on the knowledge of this difference.

The last major test which I will discuss has to do with the physical disability field. In this specialty we have been placing heavy emphasis upon muscle efficiency and enabling devices. There is a long, perilous and complex ladder to be scaled between neuromuscular efficiency and work satisfaction. The ontogenetic reconstitution of motor behavior is a tedious process and must be done step by step. It begins at the reflex muscle action stage and proceeds to the development of complex patterns of motor skills which are utilized in a rich variety of work skills. These, in turn, must be disciplined to a sustaining level of tolerance for routine labors. It is upon this broad pattern that human tolerance for working with people in people affairs is built. If any of these steps are missing, they must be refashioned and the whole pattern reshaped accordingly. The proof of the occupational therapy hypothesis in the physical disability field will depend upon how much we know about the process of restoring work capacity. It cannot be done from prescriptions based upon a narrow understanding of human productivity. It cannot be done in cramped clinics dependent upon scrap material. Nor can it be done from our present ignorance of the world of industry for which we believe we are preparing patients. The challenge to the hypothesis in this area is severe, yet provocative. The technical literature of our profession is indicating that this challenge is not being ignored.

Summary and Conclusion

In summarizing the many ideas I have touched or expanded upon in this thesis, I once again return to my original question: *Is occupational therapy a service vital and unique enough for medicine to support and society to reward?* In answering it, I have said that we have had a magnificent hypothesis to prove and if it could be proven, even to some degree, the answer would be that we are valuable to medicine and to society. The hypothesis that I presented for evidence of proof was that *man, through the use of his hands, as they are energized by mind and will, can influence the state of his own health.* I asked if this were a kind of idea that America could subscribe to and to that I replied with a resounding yes. I wondered about the stress that the terrible 20th Century was putting on this idea and worried some about the energy left to us to advance it. I suggested the hypothesis would begin its proof when we identified the drive in man for occupation and would continue as we shaped our services to fill that need. I speculated on some of the crises the hypothesis was now undergoing and left the decision not in the lap of the gods but in our own laps for us to think and act upon in our daily practice.

I have said that our profession has a magnificent medical purpose. Whether we shall fulfill it or whether it shall ever be fulfilled I have not said because I do not know. But this I can say from personal experience, that we belong to a profession that requires the mind to look at the history of man's achievements throughout civilization. It requires the spirit to respond to the wonders of what man has accomplished with his hands. It gives us a mandate to apply this knowledge and more to help man influence the state of his own health.

BIBLIOGRAPHY

1. Merton, Robert K. "The Search for Professional Status." *American Journal of Nursing,* March, 1959.
2. Lerner, Max. *America as a Civilization.* New York: Simon and Schuster, 1957.
3. Fromm, Eric. *The Fear of Freedom.* London, England: Routledge and Kegan Paul Ltd., 1960.
4. Solomon, Philip, & etc. *Sensory Deprivation.* Cambridge, Massachusetts: Harvard University Press, 1961.
5. Murphy, Gardner. *Human Potentialities.* New York: Basic Books, 1958.
6. Hendrick, Ives. "Work and the Pleasure Principle." *Psychoanalytic Quarterly,* Vol. VII, No. 3, 1943.

BIBLIOGRAPHICAL NOTES

Work has been studied from the viewpoint of economics, philosophy, sociology and psychology, and although the literature is considerable, and is being added to constantly, it is a comparatively recent focus for scholars. So far no general study of work has been written, but to some extent a student in this field need not be left entirely without guidance. He needs to remember, however, that the literature is too extensive for one individual to investigate thoroughly. This bibliography noting is designed to serve as an introductory guide. Many of the recommended writings also include full bibliographies of the topic with which they are concerned.

Anyone who seeks to be a student of human occupation should attempt first to build a historical perspective of the field. *A History of Technology*, edited by Charles Singer, E.J. Holmyard and A.R. Hall, is a massive five volume series published by Clarendon Press in Oxford from 1954 to 1958 and provides a general historical background as far as science, economics and technology is concerned. An account of the effect of labor and technology on the culture of the west is set forth in another series titled *The History of Civilization*, edited by C.K. Ogden and published in New York by Alfred A. Knopf, 1926 to 1929.

The sociological nature of work may be approached through a study of the socialization process and the field of industrial social psychology. This aspect of study is excellently covered in *The Handbook of Social Psychology*, edited by Gardner Murphy and published in two volumes by Addison-Wesley Company in 1952. A recent perceptive and illuminating view of the social and economic nature of work and the worker is presented by *Theories of Society*, Vol. I and II, edited by Parsons, Stills, Naegele and Pitts published by the Free Press of Glencoe, Inc., in 1961.

The specific classics regarding human occupations are exemplified by: Theodore Caplow's *The Sociology of Work*, (Minneapolis: The University of Minnesota Press, 1954); Eli Ginzberg's *Occupational Choice: An Approach to a General Theory* (New York: Columbia University Press, 1951); Anne Roe's *The Psychology of Occupations* (New York: John Wiley and Sons, 1956); Donald Super's *The Psychology of Careers: An Introduction to Vocational Development* (New York: Harper and Brothers, 1957) and John Darley and Theda Hagenah's *Vocational Interest and Measurement: Theory and Practice* (Minneapolis: The University of Minnesota Press, 1955).

The classics concerned with human creativity are: Viktor Lowenfeld's *Creative and Mental Growth*, revised edition, (New York: The Macmillan Company, 1952); Edwin Ziegfeld's *Education and Art: A Symposium* (Paris: 19 Avenue Kleber, United Nation's Educational, Scientific and Cultural Organization, 1953) and Harold Anderson's *Creativity and Its Cultivation* (New York: Harper and Brothers, 1958.)

The author further recommends: Robert Gagne and Edwin Fleishman's *Psychology and Human Performance* (New York: Henry Holt and Company, 1959); Ernest Schachtel's *Metamorphosis* (New York: Basic Books, 1959); Gordon Allport's *Personality and Social Encounter* (Boston: Beacon Press, 1960); Hannah Arendt's *The Human Condition* (New York: Doubleday Anchor Books, 1959); Erich Fromm's *Man for Himself* (New York: Rinehart and Company, 1945); Gerald Gurin, Joseph Veroff and Sheila Feld's *Americans View Their Mental Health: Number Four* (New York: Basic Books, 1960); and Frederick Herzberg, Bernard Mausner and Barbara Snyderman's *The Motivation to Work* (New York: John Wiley and Sons, 1959).

The 1962 Eleanor Clarke Slagle Lecture

The Challenge
of the Sixties

Naida Ackley

It is with feelings of trepidation and humility as well as pride, that I take my place in the lengthening procession of Eleanor Clarke Slagle lecturers. Although deeply honored to be the recipient of this award, I feel you have not so much honored me as an individual, as that you have chosen me as a symbol, a representative, for all the occupational therapists who have devoted their interest and professional competence to the treatment of the mentally ill.

Changing Roles

I would like to use this time to examine with you some of the current developments in psychiatry in the United States of America which have implications for us and for our future practice. Many changes are taking place in the whole field of psychiatry. Long established and accepted concepts of care and treatment are being critically evaluated; different types of in- and outpatient treatment facilities are being established; traditional roles are changing as professional and nonprofessional groups review their qualifications and patterns of operation in order to improve their current function or assume new roles. Social scientists and anthropologists are contributing new insights, and the role of the community in all aspects of the mental health problem is increasingly recognized.

These changes have vital implications for occupational therapists in psychiatric practice which we must recognize and act upon. The decisions we reach and the action we take during the next few

Reprinted from *The American Journal of Occupational Therapy*, Vol. XVI, No. 6, 1962 years will determine the future of occupational therapy. We must finally answer the question "What is the function of occupational therapy in psychiatry?" There is no concensus today; opinion and practice range from dynamically oriented treatment programs to ones which are very broad in scope and general in application. My personal and professional conviction has always been that occupational therapy is treatment. In psychiatry it is a form of treatment which utilizes activities and the relationship developed around and through these activities to assist the patient in finding more acceptable patterns of relating to others, and more mature ways of dealing with and solving his problems.

Utilizing Occupational Therapy

The education of the occupational therapist is designed to prepare personnel equipped to carry out this treatment function under medical direction, but many institutions do not use their occupational therapists in this capacity. This may be due to the orientation of the hospital itself. *Action for Mental Health* documents an impressive number of institutions which are not treatment oriented. (1) It may be due to the quality and immaturity of the occupational therapists it employs. Or it may be due to the unwillingness of some physicians to accept allied medically trained personnel as co-therapists. Whatever the reason, I wonder how much longer we can persuade young occupational therapists to enter the psychiatric area if we do not demonstrate a role and function for them which is commensurate with their professional preparation. The ability to recognize and understand factors which contribute to or precipitate disability, and the acquisition of knowledge and security in using remedial techniques is the justification for the long and expensive education of the occupational therapist. Today the need for personnel with medical or medically related professional training is so acute, that it is difficult to justify the use of such personnel in any capacity which does not utilize their professional preparation to the fullest possible extent.

Future Responsibilities

There are many situations where the occupational therapist is a respected member of the treatment team and where occupational therapy makes an important contribution to treatment. These include private hospitals, psychiatric services in general hospitals, state hospitals, Service and Veterans hospitals. Since my experience has been primarily in state hospitals I shall discuss treatment focused occupational therapy in that setting. Many influential people in psychiatry feel the state hospital will be superceded by other kinds of treatment facilities for all types of mental illness. Others, equally authoritative, feel the state hospital provides the best facilities for the treatment of major mental illness and will continue to do so for many years. There is general agreement that many changes will be made, but again there is a difference of opinion about the degree of these changes and the form they will take. I am no crystal gazer and can certainly make no predictions about the future size or specific function of the state hospital, but I feel safe in saying that the future of occupational therapy in psychiatry is in our hands as it has never been before.

We, in common with other professional groups, are being asked to review and evaluate our practice, to determine objectively which of our current functions could be delegated to less highly trained workers so that professionally trained personnel can devote more of their time to specific patient treatment. This request is predicated on the well-documented assumption that professional staff shortages will exist for a long time to come, and it is thus imperative that current professional staff be relieved of every duty, administrative or treatment-focused, which could be performed by less highly trained workers. This is in no way an effort to reduce services to patients. It is rather an effort to relieve physicians and allied medical personnel of routine or administrative duties and minor responsibilities and functions which have become associated with their positions over the years, so that they will have time and energy to use their specialized skills in more meaningful patient treatment. The request to re-evaluate professional functions also takes cognizance of the development and use of volunteer groups and the services which they render, the availability of personnel with specialized activity skills, the increasing emphasis on vocational rehabilitation and aftercare services, and the use of ward personnel in ward activity programs.

Occupational therapists should recognize the implications in this request and should act to formulate a statement of role and function which will justify the continued inclusion of occupational therapy as one of the allied medical services of the hospital. If we want the recognition and status of professional personnel we must function on that level. We must be prepared to participate actively in patient evaluation, treatment planning and disposition conferences. We must understand the concepts and terminology of the psychiatrist, psychologist and social worker, and we must be able to discuss the contribution of occupational therapy in terms that are meaningful to them. Our treatment objectives must be carefully formulated and psychiatrically meaningful if we wish to have them incorporated in the overall treatment plan for the patient. If individual occupational therapists do not feel adequately prepared to function at this level or if their institutions want to use the program for diversional activity or as a management device, the program should not be called occupational therapy but should be given another designation which does not carry treatment implications.

The continuing shortage of qualified occupational therapists makes it almost mandatory that we relinquish all activity functions which can be performed by other personnel who are more readily available. To do so will permit us to fulfill treatment responsibilities which have been too often curtailed or neglected in the effort to supply activity programs for large numbers of patients. At one time occupational therapists were almost the only group able to meet activity needs, but today this is not true. There are trained personnel in the areas of recreation, music and library; volunteers conduct many activities and make available community contacts and cultural and diversional opportunities which institutional personnel could not duplicate. The increasing recognition of the importance of an attractive stimulating ward atmosphere has emphasized the need for activity programs conducted by ward personnel. These developments should be welcomed and supported by occupational therapists as each allows us to assume more of the treatment functions for which we are prepared.

This is important as the number of qualified personnel in mental health professions is not increasing. An extensive study of manpower trends, made by Dr. George W. Albee for the Joint Commission presents a discouraging picture. He is not optimistic about solving personnel problems through increased recruitment efforts, as he relates the shortage of candidates for all mental health careers to the shortages in other categories of professional manpower. He documents the fact that there are not enough candidates to begin to meet the needs of the various professions. (2) One might say we are all fishing in an inadequately stocked pool. Those of us who hoped the population bulge would solve our staffing problems have apparently been entertaining an illusion. There may be more personnel but there will be more patients who are also part of the bulge. Since we cannot realistically expect to expand professional staff to any marked degree we must utilize those we have to the greatest advantage.

Changing Treatment Goals

Today occupational therapy has to be geared to the concepts and tempo of contemporary psychiatry. Modern treatments have radically changed the character of the mental hospital which now has a quieter, more purposeful atmosphere. More patients are receiving active treatment and many more are now accessible to and can profit from psychotherapy. The goal of a short period of hospitalization is stressed and patients are encouraged to maintain their interest in and contact with the community. Techniques and procedures which alleviate acute symptoms and promote control and the ability to function are given priority while ones based on long periods of hospitalization are being used less frequently. Generally speaking there is less emphasis on individual analytical psychotherapy but much more emphasis on group techniques of treatment. These procedures utilize the attributes of group identification and interaction to develop a degree of insight which will permit the patient once again to adjust in the community. Similarly where individual psychotherapy is used, it is often short term in nature and directed toward assisting the patient in reintegration of ego functions and the development of a sufficient degree of insight to facilitate social and work adjustment in the community.

The insidious factors in hospitalization are being identified and the more noxious are being removed or ameliorated as rapidly as possible. It is interesting to note that many of these factors are ones which occupational therapists have long recognized as being undesirable and have tried to counteract in their work with patients. They have seen the development of apathy and loss of self-respect as the patient succumbed to ward and hospital procedures which stifled him in routine and protected him from all decision-making. They have observed disturbed behavior subside in the permissive atmosphere of the occupational therapy clinic and they have fostered and nurtured any sparks of initiative and creativity which could be awakened. They have encouraged patients to accept responsibility for their own work and they have trusted them with dangerous tools and expensive equipment. These few examples among many possible ones are not recent developments in occupational therapy. They are based on insights which the occupational therapist has utilized for many years. The occupational therapist has had little difficulty in accepting the idea of a therapeutic community—in many aspects it is only an extension to the hospital as a whole of attitudes and concepts which are traditional in our clinics.

Correlating Treatment

Contemporary occupational therapy cannot exist in a vacuum or on the outskirts of medical awareness. To make an effective contribution in today's intensive treatment schedules it must correlate its treatment skills with other treatment effort, and it must contribute its observations and insight for the use of all team members. The organization of professional staff to achieve this focusing of treatment resources and knowledge will vary with the type of service but the importance of good communication in good treatment is universally recognized. Today the psychologist, social worker, psychiatric nurse and occupational therapist under the leadership of the psychiatrist, pool their collective knowledge to work out and implement effective treatment for patients assigned to their care.

The functions of occupational therapy in a dynamically oriented center are determined by the needs of the patient and the other treatments he is receiving. It may be used as a form of psychotherapy to augment psychotherapy or it may be used to facilitate the process of repression and restitution of ego functions. It may be evaluation, either initial or ongoing, used by itself or in conjunction with other diagnostic procedures, or it may be used to determine a patient's response to special treatment procedures or overall therapy. The patient may be referred for occupational therapy upon admission, at any stage of treatment or for evaluation for readiness and suitability for vocation rehabilitation, community placement or intrahospital transfer.

If occupational therapy is to discharge these functions, adjustments must be made by other services and divisions of the hospital. Large numbers of patients needing supportive activity cannot be included in occupational therapy groups where therapists are trying to establish meaningful interpersonal relationships and provide corrective emotional experiences for the active treatment of patients. The size of the occupational therapy groups have to be determined in accordance with the severity of the patient's symptoms and the goals of the treatment, and usually comprise from six to fifteen patients per therapist. The occupational therapy department has to have an adequate budget. It cannot rely on a revolving fund supported by the sale of projects, and the department should not be expected to function as an interior decorating service or the source for small items of equipment or furniture for the hospital. These functions are generally not compatible with the needs of the patients, and might be considered as a continuation into the present of the era when patient labor was basically for the benefit of the institution.

Intensive Treatment Program

Many hospitals consider the primary function of occupational therapy as work with the nonverbal, regressed patient who cannot be reached by treatments which are based on group participation or words. It is true that occupational therapists are often very effective with these patients, but I cannot agree that this is our primary function. Such patients are only one of a number of types of patients who are included in an intensive treatment program. When these regressed, withdrawn patients are referred to occupational therapy they are assigned to clinics where a small number of patients (usually 6 to 8 at one time) are treated in an atmosphere that is warm, friendly and undemanding. A limited number of activities are available but these include both those that are structured and can be used to give support and security, and those which are unstructured and projective in nature and may be used by the patient to express his problems and anxieties. Interpersonal demands are kept at a minimum, but at all times the therapist provides support, reassurance and acceptance. The patient is encouraged to participate in an activity which may provide the staff with insight into his problem, but often the complete freedom of projective techniques is too threatening. In that event structured activity is substituted. This permits guidance from the therapist and may be the first step in a meaningful relationship which the patient could not tolerate without the activity to provide the justification for instruction and guidance. If the therapist has been sufficiently accepting and undemanding, and has tried to understand the nonverbal communication, the patient will generally become more relaxed and less frightened. As this occurs he can relinquish some of his more extreme defenses and may begin slowly to establish verbal contact with the therapist. This should be quietly accepted and unobtrusively utilized to deepen the relationship. When the patient can tolerate awareness of the others in the group, or when he begins to show any interest in them, the therapist will then try to encourage a relationship with another patient or patients.

Observation and Evaluation

As the process of reintegration continues, the team may decide on other forms of therapy which may either take the place of or supplement occupational therapy. This illustrates another point in the team concept of treatment. Although all disciplines are represented, under the supervision and direction of the psychiatrist, any member of the treatment may become the dominant therapist. This role will pass from one discipline to another as the patient is able to utilize the special skills of each. This approach provides a continuous, coordinated but flexible program under medical direction which can be adjusted to meet the changing needs of the patient during his period of treatment.

Newly admitted patients are often referred to occupational therapy for observation and evaluation. The rationale for this procedure is based on the concept that all of a patient's behavior and reactions are significant and are directly related to the problems which cause his illness. Occupational therapy is one of the most normal situations which the hospital provides in which to observe characteristic behavior and patterns of defense, and the observation which the occupational therapist can supply for the use of the psychiatrist or the team in evaluating the patient's condition and determining procedures of treatment will become an increasingly important function of occupational therapy. Current emphasis on the desirability of psychotherapy for increasing numbers of patients has meant that psychologists, as one of the groups best able to meet this need, are devoting more and more time to this function, with a corresponding decrease in the number of psychological evaluations which they can provide. I do not mean to imply that information which the occupational therapist can supply is a substitute for the psychologist's evaluations which are based on standardized test procedures and protocols. Rather it is a means of evaluating the functioning level of the patient in a reality-oriented situation where he can be as active or passive in participation in activities and relationships as he chooses.

The occupational therapy clinic looks like a well-equipped home workshop, a familiar kitchen, a hobby shop or a pleasant club room such as one finds in various community centers. The atmosphere is relaxed and there is little to remind one of a hospital. In this environment the patient is invited to select and participate in an activity. The type of activity he chooses, the way he goes about the task, the nature and degree of help he seeks and his movement towards completion all indicate his habitual approach to problems and their solution. (3) Since observation and reporting of characteristic patterns of behavior is the objective of the referral, the occupational therapist cannot interfere in the situation in any way except to protect the patient or other patients in the groups from serious physical injury. He cannot offer guidance (unless the patient requests it,) he cannot protect the patient from the results of faulty judgment or patterns of behavior, for to do so would influence the patient's choice and/or normal pattern of behavior and thus invalidate the information obtained. In this type of situation the patient is exposed to the personnel, patients and available activities and allowed to proceed on his own initiative. The way he reacts in the situation usually reflects his patterns before hospitalization. If these patterns have been such as to court or insure failure, this will be demonstrated. If his behavior has been such as to invite rejection or retaliation, this will probably be forthcoming from other patients, or the occupational therapist may recognize the wish to reject or retaliate in his own feelings. Through such observations the occupational therapist will gain concrete, "on the spot" examples of the patient's usual behavior and reactions which will clarify his problems. The occupational therapist has an advantage when evaluating not generally shared by the psychiatrist, social worker or psychologist, who more frequently evaluate through interview or other techniques in a one-to-one situation. The occupational therapist, on the other hand, generally evaluates the patient in a situation where other patients are present. This permits observation of the patient's responses in situations which can generate sibling rivalry, dependence or other characteristic behavior in relating to people.

Evaluating Purpose

It is desirable to distinguish between evaluation which is a preliminary to planning treatment and the ongoing evaluative process which is an integral part of treatment. It is advisable to differentiate when occupational therapy is to be used as an instrument of evaluation and when it is to be used as treatment. When occupational therapy is used as an evaluation procedure, the therapist is as passive and nonintervening as possible. No effort is made to inhibit self-defeating behavior. The faulty patterns of relationship or performance which have created difficulties for the patient prior to hospitalization, tend to be repeated within the occupational therapy setting. This repetition of destructive or inappropriate behavior may be a detriment to later treatment, but this is not the case if the patient is placed on a type of psychotherapy designed to uncover unconscious motivations and to foster the development of insight. Patients who are receiving other forms of therapy usually appear to derive more benefit in occupational therapy from activities and techniques which permit the therapist to give them a great deal of personal attention with enough firmness and control to provide support and security in the situation.

The period of observation and evaluation is followed by the initiation of an individual program of treatment. Should this program include any of the somatic therapies it is very helpful if the occupational therapist has had an opportunity to observe the patient's pretreatment reactions, since somatic therapies tend to have a repressive effect which masks psychotic symptoms. In addition there may be organic reactions directly related to these therapies which affect the patient's response in occupational therapy. Immediate treatment objectives are limited being directed primarily to the relief of confusion, strengthening contact with reality and assisting the patient to regain self-confidence and security. Treatment procedures and activities are simple, structured and of a nature which permits and encourages frequent contact with the occupational therapist to supply the support and reassurance which the patient needs. Later the goal should be to facilitate restitution of ego function and the satisfaction of emotional needs, with no specific attempt to provide insight, since somatic therapies are not primarily designed to uncover underlying or unconscious material. This approach requires just as much psychiatric knowledge on the part of the occupational therapist as one involving the development of insight, since he must be able to recognize the dynamics which underlie symptoms, the importance of different patterns of relationship, and the way in which activities may be used to satisfy unconscious emotional needs.

If the patient is assigned to a treatment program emphasizing the development of insight, the function of occupational therapy will be quite different. I should like briefly to describe two such programs, one designed for residents of a hospital and the other for day hospital patients.

The residential program is focused around an open ward in the men's division of the hospital which is made as attractive and homelike as possible. Treatment includes group psychotherapy and occupational therapy and is supplemented by industrial assignments. Adequate library and recreational facilities are available. The psychotherapist and the social worker, who have their offices on the ward, and the ward personnel offer support and encouragement, but responsibility for planning diversional activities, meeting individual assignments and ward housekeeping are delegated to the patients. In order to maintain or develop normal social interaction, the men go for lunch each day to the comparable women's ward. At least once a week these women spend the evening on the men's ward where they play cards or converse and there are frequent dances. Activities away from the hospital are sponsored by volunteers.

Coordinating Program

Occupational therapy and group psychotherapy are closely coordinated. The psychotherapist meets once a week with the occupational therapy personnel in the occupational therapy clinic, to examine the patient's work and discuss all significant developments which have occurred in either locale. In addition a weekly meeting is held with the social worker, ward personnel and occupational therapist to share information, review and revise treatment goals and evaluate new developments. Occupational therapy is directed toward providing both individual and group experiences for the patient and facilitating his ability to appraise more accurately the demands of, and react appropriately in, both types of situations. Since the majority of these patients are psychotics with considerable variation in age and background, it is sometimes difficult to find group activities which are generally acceptable, but wherever possible they are selected by the group and worked out with the guidance of the occupational therapist.

The day hospital group is composed of patients who are primarily neurotic or borderline psychotics. The majority come from the community each day, although some inpatients are assigned for a transitional experience before complete separation from the hospital. All patients have group psychotherapy daily and most are seen in individual therapy sessions. These patients attend occupational therapy as a group and often use part or all of the session as an extension of their psychotherapy hour. In order to facilitate appropriate identification and to provide as nearly a normal situation as possible there are both a woman occupational therapist and a man who is a certified industrial arts instructor in the clinic. The personnel have to play many roles and assume many responsibilities, perhaps the most difficult being to keep the group active and therapeutically effective. The personnel must have confidence in the value of dynamic group interaction and they must not impede the group process with their opinions, advice or interpretations. There must be meaningful communication and correlation of effort between the occupational therapists and the day hospital nurse and psychotherapist. Personnel in both situations must be informed about all developments and reactions as they occur in order to maintain consistency in attitude and to frustrate the patients' efforts to manipulate the situation and embroil the personnel in dissension. Where good correlation exists, each group experience (psychotherapy or occupational therapy) enhances and strengthens the effectiveness of the other. Occupational therapy provides an opportunity for reinforcement and testing of insight, release of tension created but not expressed in the psychotherapy session, and stimulation of enough tension and anxiety to keep the patients working and talking in group therapy. The occupational therapist must frustrate the group's dependency, which is expressed by trying to force her into a position of leadership, consistently handing all responsibility for insight, opinions, judgments and solution of problems back to them as individuals or as a group.

However the occupational therapist cannot therapeutically ignore all dependency needs. Activities provide one area where the patient is justified in seeking assistance and instruction and where the occupational therapist can accept and fulfill the dependency needs, symbolically, through concern and attention expressed in her instruction and supervision. A good variety of activity should be available but there should be no overt pressure to participate. The atmosphere of the clinic and the example of other patients is usually enough to motivate the patient to start a project. Once started, the patient soon utilizes the activities in the clinic to externalize and express unconscious material. The atmosphere is one of controlled permissiveness with sufficiently defined limits to protect the patients from unrestrained acting-out. For example, patients may be verbally aggressive but they are not permitted to indulge in assaultive acting-out. They can destroy their own projects but they may not destroy other patients' work or clinic property.

Developing Insights

The occupational therapist must be constantly aware of transference reactions, interpersonal relationships and the way the patient uses, or does not use, the group and activity. The response by occupational therapy personnel to the misconceptions and distortions expressed in behavior and verbalization are determined by the patient's needs and his treatment plan. For one this might be an interpretive statement, "This is the way you would like to treat your father." Another may need to be confronted with reality, as, "But I am not your sister," while in many instances the group itself will confront the patient with an interpretation. The patient uses the clinic, the activities, the personnel and the group to work through and test developing insights, to practice new patterns of relating to people and reacting to frustration and pleasure, and to demonstrate to himself the greater satisfaction derived from more mature and objective ways of facing and solving his problems.

Evaluation Service

Following completion of formal treatment and during the state of consolidation and convalescence, occupational therapy is called upon to supply another type of service. This relates to preparing the patient for his return to work and the community. Since the "work" of most women patients is still homemaking, a unit is provided utilizing skills such as food shopping, cooking, cleaning, laundry and sewing for the home as modalities. The patients receive instruction and practical experience in such activities as budgeting and efficient home management, menu planning and food service, home decorating and personal grooming. This program has demonstrated its value in helping the patient make the transition from hospital to home duties without undue anxiety and often with increased security and competence.

This period of the patient's hospitalization is also used to evaluate suitability for vocational rehabilitation if this is needed. Occupational therapy does not provide vocational rehabilitation services but it does provide a preliminary evaluation and screening service for the vocational rehabilitation counselor which is not available from other hospital services.

Supportive Activity

I have talked about the functions of a treatment focused occupational therapy program in a dynamically oriented state hospital, but I have not mentioned two groups of patients who must receive attention, the chronic and the geriatric. I have purposely left these groups until now as I believe they need a program of supportive activity rather than specific treatment. The chronic patients have generally received all appropriate treatment which the hospital provides without evidencing sufficient improvement to permit their return to the community. Occupational therapy for these patients should be directed toward maintaining the level of improvement which has been achieved, providing the support and reassurance which encourages further progress, and preparing them to function at their maximum level of adjustment within the hospital community. The same goals apply to the geriatric patient, except that ability to function in the hospital community is often more limited.

Many occupational therapists consider that this type of program is also treatment. I cannot agree. I believe that a program can be valuable and perform an essential function within the hospital structure without having to bear the label "treatment." In fact I feel that the indiscriminate labeling of everything which occurs within the hospital as "therapy" or "treatment" has devalued the term, and has made the thoughtful physician sceptical about most nonmedical so-called "therapies." It is commonly said that we treat the whole man and that we want to return him to his community as a functioning individual with the insights gained through treatment enriching his capacity to live. Do we want to send him back to the community with the concept that his work is a treatment, his recreation a treatment, if he reads a book or attends a concert he is engaged in a form of treatment? I am of the opinion that the provision of components of normal life situations within a hospital is no more a part of specific treatment than is the provision of an adequate diet or heat in the winter time. The fact that recreation, library and music enrich our lives, and that work is an essential activity in our culture, does not make participation in them treatment per se. I am in favor of providing as many types of activity as we can for patients; all I ask is that we do not slip into the fallacy of labeling activity "treatment" just because it is carried on within the hospital boundaries.

Reevaluation

I called this paper "The Challenge of the Sixties" and I should like to restate the challenge as I see it. We, along with other mental health professions, need to reevaluate our role and function in the care and treatment of patients suffering from mental illness. We need to undertake this reevaluation in the interests of providing better treatment for more patients. Can we as a professional group meet these needs? In order to reevaluate the role and function of occupational therapy in psychiatry, we should reach a broad agreement on what our role and function is. Certainly reevaluation can be carried out on a departmental basis, but this is not resolving the confusion which exists concerning the role of occupational therapy as a professional entity. Vacillation in coming to grips with this problem and in working out a solution has in turned inhibited our ability to work towards the solution of related problems which call for action. We have all expressed the feeling that physicians should receive more orientation to occupational therapy in medical schools. Even if time were made for it in their crowded curriculum, whose concepts should be presented? We look forward to the day when we can have accreditation of clinical centers, but what will form the basis of accreditation? We wish students were better prepared for practice in the clinical area, but for which type of program should they be prepared?

Professional roles are changing. Social workers, nurses and psychologists have been engaged in studies of their role and function for some time and already changes are in evidence. Some of these came about rapidly; others have occurred almost imperceptibly. Think for a moment of nursing and what seems to have happened in the last five years. Practical nurses now perform most of the bedside functions which registered nurses used to carry out, registered nurses now perform some procedures previously restricted to physicians, and a whole new category of workers have come onto the scene as ward secretaries, cleaners, porters, food servers, and so forth.

Changes are also occurring in the physician's role. In order to meet the needs of patients who could benefit from psychotherapy there has been a rapid increase in the use of group therapy techniques and the utilization by the physician of allied personnel as co-therapists, group leaders or as primary therapists. In the capacity of team leader the physician functions as a consultant and adviser who supports his team in their work with patients. While medical responsibility for diagnosis and treatment is vested in the physician, he uses the specialized training and competence of his team to assist him in both functions, and through the team's effort more patients are treated than could be reached through the physician's efforts alone.

The greatest challenge for occupational therapy is to define our own role in terms of present day psychiatry, and to determine which of our current functions actually require professional preparation and which could be adequately performed by less expensively prepared personnel. If the function does not require professional preparation it should be relinquished. This is not going to be easy, but if we do not accept this responsibility we shall not long retain our identity as members of the institution's professional staff. Today the graduate occupational therapist is considered part of the professional medical staff in many treatment-oriented centers and service at this level should be the goal of all occupational therapists in psychiatric practice. We should utilize our training in the medical aspects of treatment and remember that at this time we are one of the few groups which have such qualification. Many psychiatrists recognize and value the contribution which occupational therapy currently makes to patient treatment and are willing to provide guidance and support if we demonstrate our readiness to accept increased responsibility. When the psychiatrist is willing and prepared to use the occupational therapist to the extent of his education and ability to assist in treating patients, there remains the problem of supplying therapists to use in this manner. If occupational therapy is to be a significant part of psychiatric treatment, we must attract with some degree of consistency competent and enthusiastic recent graduates to our centers. This can be accomplished only if we provide challenging opportunities for them to work in treatment situations which demand all of their professional knowledge. Recent graduates are not interested in nor attracted to positions which require primarily activity or even administrative skills.

Student Training

It is more than possible that disinterest or lack of attraction has its roots in the clinical affiliation in psychiatry, and what has just been said of the recent graduate is equally applicable to the student in affiliation. Indeed it is my belief, that if a student's clinical experience in psychiatry takes place in a department where occupational therapy is an activity program and where the graduate occupational therapists function only as administrators, the future graduate is already lost to psychiatric practice. The student in affiliation who has had an unfavorable experience in one clinical area generally avoids undergoing a corrective experience as a staff member in the same area.

Fortunately it should be easier to provide the affiliating student with an effective experience of occupational therapy used as treatment in a psychiatric program than it is to provide this same experience for a young staff member. The students, performing directly under close supervision by a qualified occupational therapist who serves as preceptor, desirably will observe, comprehend and practice occupational therapy as treatment through the example, discussion and constructive criticism of the occupational therapist. The staff member, on the other hand, does not often enjoy such immediate guidance and may be said to have to light his own way.

All students in psychiatric affiliation are entitled to the following positive experiences. (1) They should be shown the different ways that patients use activity to satisfy their emotional needs. (2) They should be shown how the occupational therapist not only facilitates this use of activity by the patient but can also help the patient gain insight into his feelings and behavior through his reaction to activity. (3) Students should be shown the various patterns of relationship which the occupational therapist uses to achieve treatment goals for individual patients or for the functioning group. (4) Finally students should be shown how to observe, analyze, evaluate and formulate appropriately the factors pertinent to planning or reporting treatment for a psychiatric patient.

These experiences should not be left to chance and the native awareness and skill of the student. The supervising occupational therapist should make certain that the student observes accurately the actual patients in the clinic, understands the significance of what he sees and his own reactions to it, can set realistic goals in occupational therapy for the patient and arrive at a feasible program to achieve them. The student should progress from the role of observer (by way of discussion and practice) to active participant in the therapeutic situation and finally to that of therapist, with all the responsibility that this implies. A student who has had this type of experience during the psychiatric affiliation becomes a young staff member who is prepared to administer treatment and who will continue to grow in professional skill through constant self-evaluation of his practice.

Specific mention must also be made of one other experience which is of great value to the young staff occupational therapist, which should also be shared by the affiliating student wherever possible. This is participation in conferences of the psychiatric treatment team. In this situation the occupational therapist has an opportunity to judge for himself the significance of occupational therapy's contribution as it is seen by other disciplines. Moreover, there is no better preservative or restorative of the sense of proportion than genuinely working with members of other professions in treating the same patient or group of patients.

Conclusion

My summary is not lengthy but it is as sincere and heartfelt as anything I have ever said in my lifetime as an occupational therapist in psychiatric practice. We occupational therapists in psychiatry must now make a decision as to our future course. On one hand we can strive to turn out many occupational therapists to be the personnel responsible for carrying out or supervising programs of activity for large numbers of patients as an instrument of patient management. Unfortunately it does not seem realistic to anticipate the necessary numbers of these personnel resulting from the current educational pattern of the registered occupational therapist. On the other hand we may work to produce a more limited number of occupational therapists who will perform a strictly treatment role for selected patients, having relinquished nontreatment or routine treatment aspects of previous occupational therapy functions to other personnel (even including supervision of nonoccupational therapists). These specialists will find that their practice utilizes all their professional preparation and indeed demands continually increasing competence. Young persons who are considering a career of service in a health-related profession respond to challenge, and it is with confidence that I predict an adequate, although always limited, supply of good students and recent graduates to meet the demands of the psychiatrist who uses occupational therapy as treatment. In the last analysis, continuance of a profession depends upon the generation to come. So long as occupational therapy in psychiatric practice continues to attract vital recruits, so long will it maintain the worthy tradition of service to patients laid down by pioneers like Eleanor Clarke Slagle.

REFERENCES

1. Joint Commission on Mental Illness and Health. *Action for Mental Health*, 19-23.
2. Albee, George W. "Mental Health Manpower Trends—1959." *Action for Mental Health*, 154-158.
3. Ellis, Madelaine and Arthur Bachrack. "Psychiatric Occupational Therapy: Some Aspects of Role and Functions." *American Journal of Psychiatry*, 115: 319-322, 1958.

The Development of Perceptual-Motor Abilities: A Theoretical Basis for Treatment of Dysfunction

A. Jean Ayres

Central to the concept of occupational therapy are the evaluation, enhancement and use of skilled motor actions. While many central nervous system processes are involved in skilled movement, one aspect of sensorimotor function has come under particular attention lately as a large determinant of fine motor facility. That aspect is perceptual-motor functions, formerly called "eye-hand" coordination. Deficits in this domain are most easily and frequently observed in the patient who can accomplish simple grasp and release with apparent ease yet who cannot accomplish with comparable dexterity such tasks as tying shoes, handling tools or manipulating objects. The possible nature of that dysfunction is described in this paper and hypotheses presented regarding related developmental processes.

One of the more generally accepted postulates on which treatment of motor dysfunction is based is the recapitulation of the sequence of development. Accordingly, theories regarding the ontogeny of perceptual-motor abilities provide a basis for treatment of dysfunction in this area of human behavior. The data to which the theoretical system is anchored come largely from a research project conducted at the University of Southern California. (This investigation was supported in part by a PHS research grant MH06878-01 from the National Institute of Mental Health, Public Health Service.) Results of published research by neurophysiologists have served as additional sources of knowledge. Although well supported with scientific facts, the highly provisional nature of the theoretical frame-

Reprinted from *The American Journal of Occupational Therapy*, Vol. XVII, No. 6, 1963.

work must be kept in mind. It has been necessary to force considerable structure onto the data (largely by omission of detail) in order to make them manageable. As our conceptual formulations become more familiar and secure, we will undoubtedly find that they have oversimplified the true nature of perceptual-motor function and it will be necessary for us to restructure them on a more complex basis.

Method of Obtaining Information

A brief review of the method by which the major research data were gathered is needed for their interpretation. One hundred children of approximately six and seven years of age who were suspected of having perceptual deficiencies were administered a battery of tests covering visual, tactile, and proprioceptive perception and some motor skills. Auditory and language functions were not included. None of the children carried a medical diagnosis of cerebral palsy; all of them had or had had learning or behavioral problems. The battery of tests was selected on the basis of descriptions in the literature of areas of perceptual-motor dysfunction. The scores made by the children on the tests were correlated and then subjected to R-technique factor analysis in order to determine the possible existence of associations among symptoms that would justify hypothesizing the presence of taxonomic categories or syndromes of dysfunction. Establishment of factors is a means of summarizing and simplifying masses of confusedly interrelated observations, a function not possible by the human brain alone. A factor is a process which accounts for differences in a domain of behavior under observation—the domain in this case being perceptual-motor function. For example, among cerebral palsied children, certain neurophysiological processes account for the behavioral manifestation called spasticity, different processes determining athetosis, and another type of dysfunction causing ataxic behavior. These different neurophysiological processes are used to identify the neuromuscular problem of the patient. Understanding the process has served as a basis for establishment of treatment procedures.

In essence, this study has attempted a comparable categorization of a domain of neurological dysfunction, with reliance not upon subjective human judgment, but the objective accuracy of statistical computations. Nevertheless, a major limitation to this type of study lies in the fact that the emergence of a syndrome and its nature is dependent upon the type of data gathered. A serious omission in data collection will result in a gap in the results. Consumers of the information must be alert to this limitation.

Since the data were gathered from children with learning or behavioral disorders, we can expect to find similar syndromes of dysfunction among other children with comparable difficulty. Although cerebral palsied and definitely mentally retarded children were not included in the sample population, it is not unreasonable to expect these data to apply to children with those disorders. Caution must be used, however, in assuming that comparable clinical syndromes might be manifested in the individual sustaining brain injury as an adult.

Areas of Perceptual-Motor Function

Some of the types of perceptual-motor functions covered in the test battery are shown in the accompanying diagram. In some instances, an area of function represents several tests. In these cases the mean factor loading of a group of tests was obtained by taking the square root of the mean of the squares of the factor loadings of several tests, all of which had significant loadings on that factor.

Motor planning was evaluated by (1) how well a child could draw a line with a pencil on top of another line, (2) the degree of quickness and accuracy with which the child could assume a posture demonstrated by the examiner and (3) the ability to manipulate an object. Finger identification was evaluated by the identification by the child of which of his fingers the examiner touched. Tactile perception was based on (1) the accuracy with which the subject could localize a tactile stimulus on hand or forearm, (2) his ability to discriminate between one and two tactile stimuli in the finger tips, (3) the degree to which he could perceive two simultaneously administered tactile stimuli to cheek and/or hand, and (4) his accuracy in identifying simple figures drawn on the back of the hand. Manual perception of form was tested by visual recognition of a geometric form held in the hand. The accuracy with which the child could return his hand to a position previously assumed with the help of the examiner was the basis for the score on kinesthesia. Visual perception of form and space included Frostig's tests of form constancy,

FACTORIAL CONTENT OF FIVE MAJOR CLINICAL SYNDROMES OF PERCEPTUAL-MOTOR DYSFUNCTION

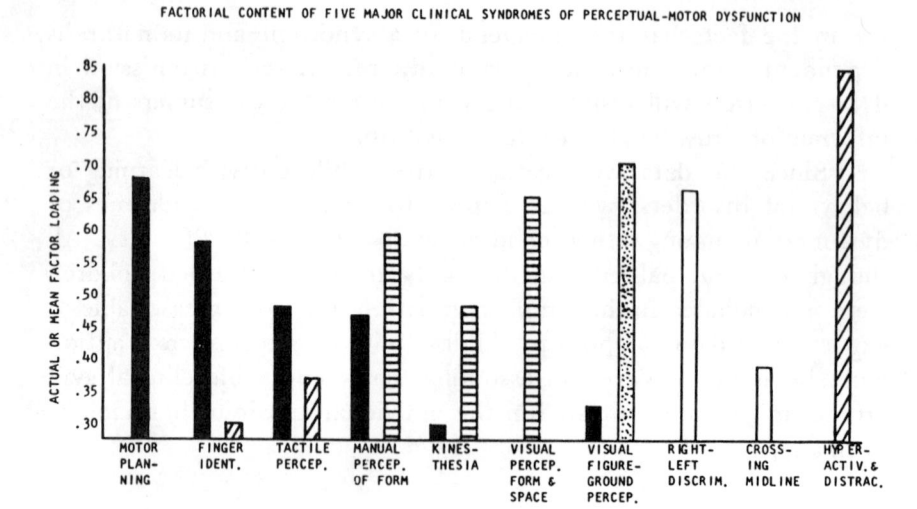

AREAS OF PERCEPTUAL-MOTOR DYSFUNCTION

LEGEND FOR SYNDROMES

- ■ APRAXIA
- ▤ PERCEPTUAL DYSFUNCTION: FORM & POSITION IN SPACE
- ▢ INTEGRATION OF SIDES OF BODY
- ▨ PERCEPTUAL DYSFUNCTION: VISUAL FIGURE-GROUND
- ▧ TACTILE DEFENSIVENESS

position in space, and space relations. Ability to identify superimposed and imbedded pictures of objects made up the test of figure-ground perception. Right-left discrimination refers to the child's identifying his right and left sides as well as those of the examiner. Reluctance to cross the midline of the body was evaluated by whether or not the child would spontaneously put his hand on a part of the body on the opposite side and, in addition, pick up objects placed on the other side of the body's mid-line. Hyperactive, distractible behavior is self-explanatory.

The Major Syndromes and Their Hypothesized Development

The statistical analysis of the data gathered by the method described above (and to be described in statistical detail elsewhere) leads to postulating the existence of five major syndromes of perceptual-motor dysfunction. These syndromes, which emerged from the analysis as factors, and the mean or actual factual loadings of the tests of perceptual-motor function on each factor are shown in the diagram. The most important general observation to make is that different syndromes are represented by different constellations of deficits of function. This fact provides the basis for categorizing symptoms into syndromes. The structure of the constellation of areas of dysfunction also directs our reasoning in theorizing about the nature of perceptual-motor development and dysfunction. Each factor will be discussed individually.

Apraxia

Because a deficiency in the ability to motor plan is the primary characteristic of one of the categories of dysfunction, it is suggested that it be called "apraxia" or "developmental apraxia." A child with this disability has difficulty directing his hands or his body in performing skilled or unfamiliar motor tasks. His major perceptual deficiency lies quite clearly in tactile functions. According to the data gathered, kinesthetic and other proprioceptive sources of information play a less important role in apraxia than do tactile sources. Of the conditions which are usually considered aspects of body scheme disturbance (which is often considered to be associated with apraxia) only diminished finger identification appears closely linked with apraxia, as defined here.

The close relationship between deficits in motor planning and tactile perception suggests the primacy of tactile functions in the maturation process. It is hypothesized that the development of central nervous system processes of organizing, inhibiting, and augmenting tactile impulses in association with meaningful experiences must precede the ability to perform skilled motor tasks. Emphasis is placed on the word "precede," for concomitant tactile perception during a motor task is not a sufficient basis for motor planning. It seems that the continuous flow of tactile sensations, if meaningful, lay down in the brain the body scheme upon which all future motor planning is based.

Skill in all motor activity involving the hands is dependent upon finger gnosis. The close linkage between finger identification and tactile perception has invited the hypothesis that finger agnosia is, at least partially, a function of a disordered tactile system.

Our approach to treatment of the child with apraxia must focus on normalizing the tactile functions as well as training in motor skill.

Perceptual Dysfunction: Form and Position in Space

Another important syndrome reflects a deficit in perception of form and position in two-dimensional space. As shown in the diagram, perception refers, here, not only to visual perception, but also to tactile perception of form and kinesthetic perception of the position of the hand in space. It is the grouping of these three sensory modalities that provides us with a major clue regarding the development of visual perception. It is hypothesized that the visual perception of form and position in space is preceded developmentally by the purposeful response to tactile and kinesthetic sensations carrying information about form and space. If a child feels with assurance where his hand is, how his fingers are positioned, and what they are holding, he will be better able to visually cope with form and space, such as is required in tasks as simple as setting a table or as complex as drawing designs, reading, or assembling an object on the production line. The relationship may not be an inevitable one, however, for relationships among perception of form and space in the three sensory modalities may be a function of a common neurological process.

The implication for treatment, again, is to first normalize, as much as possible, tactile and kinesthetic sensation, followed by the enhancement of perception in these modalities and of visual stimuli.

Deficit of Integration of Function of the Two Sides of the Body

From the research data emerged a syndrome with characteristics to which reference has been made in the literature for many years. However, the grouping of symptoms into a single dimension of central nervous system development and organization appears not to have been suggested prior to this time. The two most distinguishing aspects of behavior of this syndrome are a tendency of the hands to avoid crossing the midline of the body when engaged in motor tasks and difficulty in learning to discriminate and identify the right and left sides of the body, the latter type of behavior being the best representative of the syndrome. It is possible that there are other, more effective means of identifying this type of dysfunction. Studying those aspects of perceptual-motor dysfunction which showed close association with crossing the midline and right-left discrimination suggests a basic clinical syndrome of inadequate integration of the two sides of the body. Whenever the motor function of one side of the body is related to activity of the other side, the function of the two sides requires coordinating by a central nervous system mechanism of unknown type which is clearly vulnerable to disorder. Thus, successful participation in rhythmic activities requiring a temporal interrelationship of the two hands or two feet is partially dependent upon this central nervous system mechanism even though the midline is not crossed. Similarly, jumping with both feet simultaneously and performing reciprocal motions with the extremities are affected. It even seems likely that having to draw on one side of a page a duplicate of a design appearing on the other side of the page involves integration of the two sides of the body. The ability of the eyes to cross the midline of their respective ranges of motion is part of this behavioral dimension.

The sensory component of the syndrome is obscure, but, again the significant correlations between scores on tests of tactile perception and crossing the midline or right-left discrimination suggest the importance of tactile stimuli in the developmental process. It is hypothesized that crawling or creeping has found favor among therapists and psychologists as a therapeutic process partly because it is one of the most basic and ontogenetically early sensorimotor patterns requiring and enhancing integration of function of the two sides of the body. It is interesting to note that at the age of six or seven years, the degree to which the right and left sides could be correctly identified was apparently a function of the maturation of a specific area of sensorimotor development, as contrasted with verbal skill. This syndrome is deserving of much attention from the occupational therapist. As in the case of most of the other syndromes, it requires treatment with controlled sensation and bilateral motor activity. The effect of some of our bilateral activities begins to take on new significance.

The fact that diminished body balance is associated with poor integration of sides of the body leads to wondering whether there is a neurophysiological deficit basic to both balance and body side integration or whether balancing on one foot involves the kind of neuromuscular integration diminished in children with inadequate functional interrelationship of the two symmetrical halves of the body.

Identification of the pattern of dysfunction in the cerebral palsied child may be very difficult. It is not likely that it would have been detected statistically in a cerebral palsy population. Our inability to detect it does not preclude its presence, and we must be alert to its manifestation and response to treatment.

Perceptual Dysfunction: Visual Figure-Ground

Deficiency in visual figure-ground perception has been identified as a clinical condition for many years. The disability emerged from the research data as a specific and independent syndrome, although some of the children with apraxia also demonstrated disturbance in figure-ground perception. Inspection of correlations between scores on tests of visual figure-ground perception and other perceptual-motor tests suggests that the neurological process basic to figure-ground perception is also basic to all other types of perceptual-motor ability. Somatic perception is closely associated with visual figure-ground perception, the latter even appearing within the apraxia syndrome. The relationship may lie in mutual dependence upon the discriminatory functions of the non-specific processes of the reticular formation and thalamus. The developmental process underlying visual figure-ground perception is far from clear.

A neurophysiological approach to treatment of this syndrome remains to be investigated. The most fruitful approach will likely be through influencing the function of the nonspecific reticular system by control of sensory input. If we can enhance the discriminatory function of the general system, figure-ground perception will likely improve. The area is a fertile field for investigation by therapists.

Tactile Defensiveness

The last major syndrome to be described is one brought to our attention for the first time by our research at the University of Southern California. It is characterized by deficit in tactile perception, by hyperactive, distractible behavior, and by a defensive response to certain types of tactile stimuli. It is interesting to note that hyperactive and distractible behavior carried a significant loading on only one syndrome, suggesting that this troublesome behavior problem may, in these children, be linked to a specific neurophysiological mechanism. The syndrome is closely and directly associated with emotions. These data, when taken into consideration with other neurophysiological information, have led to a fruitful theory described in detail elsewhere. In essence, the developmental process suggested by the syndrome reflects the phylogenetic primacy of tactile stimuli as messages warning the organism of danger and to prepare to flee or fight. This type of interpretation of tactile stimuli leads to the over-alertness of distractibility, the flight-like behavior of hyperactivity, and a tendency toward negative affect (fight). The presence of the syndrome interferes with the development of perceptual-motor ability. It was found primarily in association with the other syndromes and not as an isolated condition.

Identification, at least hypothetically, of a neurophysiological basis for certain types of hyperactivity gives us a cue for another approach to treatment of the dysfunction—the approach being a normalizing of tactile functions.

General Discussion

Attention must be drawn to the fact that the five syndromes may not be expected to appear in pure states in any child. Correlation among scores on perceptual-motor tests warrants the expectation that a child who is perceptually deficient in any one area is likely to be deficient in all other areas but he is not necessarily so. From the statistical analyses, emerged many other syndromes of lesser clarity and accounting for less of the source of variance among the children. Additional research may indicate their significance.

Although tactile functions emerged as highly significant, the apparent comparative lesser role of the proprioceptors may be purely a matter of inadequate evaluation of their function or an inability to interpret the results.

While emphasis has been placed on a neurophysiological understanding and approach to treatment, the cognitive approach is certainly not excluded as an important aspect of treatment. The two approaches are really ends of the same continuum. It is strongly suggested, however, that treatment based primarily on influencing basic neurophysiological integration, through control of sensorimotor behavior, and secondarily on intellectual processes will be the most effective approach. There is a long gap between these basic research data and the assurance that a treatment procedure is effective. We need many studies to test, scientifically, the hypotheses suggested by the theories.

Learning as a Growth Process: A Conceptual Framework for Professional Education

Gail S. Fidler

An honor such as that which is mine today seldom represents the single achievement of one individual but rather a synthesis of the knowledge, ideas and experiences of many. I am deeply indebted to associates and others in related fields but particularly to those colleagues and students with whom I have been privileged to work and whose creative thinking and imaginative experimentation has contributed so much to my knowledge and to the development of occupational therapy. What I shall say regarding the nature and scope of professional education is neither new nor unique but is an attempt to relate these theories to the education of the occupational therapist in such a way as to hopefully increase our skill and knowledge as therapists and educators and enhance our growth into a profession.

The rapidly changing, complex world of today creates new and increasing demands upon and expectations for the professions. The development and maintenance of a vitality essential to the existence of a profession and to the fulfillment of its obligation to society is inextricably bound to its philosophy of education and those processes directed toward attaining professional competency.

In a changing society, roles need to be constantly assessed and a profession must continually ask itself how it may impart to the learner a given body of knowledge and nourish the development of skills in such a way as to motivate the developing professional to creatively elucidate and expand concepts; develop and test new

Reprinted from *The American Journal of Occupational Therapy*, Vol. XX, No. 1, 1966.

hypotheses; continually enhance and refine skills and thus contribute to the growth and maturation of that profession.

It is axiomatic that the scope and function of a profession, its role and definition determine its educational objectives. Since educational objectives are delineated in relation to the scope and function of a profession, they can be defined and pursued only in so far as the nature and role of that profession is clearly conceptualized.

Professional roles are set forth by the needs of the society to be served, circumscribed by the profession's delineation of the extent to which it may be expected to fulfill such needs. It therefore follows that the responsibilities assumed by a profession define the nature and quality of the particular knowledge and skills required of its members.

Assumption of professional responsibility involves both privileges and obligations and it is these which constitute a professional identity and provide a basic frame of reference for those learning experiences which may be expected to prepare the student to fulfill such obligations. A profession is characterized by the nature and quality of its body of knowledge and skills, the capacity to discern when the application of such knowledge and skill is indicated and the ability to make reasonable predictions regarding the outcome of such application.

A second identifying characteristic of a profession is the existence of a definable set of principles, concepts and attitudes basic to its functions but which also transcend the confines of that profession to the extent that the professional is able to share with others a concern for and dedication to the welfare of all peoples and thus to share freely and work collaboratively with others in the service of human welfare.

An infinite commitment to the advancement of learning, to research as an attitude and to the maintenance of critical, evaluative and creative thinking, is still another criterion of professional identity. Furthermore, a service profession is characterized by its inherent belief in the integrity of man, in the capacity of the human being for growth and change and in those attitudes and feelings which make possible appropriate and satisfying interpersonal relationships. A fifth criterion may be stated as a deep and objective commitment to the growth of the profession as a human welfare service and to the maintenance of the unique identity of that profession.

Finally, a profession is identified by a practice wherein authority and privilege is derived from the requirements which the profession sets regarding knowledge and practitioner skills. Thus power and privilege stem from the profession itself and exist in relation to the standards of that profession rather than emanating from sources outside itself.

Such criteria suggest that more is at stake in educating for the professions than the accumulation of facts and data or the teaching of skills per se. Professional preparation requires that the educational process be concerned with teaching a body of principles and concepts rather than routine skills or "slide rule approaches." Ralph W. Tyler (1) warns against cluttering professional curriculum with activity courses that can be learned on the job. He emphasizes that a profession must base its technique of operation upon principles rather than rule of thumb procedures or routine skills. Charlotte Towle (2) in discussing the general objectives of professional education states that, "it is characteristic of professional education that it teach a body of principles and concepts for differential use. In short, it endeavors to set in operation a learning process that will endure and wax strong throughout the years of professional activity. Such a focus makes possible the achievement of self-dependent, professional thinking and functioning rather than the more limited technical 'how or what-to-do' approach."

A second aim of professional education is to develop in the student the capacity and drive to learn; the ability to think critically, creatively and analytically; to teach the process of logic and thus to enable the learner to develop and refine problem-solving and decision-making skills. An attitude of scientific inquiry, the ability to analyze, synthesize and generalize requires an open mindedness, a freedom to explore and accept new ideas and different ways of thinking. The educator and thus the educational process must then be committed to change as the outcome of learning providing the incentive and opportunity for such change. Furthermore, such perspectives place high value on the ability and right of the individual logically to arrive at his own conclusions. Thus sound professional education needs to provide the opportunity to develop capacities for independent thought and action. Walter Lifton (3) speaking to this point warns against teaching a repertoire of typical responses and suggests that, "it is only when we are not sure that our answer is best that we fear having a person seek his own best solution."

A third objective in the advancement of learning is to nurture a set of attitudes and feelings which will enhance the student's capacity to think and function appropriately. Such an objective points up the importance of understanding self and others and emphasizes the need for learning experiences which provide opportunity for the student to become aware of his attitudes and feelings, how these influence his own behavior and the response of others and finally to work toward necessary attitudinal changes.

Students bring to the learning experience a variety of attitudes, values and previously learned responses. Some of these will need to undergo change, others be enhanced and broadened if the learner is to achieve the personal growth and the critical human perception essential for meeting the requirements of a profession. The capacity to effectively alter or change attitudes is dependent upon being able to look at one's set of values and beliefs critically and objectively, to come to have some understanding of self, developing an identity and integrity sufficient to enable learning and growth to occur. Thus learning needs to occur within a setting and in such a manner as to support and foster these perspectives and concomitant growth. Self awareness for the sake of self awareness is never an aim of professional education but is the means whereby a student may develop those capacities and that breadth of knowledge essential for professional fulfillment.

Another goal in training for the professions is the development of a capacity to engage in appropriate, mutually satisfying interpersonal relationships. The ability to work collaboratively with others, to establish and sustain relationships is in proportion to one's understanding of and respect for self and others. Achievement of such understanding and respect emanates from a receptivity to self awareness and understanding and thus the educational process aims to increase such receptivity and to provide interpersonal learning experiences which will enable the student to use this appropriately and productively.

In addition, a sense of security and integrity generated by an increasing capacity to think logically and independently and comprehension of the basic set of principles indigenous to the profession contributes immeasurably to collaborative and interpersonal skills. In essence, the capacity to establish and maintain interpersonal relationships represents the ability to think and feel appropriately and evaluatively with minimal biases regarding self and others. Charlotte Towle (4) succinctly describes what is involved in such relationships when she states: "Decisive also in establishing and maintaining purposeful working relationships will be the readiness to assume and sustain responsibility, the capacity to meet the dependency of others without taking the management of affairs out of their hands, the willingness to play a minor or subordinate role as well as a major one and the ability to separate one's self from another so that one's own feelings, attitudes and needs are not blindly projected onto others."

Finally, professional education must teach a perspective regarding the place of the profession in society and its service to the individual in relation to that society. This perspective should make possible firm commitment to the maintenance of the professional identity but also generate an ongoing constructively critical evaluative attitude regarding that profession. While a profession is recognized by a given body of knowledge which makes possible a distinguishable service, objective appreciation of its unique contributions, as well as its limitations, can be achieved only through an understanding of the significance of other professions and the needs which they serve.

Attainment of these educational goals can become a reality only insofar as the learning experience is conceptualized as a growth process directed toward the development of a professional person. Within this context, the educative process stresses integrated learning in preference to cognitive as the means whereby new functions are integrated and growth and change consolidated. This frame of reference brings the teaching-learning experience into focus as a dynamic human relationship and underlines the need to evolve an effective teaching-learning theory.

Development of a dynamic teaching-learning theory requires understanding the nature of the integrative learning process, perceptual organization and the way in which a function becomes an integral part of the self.

Pearce and Newton (5) define growth as the integration of a new function or the expansion of a function. They emphasize that in order for new learning to become an integral part of the self system such learning, including a synthesis of prior and current experiences, must come clearly into awareness at the time of integration and be consensually validated with a person or persons of significance. This concept of growth points up the importance of bringing all aspects of new learning experiences into clear awareness and building a student-teacher relationship which will maximize the necessary synthesis and consensual validation. The implications of these theories for the teaching-learning relationship have been outlined in an earlier paper which explores concepts relating to professional learning and defines a frame of reference for such learning and growth. (6)

Identifying growth and change as the ultimate aim of education, Leland P. Bradford (7) points out that a deeper and broader goal than cognitive learning must exist if growth and change are to occur. He comments that learning which remains merely cognitive and does not become part of one's internal systems and external behavior, becomes compartmentalized and of little value. He stresses the importance of consensual validation in the learning process emphasizing that one learns under conditions in which relevant, accurate and acceptable feedback is provided.

An effective teaching-learning process requires understanding of the role of the learner and of the teacher, what each brings to the transaction and how each influences that transaction. The needs, attitudes, biases and expectations of both student and teacher regarding learning, knowledge and growth play a significant role in defining the nature and quality of the learning experience. What are the learner's concepts regarding himself, how does he conceptualize his potential for learning, for growth? What does learning mean to him and on the basis of his past experiences what expectations does he bring to the transaction?

The teacher needs to be aware of his own particular needs and attitudes. Arthur Jersild (8) suggests that the teacher needs to deal with his anxieties relative to his role of authority and/or benefactor. Bradford (9) articulately defines the importance of the teacher's awareness and understanding of his own needs and motivations when he asks, "to what extent does the teacher's need to control people, to maintain dependency upon himself or to seek love and affection distort and disturb his function and thus the learning transaction? To what extent does his fear of hostility develop repression in the learner so that healthy conflict as a basis of learning is lacking? To what extent does his fear of relationships with people keep the learner at arm's length and thus reduce the possibility of an effective teaching-learning transaction?"

Recognition of the significance of human needs, respect for the integrity of man, belief in his capacity for growth, change and self-dependent functioning are essential ingredients for an effective teaching-learning relationship. Productive learning will in good measure be determined by the extent to which these attitudes are an integral part of the teacher's self system and become evident in his transactions with students.

Theories concerning the nature of the learning process need also to relate to resistance to learning. The importance of anxiety both as a change-inducing agent and as a response to the threat of change must be recognized. The new and unknown, the expectation that old safe patterns and attitudes will need to undergo change and alteration is understandably anxiety provoking. Anxiety associated with change, however, is at the same time in conflict with man's innate drive toward growth. The teacher needs to understand the nature of this dilemma and through such understanding provide the appropriate measure of support to diminish blocks to learning, nurture receptivity to changes and guard against intellectualization or cognitive rote learning as a defense.

Finally, an effective teaching-learning theory recognizes the dynamics of the group and the dyadic relationship as forces for learning, as interactional, growth-inducing processes.

Generative engagement in the teaching-learning transaction requires more than knowing about human behavior and learning theories. It demands a sensitivity to ongoing relationships and skill in using this perception in creating a culture conducive to integrated learning and more concretely in directly facilitating the integration of a function. The teaching-learning relationship must provide sufficient freedom and help to enable the student to learn to reason and function independently and collaboratively; to increase his capacity for creative original thinking; to translate such thinking into productive action; to assume responsibility for making decisions as well as the results of such decisions and finally to make mistakes and find support in learning from these.

Teaching then is conceptualized as the process of making opportunities available for the development of a body of knowledge, skills and attitudes in such a way as to enhance the learner's capacity to function creatively, with skill, understanding and discernment; the nature of such a process constituting an interpersonal transaction conducive to growth and concomitant change.

Such a definition of teaching also rightfully describes the nature and goal of the therapist-patient interaction, for if we are to teach students to become skillfully engaged with patients or clients in a helping-growth process, the students' learning experience must itself then be a helping growth process.

Appreciation of learning as a growth process inevitably points up the need to reexamine and carefully scrutinize our methods of education, both in the didactic and clinical spheres. First, however, we must define our expectations regarding educational experiences. What are we to teach in occupational therapy? What growth do we hope for; what knowledge, skills and attitudes do we expect the learner to integrate? Are we willing and able at this time to commit ourselves to the development of occupational therapy into a profession? Or, is such a commitment incongruous to our definition of its role and function? Professional responsibilities cannot be compromised. As Charlotte Towle so aptly states (10) "there cannot be an admixture of limited goals and high goals. Professional education cannot be designed to train a few to lead, many to follow and others to permanently serve under the guidance of more competent members. It is to be remembered that a profession's leaders cannot advance it beyond the level of its common practice."

Answers to these questions will define the nature and quality of the learning experiences we structure for our students. If we can consensually define our goal as the growth of occupational therapy into a profession and if we are willing to accept the responsibilities inherent in such a decision, we must then clearly define our professional role and scope and reassess those procedures and experiences which we provide as the developmental process for the occupational therapist.

Expectancies for undergraduate and graduate learning will need to be redefined within the context of the level at which one can train for professional competency. It is perhaps understandable that as a young, developing discipline, education in occupational therapy has had to be primarily concerned with the needs for a multiplicity of subjects at the sacrifice of depth of content and dynamic teaching-learning theories. It has, however, been evident for some time that adequate preparation of the occupational therapist for today's practice requires graduate level education. One must seriously question the concept that education to fulfill professional expectations can be achieved at an undergraduate level, regardless of the nature of that profession. As disciplines or quasi-professions have moved toward professional roles each has found this to be evident. The depth and breadth of specialized knowledge and skill required of today's professional cannot be achieved at the undergraduate level and development of occupational therapy into a profession is contingent upon recognition of this fact. Undergraduate experiences may be structured to provide a broad base upon which professional education may build but they can no longer be perceived as professional preparation.

Learning occurs at several different levels and should progress from the perceptual to the most complex one of conceptual integration. Education for professional responsibility requires that learning proceed through each stage and be integrated at each organizational level. It is this process which differentiates cognitive from integrated learning and makes self-dependent, continued learning possible. By and large, the average educational experience does not train for perceptiveness and there are few disciplined opportunities for developing sensitivity awareness. The ability to conceptualize and to make theoretical constructs operant has its foundation in learning at the primary level of perceptual organization. Thus we might perceive our undergraduate education as learning experiences preparatory to professional education, with a focus on teaching the young student to become more acutely aware of sensations and building skill in perceptual organization process. Professional education could then rightfully place greater emphasis on learning at higher levels of integration.

These frames of reference relating to professional identity and education suggest that the classroom needs to be viewed as a potential for dynamic human interaction and thus for learning in an experiential way the perceptiveness, the human interactional skills and the principles and concepts genetic to theories of occupational therapy. The practicum is conceptualized as a continuing growth process, as a laboratory for integrating, consensually validating and consolidating those functions inherent in professional competency. Within this context, it would seem useful to briefly explore learning

experiences both in the classroom and practicum which may comple-
ment such definitions.

Traditional lecture methods have generally been the procedure
of choice when didactic material needs to be mastered, while group
discussion has been reserved for dealing with content relating to
feelings and attitudes. It would seem that such is the case since too
frequently the seminar or group discussion is perceived as a permissive, unstructured experience concerned primarily with opinion sharing and attitudinal change. Such criticism should in no way be perceived as generally applicable to the small group experience wherein
group process is used to facilitate personal growth and attitudinal
change. Such groups have been used and studied extensively and
there is little doubt that with skillful leadership they are effective,
growth-inducing experiences. However, mastery of didactic material
presents a somewhat different problem.

Learning complex didactic material is not maximized by permissive unstructured approaches. However, when skillfully planned, the
classroom discussion group can become an effective, dynamic way of
learning even the most difficult material. It is essential to recognize
that in using the classroom discussion group approach the teacher is
involved with group process skills as well as subject matter teaching.
Thus the teacher needs to acquire facility in group work skills if the
classroom is to provide experiential learning concomitant with mastery of didactic material.

William Faucett Hill has developed a creative and functional
method for structuring the classroom discussion group to achieve this
goal. His monograph, "Learning thru Discussion" (11) including his
cognitive group map presents well organized and lucid guidelines for
dynamic learning experiences within the classroom. The cognitive
group map provides a procedural outline for didactic content analysis
and group interactional processes. This method enables mastery of
subject matter using group process as the milieu, wherein integrated
learning of didactic material becomes possible and group development is used simultaneously as a learning and growth experience.
Presenting the rationale for such an approach, Dr. Hill emphasizes a
well known fact of learning theories that isolated, unassociated facts
are the first to be forgotten and that knowledge must not only be
accumulative and integrated but also have personal value and significance to the student. He states, "Subject matter mastery should

enhance feelings of ego mastery. Acquired knowledge that is not internalized and remains ego-alien is either readily forgotten or if it is retained results in the creation of arid scholasticism or mere pedantry." The lecture method approach frequently encourages little more than cognitive learning.

In addition to the use of Hill's cognitive group map procedure, other methods have been found to be effective in maximizing the potential of the classroom group as a setting for learning and growth. Role playing and use of the critical incident provides opportunities for students to test the efficacy of newly acquired knowledge and concepts, practice problem-solving and diagnostic skills and synthesize that which is being learned. When other students function as observers or alter egos to the role playing or critical incident analysis, additional experience is provided for synthesizing as well as developing insight into the influence of feelings on perception, thinking and behavior. These techniques have been especially useful in helping the student develop a perceptive understanding of the dynamisms of interpersonal and group transactions, evaluative and observational procedures and many other facets of the occupational therapy experience. However, carefully structured, well organized planning is essential if mastery of subject matter is to be achieved. Too frequently role playing, like the group discussion or seminar, is too loosely structured and permissive to teach complex material or depth of content.

The spontaneous panel offers additional opportunity for integrating complex theoretical material, dealing with content analysis in a personally significant way and developing vital skills in verbal communication. These experiences are most effective when panels are formed spontaneously and the students expected to discuss and think through a given problem or issue without preplanning their presentations. Such methods facilitate conceptualization of occupational therapy theories and provide essential experience in the use of logic and analysis.

If we are to teach a set of principles from which critical discernment and professional skill may emerge then our methods of teaching must be analogous to content so as to firmly consolidate an appreciation of the reciprocal relationships among theories and functions. There are inherent correlations between interpersonal theories and skill, group process, self awareness, psychiatric theory and the

meaning and use of objects. Our teaching needs to conclusively demonstrate the dynamic interrelatedness among these and others and
thus guard against learning isolated facts or skills per se.

Adaptations of a technique used by Blake and Mouton (12)
have been effective in combining the learning of didactic subject
matter and group process skills. This method requires that each student prepare a solution to a given problem or critical incident, presenting this to his small discussion group. The group is then expected
to arrive at one solution after which each student's answer is given a
numerical scoring by the group. Ratings are based on content mastery and process of logic. Finally each group is asked to critique how
it functioned as a group in arriving at a consensus regarding both a
solution and individual scoring. Total classroom discussion then centers around the accuracy of solutions and group interactional processes.

Use of the task-oriented group pattern is still another procedure
for maximizing the potential of the classroom as a dynamic setting
for experiential learning of didactic material as well as interpersonal
and group process skills. This procedure calls for the formation of
small working groups whose membership remains constant throughout the course. Each group is responsible for completing several content related assignments and presenting these to the class group for
critique. Each group is also expected to present at the end of term a
process analysis of their group. It has been found that in addition to
actively engaging the student in learning content, these leaderless
groups provide an excellent experience in group development and
constructively increase awareness of the impact of one's feelings and
behavior on others.

An awareness of oneself as an interacting, dynamic force in all
human transactions and the capacity to develop and use this potential is fundamental to professional competency. Thus throughout our
educational program, appropriately related opportunities need to be
provided in order to enhance self-awareness and give impetus to
growth and change.

Personal diaries or logs in which feelings and responses to learning experiences are recorded provide a means for self-evaluation and
an opportunity to increase one's understanding of self and others,
perceive changing attitudes as well as blocks to learning and growth.
Personal diaries have been used by many persons, in a number of

settings to enhance self-awareness and sharpen perceptiveness of cause and effect relationships. Two well formulated discussions of this method may be found in the works of Lifton (13) and Wechler and Reisel. (14) The use of such diaries in conjunction with the occupational therapy classroom seminar and the task-oriented group experience has demonstrated their value in helping the student to consolidate new insights, attitudes and concepts.

The use of students as process observers during classroom sessions creates opportunity for learning techniques of observation, for increasing awareness of interaction and enhancing the student's ability to identify pertinent and related occurrences. Consensual validation and practice of communication skills is possible when the student-observer reports his observations to the class for discussion.

The activity laboratory is an experience which helps to develop an appreciation for and understanding of the meaning of objects and activities and the impact of these on feelings and behavior by engaging the participant in a sequence of activities and object creations. As the activity is pursued, students are encouraged to identify feelings which occur, explore the specific characteristics of both the action and objects which seem to elicit such feelings and discern how feelings are manifested in behavior and in the content of productions. Involvement such as this teaches in a personally significant way the very basic concepts of occupational therapy, initiates a receptivity to self-awareness, sharpens sensitivity and understanding and thus creates the basis for an ultimately more accurate and sensitive appreciation of patient response.

Teaching methods need always be related and appropriate to the material being taught. They also reflect basic attitudes regarding ourselves, our students and growth. If we are to approach the aims of professional education, our teaching theories must indeed mirror such objectives and our methods facilitate rather than obstruct or dull the innate drive of the student to learn and grow.

One student commented in her diary, "I wonder sometimes if this course is not to teach us so much as it is to make us able to learn—it would seem that what I am learning is how to learn and teach myself—this conviction grows stronger each week."

A second student wrote, "I'm beginning to get the impression that Mrs. ——— doesn't really care half as much about what we think as that we think." Another commented, "It's infuriating! Think and reason, think and reason—I'm sick of these words! Seven weeks and no hard cold facts! The assumption that students can answer their own questions is ridiculous. Why do we come to college in the first place?" Near the end of the semester this same student wrote, "It's taken a long time but I finally seem to be getting the message—things are beginning to fall into place and what's so exciting is that *I* have put them there—not some teacher who *'told me!'*"

The practicum or clinical experience is an additional opportunity for growth, for learning to apply knowledge, develop and test clinical skills, consensually validate and thus consolidate those functions which comprise professional competency. Within this frame of reference self-dependent thinking becomes a primary objective. A sense of professional responsibility needs to be created and decision-making skills developed by allowing the student to assume realistic responsibilities with sufficient freedom to make decisions rather than limiting these on the basis of unrealistic expectations. Collaboration with others is best taught by expecting and supporting collaborative roles rather than passive-dependent ones. Latitude to think and function in this manner, however, will be consistent with theories and goals of the professional educative process only if supervision is an integral part of the learning-growth process. Time and a multiplicity of experiences are not the primary agents for growth but rather skillful teaching which nurtures the development of the professional person.

Generally the concept of supervision seems to be in the literal sense of Webster's definition, "to oversee, to direct or inspect with authority." However, as a growth process in professional education, supervision is conceptualized as a dynamic teaching-helping relationship committed to the learning and growth of the student or supervisee. This learning experience has as its focus the exploration, analysis and synthesis of the ongoing functions of the learner to the extent that theoretical knowledge may emerge as professional skill. It exists on the basis that learning must be a conscious process in order for integration to be maximized and that self-awareness and understanding is the substructure of professional maturation and competency. Supervision in this sense then becomes the primary modus operandi in fulfilling the educational aims of the clinical experience and such is the contract which binds supervisor and learner together.

Frequently individual supervisory sessions are perceived as

occurring only when specific problems or questions arise. However, this helping-teaching process needs to be an ongoing occurrence, regularly scheduled and proceeding in a logical sequence related to the learner's individual capacities and what is to be learned. Although what the student brings to the learning experience has an influence on the transaction, fulfillment of the supervisory contract will depend in great measure upon the attitudes and skill of the supervisor. The teaching-helping relationship, in the context of preparation for meeting professional expectations, has as one of its major goals increased self-awareness and understanding—perception and understanding of self not as a goal in itself but for the purpose of developing a coherent, definable set of constructs concerning the dynamics of interpersonal relationships and the assimilation of these into basic attitudes and modes of functioning. The supervisor therefore must be sufficiently secure and free from biases to be able to approach situations realistically. He must possess an openness and receptivity to looking at feelings and their impact on behavior and have enough self-awareness and understanding to provide the assurance and objectivity so necessary to exploring and understanding ongoing function and catalyzing appropriate change.

In conceptualizing supervision as a learning-growth process, it is important to understand the difference between this experience and therapy. Therapy is that process which has as its primary focus the alteration or diminution of psychopathology and thus is frequently concerned with the unconscious and genetic forces motivating pathological thinking and behavior. Supervision is directed toward learning and explores feelings and behavioral responses only in relation to the facilitation of learning and the development of professional skills. Extensive or depth exploration of personal feelings and their causative factors has no place in supervision. Personal problems which seriously interfere with learning and growth may well need to be worked through in therapy before the goals of supervision can be realized but the supervisory session is not therapy and the resolution of these problems belongs in another setting. For example, a student who has difficulty in helping a patient deal with his angry, hostile impulses, needs to explore with the supervisor the nature and quality of the problem and come to have some understanding of how his own attitudes regarding such feelings have an impact on what transpires between himself and the patient. However, the personal, historical basis for such attitudes on the part of the student and working these through in depth does not belong in the supervisory session.

Charlotte Towle (15) presents some excellent formulations on the nature and scope of the supervisory relationship and Margaret Williamson (16) in her description of supervision makes useful comparisons between such processes, psychotherapy and counselling.

The terms administration and supervision are frequently used interchangeably. However, the concept of supervision as presented here emphasizes that the two, although related, are essentially different processes. Supervision is a dyadic relationship committed to the learning and growth of the individual. Administration is perceived as those procedures which are directed toward creating a milieu or culture, an organizational pattern, which may be expected to maximize attainment of the goals of a given institution or organization. Supervision is concerned with the professional development of the individual, administration with maximizing goal achievement of organization. Such a differentiation points up the relatedness of these two processes and at the same time brings into focus an appreciation for the different modes of operation within each. While the needs of the learner are served by each it is important to understand their particular differences in order to keep in focus the set of values and frames of reference unique for each setting in which learning occurs.

Development of the learner as a professional person requires that the teaching-learning process be perceived and understood as a dynamic human interactional growth process. In order for a profession to fulfill its obligations to the society it serves, learning must be a continuing, ongoing process. Education for the profession does not stop at the time of graduation. We must teach in such a way that learning will result in a research attitude; a way of thinking so that questioning, investigation and constructively critical evaluation becomes a way of life and thus learning and growth a continuing process. In addition, professional education should assure the maintenance of change, the learning transactions being of such a nature as to provide the developing professional with a sense of ego mastery so that his new set of values and concepts are not dangerously compromised once the teaching-helping relationship has been terminated.

Perhaps at no other time have there existed for us the opportunities we face today. Modern medicine with its developing sociologic focus creates new and exciting expectations for all professions. The concept of the whole man as a social interacting being brings more sharply into focus the significance of those concepts and practices indigenous to occupational therapy. Man's innate drive to fulfill his needs for self identity and self realization through productive transactions with his object and interpersonal world is and has been the corner stone of occupational therapy.

It is the privilege and responsibility of a profession to define the kinds of learning which will develop its student's potential for the fulfillment of its educational aims. May we have the courage, the knowledge and the sensitive discernment to measure up to the greatness of this challenge and to prepare professional leaders for tomorrow's practice.

REFERENCES

1. Tyler, Ralph W., "Educational Problems in Other Professions," in Bernard R. Berelson (ed.) *Education for Librarianship*, Am. Library Ass'n. 1949.
2. Towle, Charlotte, *The Learner in Education for the Professions*, Univ. of Chicago Press, 1954, p. 5, 10.
3. Lifton, Walter, *Working with Groups*, John Wiley and Sons, 1961, p. 5.
4. Towle, Charlotte, op. cit. p. 10.
5. Pearce, Jane and Newton, Saul, *Conditions of Human Growth*, The Citadel Press, 1963.
6. Fidler, Gail S., "A Guide to Planning and Measuring Growth Experiences in the Clinical Affiliation," *AJOT* Vol. XVIII, No. 6, 1964.
7. Bradford, Leland P., "The Teaching-Learning Transaction," in *Forces in Learning*, Selected Reading Series Three, Nat'l Training Laboratories, Nat'l Ed. Assn., Wash., D.C., 1961, p. 8.
8. Jersild, Arthur, *"When Teachers Face Themselves,"* N.Y. Bureau of Publications, Teachers College, Col. Univ., 1955.
9. Bradford, Leland, op. cit.
10. Towle, Charlotte, op. cit.
11. Hill, William Faucett, *Learning thru Discussion*, Youth Studies Center, Univ. of Southern California, 1962.
12. Blake, Robert R., and Mouton, Jane Srygley in Weschler, Irving R., and Schein, Edgar H., *Issues in Human Relations Training*, NTL Selected Reading Series, No. 5, 1962.
13. Lifton, Walter, op. cit.
14. Weschler, Irving R., and Reisel, Jerome, *Inside a Sensitivity Training Group*, Institute of Industrial Relations, Univ. of California, 1960.
15. Towle, Charlotte, op. cit.
16. Williamson, Margaret, *Supervision—New Patterns and Processes*, Association Press, 1961.

Authentic Occupational Therapy

Elizabeth June Yerxa

In the spring of 1963 I attended the "Workshop on Graduate Education in Occupational Therapy" held in the Ozark mountains of Missouri. The air was heavy with the fragrance of a million dogwood blossoms. I was just settling into a mood of peacefulness when my tranquility was abruptly shattered by Earnest Brandenburg, dean of the University College of Washington University. Dean Brandenburg said, "It is my candid judgment that the field of occupational therapy in 1963 is *not* regarded and probably should not be identified as one of the professions." (1)

What image do you see when you think of a professional? A person who always wears clean white shoes or someone who can spout off the origins and insertions of every muscle in the body or one who can discuss Freudian theory with a psychiatrist? No, professionalism is much more than appearance and intellectual accomplishments. It means being able to meet real needs. It means being unique. It means having and acting upon a philosophy. It also means being "authentic."

Steps Toward Professionalism

In 1966, occupational therapy is moving with speed and accelerating self-confidence toward true professionalism. In the past we often dwelled upon our insecurity about who or what we were to the point that we were paralyzed into inaction. Remember how much

Reprinted from *The American Journal of Occupational Therapy*, Vol. XXI, No. 1, 1967.

time we used to spend in masochistic soul-searching? One of my favorite cartoons from the *Saturday Review* shows two bearded mediators sitting side by side on a mountain top. One says to the other, "There must be more to life than pursuing the meaning of life." Our growth toward appropriate confidence as professionals indicates that we have discovered there is much more to occupational therapy than contemplating its meaning.

What are some of the significant steps we have taken toward professionalism? In discussing the characteristics of a profession, Dean Brandenburg emphasized that a body of knowledge is essential. This body of knowledge must be based upon accepted research. Occupational therapists are becoming increasingly involved in planning, conducting and publishing the results of their own research studies. Clinicians are developing unique tools of evaluation and specialized methods for recording data. Treatment programs have thus not only become based upon sounder thought but have been sufficiently organized and objectified to be studied.

A few years ago our conferences relied primarily on physicians and other professionals from outside our field to identify what was important to our practice. Now our annual conferences plus workshops, seminars and study courses are loaded with excellent papers conceived and presented by occupational therapists. We have learned to look within our field for provocative thought and inspiration. We have found it in abundance.

Perhaps most significant for the future development of our body of knowledge is the increased awareness that the scientific attitude is not incompatible with concern for the client as a human being but may be one of the best foundations for acting upon that concern. This awareness is demonstrated by our students of today who are much more critical of the thinking of their elders, much more objective in assessing their own performance and much more likely to be able to frame a question which can lead to research than the students of ten years ago. Yet, if anything, today's students have gained in their capacities to care about the client.

The development of a body of knowledge in a professional carries with it considerable personal responsibility for making both rational (scientific) judgments and intuitive (artistic) decisions according to Dean Brandenburg. Occupational therapists are accepting greater responsibility to contribute to the pool of knowledge about the client, to exercise judgment as to how our skills can best be used to fulfill his needs, to assess the client's responses and communicate our unique findings to other professionals who need them in order to fulfill their responsibilities. The written prescription is no longer seen by many of us as necessary, holy or healthy. Instead our relationship to the referring physician is becoming much more communicative and collaborative. The pseudo-security of the prescription required that we pay a high price. That price was the reduction of our potential to help clients because we often stagnated at the level of applying technical skills.

Dean Brandenburg suggested that in order for occupational therapy to merit recognition as a "true" profession we needed to carry out a continuous evaluation and revision of our educational curricula. Do you realize that the past three years have constituted an educational revolution in occupational therapy? Since 1962, when we published the findings of our own curriculum study, we have engaged in an overwhelming amount of educational revisions of our curricula. For example, we held a workshop on graduate education in occupational therapy, revised the Essentials of an Acceptable Curriculum in Occupational Therapy, completed a study on the implications of the curriculum study including the formulation, for the first time in history, of a thought-provoking set of proposed educational objectives for occupational therapy. Two of our curricula have started pilot programs by which students can become registered occupational therapists and earn their master's degrees simultaneously. For a profession which frequently perceives itself as moving slower than a snail going uphill against the wind, this is astounding educational progress made in three years. If I were a faculty member I think I would be tempted to say to my students, as I stood before the class, "Don't worry about today's lesson, what you will learn in tomorrow's will make all of this obsolete."

The real significance of our educational progress lies on a deeper level than studies completed and changes initiated. Clinicians and educators have worked more closely together on this process of educational self-assessment than at any time on our past history. As a result, each has learned to respect the contribution of the other. It is as if theory and practice have finally touched hands and found that they respect and need each other. This unity will lead to basic education for our students which is a unified and continuous process.

Many of these changes have been hammered cut through vigorous argument and the obstinate patience of occupational therapists who defended their educational philosophies in meetings lasting far into the night. I am certain at such times many of them longed, in their secret hearts, to rely upon some outside "authority." But they did not choose the easy way. As a result we can point with pride to the fact that *we* have taken the initiative and responsibility to evaluate and upgrade our total educational system using our unique resources. As Dr. Mary Reilly put it, "Like Rumpelstiltskin, we have taken the straw and woven it into gold."

A profession obtains wide recognition of the need for the services which it can perform. How widely is the need for occupational therapy recognized? Remember how we used to laugh, rather painfully, about the persons who would smile politely and say "oh isn't that nice" when we told them we were occupational therapists? For we knew they had no idea of what we did. To make matters worse we were not at all sure that we could tell them. We still experience similar responses but they occur less and less.

More significantly, the people and agencies who can recognize the need for our services and *do* something about it are well aware of how much they need us. The Medicare bill and corresponding state legislation recognize the need for occupational therapy in hospitals, home health services and extended care programs. These bills and regulations write our profession into the law as one criterion for an acceptable program. For the first time in history, these bills recognize our own registration process and graduation from an acceptable curriculum as the criteria for professional qualification.

Convalescent homes, outpatient facilities, rehabilitation centers and schools are clamoring for our services. One of our greatest problems of the future is not going to be how to bring about a greater awareness of the need for our services but rather to provide for the need which already exists with a level of service of which we can be proud.

An organization for a profession is also widely recognized, Dean Brandenburg stated. How widely recognized is the American Occupational Therapy Association? Our leaders have been sought for advice and counsel in writing the regulations for Medicare. Many professions are most cognizant of the educational and organizational changes we have instituted, including our pilot programs on a master's level. A physician said to me recently, "You are far ahead of many other health professions educationally. Your organization is progressive. It looks toward the future." At a recent workshop for faculty members from schools of social work I was astounded at the reaction of intense interest and admiration for our foresight in both developing and having in operation certified occupational therapy assistants training programs.

Since 1963, occupational therapy has made important progress toward true professionalism by further identifying and substantiating our body of knowledge, developing the research attitude and tools for research among practitioners and students, accepting the responsibility for using judgment and making scientific and intuitive decisions, obtaining increasing recognition of the need for our services, maintaining standards for admission to the profession and obtaining legislative recognition of our own registration process as the criterion of professional qualification and undertaking a continuing evaluation and revision of our educational curricula.

This substantial progress does not mean that we have made it. For professionalism, by its very nature, requires our continual efforts to progress in all of these areas, particularly in identifying our own body of knowledge. Through our faith in the efficacy of our practice we have resisted pressures that would regress us to the level of technicians, pressures to drop our dual educational emphasis upon the behavioral and biological sciences, pressures to disavow in practice what we were unable to prove at the moment. In resisting these pressures we have acted in the present while maintaining a vision of the future.

Purpose of Occupational Therapy

It is all fine and good to talk about our steps toward true professionalism but what is the purpose of occupational therapy? I believe that our broad purpose is to produce a reality-orienting influence upon the client's perception of his physical environment and his social and psychological self, to the end that he can function in his environment with self-actualization. This purpose is certainly not unique to occupational therapy. It is shared by many professional groups who are motivated to provide altruistic service to the client.

If this broad purpose is a shared one, then how are we unique?

When it comes to identifying even a part of the uniqueness of occupational therapy we frequently behave as though we belonged to
the school of Chinese philosophers called Taoists. Substitute the
words occupational therapy for the word Tao, in the following poem
and you will see the parallel. "The thing that is called Tao, is elusive,
evasive. Elusive, evasive, yet latent in it are forms. Elusive, evasive yet
latent in it are objects. Dark and dim yet latent in it is the life
force." (2) We are often afraid that by defining our own elusive,
evasive qualities we shall make our profession too small in concept.

For the purpose of provoking your thought and in full awareness of the dangers of limiting us, may I propose a concept? Occupational therapy is unique because we use the choice of self-initiated
purposeful activities to produce a reality-orienting influence upon
the client's perception of himself and his environment so that he can
function. Let us examine four key phrases which help identify our
uniqueness: choice; self-initiated, purposeful activity; reality-orienting; and perception.

Choice

First, the factor of *"choice."* Occupational therapy has been
unique, historically, because of the client's participation in his own
treatment. Choice has been so fundamental to our thinking that we
have questioned whether procedures which are done *to* the person,
over which he has no control, should be called occupational therapy.
Choice has been encouraged in the client's selection of media, his
unique interaction with our media and, most importantly, in setting
the objectives for his treatment program.

Since self-initiated activity is our "stock in trade" and since it is
impossible to force any human being to initiate without his choosing
to do so, choice is one of the keys to our unique therapeutic process.
It is also a necessity if we are to achieve the ultimate goal of occupational therapy, that is, the ability of the person to function in his
environment with self-actualization. For no matter how well-con-
ceived the therapeutic program, the resulting achievement of the
client's function depends both upon his capacities and his *choice* to
use them.

Our everyday vocabulary reveals our attitudes. We ask, "What
would you like to accomplish with your arm brace?" or, "Would you

prefer to plan your kitchen today or concentrate on bathing the baby?" We say we "work with the client." We do not "do" the client or "care for" the client or "manage" him.

Does the emphasis on choice mean that occupational therapists abdicate responsibility for the client's welfare, that our milieu is one of anarchy or that we are less knowledgeable than other professionals who "know" what is best for the client and treat him accordingly? Not on your life! Our client's choice is based upon exposure to our therapeutic process which encourages him to make a series of decisions leading to progressing degrees of independence.

Occupational therapists use their knowledge, skills and personalities to enable the client to experience his possibilities. He must be given the chance to choose on the basis of reality, not fantasy. He is not adequately informed to make choices until he can anticipate the results of his choices.

The occupational therapist identifies the small steps necessary to attain the client's larger goal, the purposes of the media and what the client might expect to accomplish or fail to accomplish, depending upon his choices. The occupational therapist's personal conviction may be an important means of eliciting the client's participation in an activity which he initially rejects because the experience of success, which the therapist knows he can attain, is not initially a fact to him. Many "motivation" problems occur because the client is afraid to fail and cannot anticipate the gratification of success.

This active role of the occupational therapist in helping the client delineate his choices takes more knowledge, skill and sensitivity plus more faith in the individual than an authoritarian role of "you must do this because it is good for you."

Rose Meyer, medical social worker, in her article "Dependency as an Asset in the Rehabilitation Process" said, "the rehabilitation process may be a long and dynamic struggle that influences and is influenced by the dependency-independency conflict." (3) She felt that the patient's ability to *use* his initial physical and psychological dependency could move him increasingly toward independence, similar to the evolution of his earlier life. Miss Meyer gave the following case history of a forty-year-old engineer who had recently become paraplegic: At first the patient rejected the dependency created by his injury. He tried to master his situation by learning all about his condition, his prognosis and how he could immediately participate in his own care. His aggressive, though reasonable attitude was overbearing to the nursing staff, for the progress he desired was always a bit ahead of reality. His behavior deteriorated to stubbornness and disinterested compliance. By the time he started his occupational therapy program he was threatening to leave the hospital in order to carry out many of his own ideas for developing independence. He was frustrated by the lack of opportunity to participate actively in his own program. When given the opportunity by the occupational therapist to make a choice for his treatment from several modalities for an explained purpose, he found structure for his move toward independence, not only in his own treatment but in his investment in the program of other patients for whom he designed appliances and work projects. As Miss Meyer stated, "He could depend upon the occupational therapist's knowledge and skill to act as a catalyst for his own creative investment."

The occupational therapist thus serves as a catalyst by which the client moves toward increasing self-direction. The process begins with the client's acceptance of a reasonable degree of dependence upon the therapist's skill and knowledge, moves toward his understanding of the reality of his condition, his formulation of goals based upon that reality and his selection of media within a category of choices appropriate to the goals.

But what about the patient who is too incapacitated, physically and/or emotionally, to make *any* choice. Sister Madeline Clemence, in her moving essay, "Existentialism: A Philosophy of Commitment," dealt with this question in relation to nursing. "Whenever the nurse takes an initiative which should have been the patient's, she should understand that it is only a temporary measure and that it should be ratified by the patient." (4) The same principle applies to the occupational therapist.

Self-Initated Purposeful Activity

The second key phrase in investigating our uniqueness is *"self-initiated, purposeful activity."* Self-initiated refers not only to psychological choice but to sensory-motor participation. Dr. Karl Smith, professor of psychology at the University of Wisconsin has criticized behavior theory for its past emphasis on physiological drive states as the basis for human motivation. He states, "Yet much of ordinary human behavior—verbal and graphic skills, patterns of work, artistic and recreational pursuits—which we observe in ourselves and others seem to bear little relation to hunger, thirst, sexual drives and the like." (5) Dr. Smith feels that perceptual motivation or activity motivation should be considered of primary importance in behavior organization. "The nature of this motivating force can be described specifically in terms of the intrinsic make-up of the regulatory mechanisms of motion, for the neurogeometrically organized motion systems drive the individual to action as relentlessly and more consistently than hunger or thirst."

Self-initiated activity, specifically verbal and graphic skills, patterns of work, artistic and recreational pursuits—activity of concern to occupational therapists—is of primary importance in human motivation, if we accept Dr. Smith's theory.

Motion is patterned according to the spatial and temporal demands of the environment as the individual reacts to differences in stimuli. In resolving these differences, the individual continually and by his own movements, produces new differences to which he must react. Thus self-initiated activity is both a response to sensory stimulation and a source of additional stimulation by which the individual develops patterns of adaptive behavior. Passive movements apparently do not result in the same degree of adaptation. (5) The individual must respond dynamically to changed stimulus relationships in order to adapt.

Dr. Jean Ayres called occupational therapy's emphasis on purposeful activity the factor which unites our profession in its practice for patients with emotional as well as physical conditions. She said, "If purposeful activity is one of the distinguishing functions of occupational therapy, it might well be asked if it is necessary for the treatment of motor disability." Then she answered, "In the life of the neurologically normal individual, activity is not random but purposeful, *i.e.,* directed toward the accomplishment of a goal. It is generally this *goal* that is the basis for activity in the central nervous system and therein lies its value." (6)

A year ago I helped evaluate a brain damaged client's function. She was asked to open her hand. No response occurred, except that she was obviously trying. Next she was moved passively into finger extension while the occupational therapist demonstrated the desired movement. This time the client responded with increased finger flexion. In frustration she cried, "I know, I know." Finally she was offered a cup of water. As the cup was perceived, her fingers opened almost miraculously to grasp it. Only the factor of purpose could produce the desired response.

Purposeful activity is activity which has meaning to the client, not just to the occupational therapist. Our clients are individuals who have differing ideas of purpose. Some individuals are deeply imbued with our cultural admonition that "work is virtue." Such persons may respond with greater motivation to resistive exercise than to an elaborately adapted craft activity given for the same reason. For persons with lower motor neuron disease for whom the objective is increased muscle strength which will be translated into function, such exercise, providing that it constitutes purposefulness for the client, may be the most effective physiological and psychological method for producing the desired result.

Conversely and most particularly for patients with central nervous system impairment, straight exercise might not only be purposeless to the client but through its demand for attention upon the movement and not upon the goal, might produce an undesirable response. Craft activities or other creative, goal-directed pursuits may, in such instances, elicit a neuromuscular response which cannot be attained through other means. These activities also have the advantage of distracting the patient's attention from pain thus reducing the muscular splinting or neuromuscular alienation that often accompanies pain.

Reality Orientation

Third, the factor of *"reality orientation."* In occupational therapy the patient experiences the reality of his physical environment and his capacity to function within it. Our clinics may be chambers of horror for some individuals as they confront their physical disability for the first time by trying to do something, perhaps as simple as self-feeding. Yet, if the individual is to function with self-actualization he must discover both his limitations and his possibilities. We meet our responsibilities to the client when we provide him with opportunities to readjust his value system through the development of both new capacities and the ability to substitute for some lost capacities. We are like mirrors which can reflect, without the distortion of wish-fulfillment or self-deprecation, a true image of the client's potential.

Perception

Fourth, *"perception."* Occupational therapy produces a reality-orienting influence upon the client's perception of his physical environment as well as his psychological and social self. In the area of physical perception our media produce sensory stimuli which are perceived and reacted to by the client. Our professional literature is presently concerned with identifying syndromes of perceptual-motor dysfunction, the development of evaluation tools for identifying specific problems of perceptual-motor function and the development of theories upon which to base treatment programs to improve these functions. Because our media require the use of postural movements, transport and fine manipulation and because they allow us to stimulate many sensory modalities, we are appropriately and deeply concerned with perceptual-motor function. Dr. Ayres and others from our profession have contributed significantly to the available literature in this area.

It has been found in experiments of displaced or delayed sensory feedback, that many normal individuals react to their resulting perceptual-motor discoordination with considerable emotional disturbance. (5) Similarly, persons with perceptual-motor dysfunction may exhibit severe behavior problems. Psychotic episodes have been associated with the use of such perception distorting drugs as LSD. These findings indicate the existence of a link between perceptual-motor function and emotional responses. This link, with further study, might serve to bridge another apparent gap between our practice with the physically disabled and that with the emotionally disabled person. We are one of the few professions whose education prepares us to visualize the perceptual-motor function of man as a psychobiological unity.

In addition to perception of a neurophysiological nature, the individual also perceives himself as a psychological entity and a social being. Occupational therapy provides an everyday environment in which the individual can determine, through choice, his own particular identity.

The following is an example of the kind of self-perception we sometimes deal with:

Look at me, look at me
What do you see?
A thing made of plaster, metal and skin.
Look at me, look at me
How can this be?
They make me exist in the place that I'm in.
Look at me, look at me
Help me to flee
From this world of blindness to that of the seeing.
Look at me.

This young lady, who is severely paralyzed, is pleading for help to escape from her own self-concept into the world of the "seeing," that is, a world in which she would perceive herself as being recognized, not as a "thing" but as a feeling, thinking, valuable human being.

Exposure to our media means a confrontation with objects and an opportunity for the individual to discover what he can and cannot do with them. Exposure to our professional spirit means that the individual confronts both our knowledge of his capacities and our faith that he has the right to control what happens to him.

Being a "thing" leads to social relationships based upon dependency, hostility or pity. As James Colbert, a paraplegic, said in his essay *A Study Establishing the Disabled as a Minority Group,* "pity can be referred to as a sort of sequence mechanism: disease or accident—hospitalization—disability—I am very sorry." Jim observed, "This attitude may, in fact, be responsible for motivating the disabled to stay apart from their [previous] social group and to act and interact mainly with their own [disabled] group." (7) Pity implies the socially-sanctioned classification of the disabled into a minority group and with that classification comes dismissal from the stream of "normal" society. Occupational therapy which leads to the client's ability to function in his environment can help alter other people's perception of him as the object of pity and reduce their need to classify him apart from themselves.

Occupational therapists, in my experience, are remarkably free of the sort of cynicism and expediency which might result in the client perceiving himself as a "thing." Our positive attitude has been characterized as "regulated optimism" by one occupational therapist. Another fine occupational therapist said, "Occupational therapy begins when everyone else has given up." She meant it humorously. But like most humor it had a strong core of truth. Both of these statements reflect our faith in the client.

Being able to help the client confront himself is perhaps the most sensitive, personally and professionally demanding task of the occupational therapist. For it requires courage on the part of the client, emotional support on the part of the occupational therapist and a continual mutual testing and communication of what reality is.

Just as our emphasis on "purposeful activity" unites our practice for patients with emotional as well as physical conditions, so does our emphasis upon helping the patient grasp the reality of his life situation in order to move toward increasing degrees of self-direction. For even in such a seemingly physically oriented activity as teaching a patient to dress himself, our ultimate goal is a psychosocial one. That is, by increasing the client's capacity to be independent we help him perceive himself as possessing worth. He is not a "thing" to be manipulated helplessly by others but is a human being who can exercise some control over his environment, even in being able to put on whatever shirt he wants to put on when he wants to do it.

Occupational Therapy's View of Man

The psalmist phrased the question: "What is man that thou art mindful of him?" (8) That question has been repeated over the centuries. Although fragment by fragment has been added to our knowledge of man's nature, through the sciences and historical experience, our understanding remains incomplete. For man is mysterious. He defies definition.

Yet, in spite of this mystery, our profession has chosen unique methods to help the client function with self-actualization. Both our methods and our goals imply that we have a point of view regarding man's nature. For if we are to be helpful to him, we must conceive of what is valuable to him. This takes us into philosophy.

Our particular view of man agrees considerably with that of some existential thinkers. Unfortunately, existentialism has been associated with anti-intellectualism, egocentricity, irresponsibility and anarchy. It therefore frequently conveys mental pictures of bearded beatniks who wallow in pools of self-pity, bewailing the meaninglessness of the universe, while regularly collecting their unemployment insurance checks. These associations are superficial.

According to David E. Roberts, (9) existentialism is not an organized philosophical system but rather it represents a protest against all views which tend to regard man as though he were a *thing*, that is, only an assortment of functions and reactions. It stands against philosophies or social theories in which the mass mentality stifles the spontaneity and uniqueness of the individual person. In occupational therapy's recognition of the client as one who ought to participate in his treatment and be given the opportunity to make choices, we are as Martin Buber would say, "taking a stand" in relation to him. We are viewing the client, not as an object or thing to be manipulated, controlled or made to conform but as a unique individual whose very humanness entitles him to choices in determining his own destiny. For if the client interprets himself as a thing (one thing among others in the world) he might sacrifice his selfhood and neither recognize nor realize his potentials.

Existentialists see man as involved in the process of becoming. What he becomes is shaped by himself, in response to his life experiences and relationships to others. Heidegger, the philosopher who contributed significantly to existential thinking, made a distinction between "authentic" and "inauthentic" existence. He felt that in the world of everyday experience man comes to terms with what he is only by coming to terms with his possibilities or potentialities. If he lives mainly in terms of 'what one does' or what one 'does not do' and is therefore merged in conventional mass reactions, he is emerged in inauthentic existence. Authenticity is achieved to the degree that the individual reaches true selfhood by rising out of mass reactions, taking the initiative in discovering the meaning of his own existence and disposing of his own potentialities accordingly. In order to achieve authentic existence man must have resolve to become his true self.

For the client who is hospitalized, the institution may inadvertently represent the "mass mentality" with its pressures of what 'one does' or what 'one doesn't do'. Louis Worth, the sociologist, once remarked that the only good institution is a dead institution. (10) His comment was provoked by the common tendency of institutions, implicitly or explicitly, to regard their own survival as a major goal thus losing sight of the client's individuality in the process.

Bill was the "ideal" patient. He kept all of his appointments religiously and worked diligently on every aspect of his treatment. He accepted the wisdom of the physicians who directed his rehabilitation program. He carried out his therapeutic activities without question. He used every piece of self-care equipment which was ordered for him. He attained an amazing degree of physical independence prior to discharge to the point that he became an example to inspire other patients. Six months after his discharge he came back to the hospital for a clinic visit. His facial expression was passive and lifeless. He had gained thirty pounds, had developed a pressure sore and had become dependent in all activities except for minimal self-feeding. Obviously Bill had conformed to the hospital's value system temporarily but once out of the institutional environment had become primarily a dependent and passive being. In that sense he had lived an "inauthentic" existence while hospitalized. Instead of encouraging his adherence to the value system of the institution, how much better it would have been if his behavior had been recognized as conformity. The occupational therapist might then have provided him with opportunities to question, complain and become emotionally involved in his rehabilitation program. Often the clients who distress the hospital staff the most by not behaving as "patients" become the most self-directed after discharge.

Earlier I mentioned the client's confrontation with the reality of his disability in occupational therapy. This confrontation with pain, suffering, loss of function and the high anxiety associated with it are realities about which he can begin to determine the meaning of his life's experiences. In other words, the pain and deep stresses of such an experience may lead to resolve. For such traumatic experiences, which cannot be ignored, can transform the individual's existence from that of a day to day contact with superficial, meaningless events to a "mind and heart" involvement in being. Instead of regarding himself as surrounded by circumstances and chance events, he can begin to see himself in a situation which is something to be mastered. Action on his part can become instead of mainly a series of external, practical activities, a development of inner resources which can be stronger than mere happenings.

The particular reality of the occupational therapy clinic involves not only the client's disability but his opportunity to make the kinds of choices by which he can discover, for himself, the meaning of his own existence and realize his potentials in accordance with that meaning. Our clinics are one of the few environments within institutions in which the client can make such choices.

Existentialism also makes a firm distinction between subjective and objective truth. It does not deny that through common sense, science and logic men are able to arrive at genuinely objective truth. But, it insists that in connection with ultimate matters it is impossible to lay aside the impassioned concerns of the *individual*. In the search for ultimate truth, the whole man, not just his reason and intellect, are involved. His emotions and his will must be aroused and engaged so that he can live the truth he sees. As Heidegger put it, "The scientist pursues one legitimate way of studying what is, but he makes an extra-scientific assertion when he adds, 'That's all there is. There isn't anymore'."

In occupational therapy we are providing a milieu in which the total man, not just his reason, is involved. Our purposeful media, our emphasis upon the discovery of the client's potential, the necessity for him to act in occupational therapy and his relationship to us deeply involve his will and emotions, providing that we can be authentic in relation to him.

Authentic Occupational Therapy

What then, is authentic occupational therapy? Authentic occupational therapy is based upon a *commitment* to the client's realization of his own particular meaning. The authentic occupational therapist recognizes that although initial dependency might require a temporary suspension of the patient's right to choice, the therapeutic experience is primarily an opportunity for self-actualization. Therefore, the occupational therapist does not force his value system upon the client. But rather, through using his skills and knowledge, exposes the client to a range of possibilities which constitute his external reality. The client is the one who makes the choice.

Authentic occupational therapy means *involvement* of both the client and the occupational therapist. Through the use of media the client is involved intellectually and emotionally in discovering what is purposeful to him. He is also involved in relation to objects, actions and persons. Through these relationships he is helped to come to grips with his particular reality including his disability, his emotional reactions, his will and his potential.

Professional authenticity in occupational therapy means that the occupational therapist in every professional *act* defines the profession. For example, he may believe that it is important to perform clinical research but that belief has no meaning until he *acts* upon it by initiating research activity.

As a professional, the authentic occupational therapist recognizes his responsibility to be a life-long student and to contribute to the body of knowledge. He also recognizes that an important part of what he will learn and contribute will be subjective, that is, concerned with feelings and human motivation. He will not expect science to provide him with all the answers but he will respect what science has to contribute.

Personal authenticity as an occupational therapist means that the therapist allows himself to feel real emotion as he enters into *mutual* relation with the client. In a mutual relationship as Martin Buber said, "My thou affects me as I affect it. We are molded by our pupils and built up by our works." (11) The authentic occupational therapist is involved in the process of caring and to care means to be affected just as surely as it means to affect.

William Barrett in his superb book *Irrational Man* cites the example of the successful businessman who flies to the country for the weekend, is whisked off to golf, tennis, sailing; who entertains his guests successfully, all on a split-second schedule and at the end of the weekend flies back to the city without ever having the desire to lose himself by walking down a country lane. Such a man, we say, is marvelously organized and really knows how to manage things; but the point is that he has mastery over beings but not Being. "He never has contact with Being. He goes to the country and returns without ever *really* being there." (12) We cannot really help clients unless *we are there*; that is we feel, we encounter, we take time, we listen and we *are* ourselves.

The authentic occupational therapist is open to the client's ideas and feelings and real in responding to them. He does not give in to the temptation to insulate himself against feeling because if he does so he will lose his capacity to be there. "Being there" also means being able to separate his feelings for the client as a human being from projections of how *he* would feel if he had experienced the client's disability. For the authentic occupational therapist knows that the client is the only one who can discover his own particular meaning. Stephen Becker in his essay *On Being a Patient* put it this way. "One man's hangnail is another man's broken neck." (13) He went on to say that once the disabled person has decided to live he must stop asking "why me?" He must reject pity and singularity with equal and absolute indifference. Mr. Becker, as a result of his experience of being a patient, reaffirmed his philosophy that nature never rejoices and never mourns.

In the new dimension of 1966, occupational therapy is becoming a true profession. This is a time to be proud of what we have accomplished. Our service to the client is unique in its application of choice, self-initiated, purposeful activity and its emphasis upon the goal of function with self-actualization. Our media have been identified as those activities which are at the very source of human motivation. Philosophically we do not see man as a "thing" but as a being whose choices allow him to discover and determine his own Being. Our media, our emphasis upon the client's potentials, the necessity for him to act and the mutuality of our relationship with him provide a milieu in which his suffering can be translated into the resolve to become his true self.

This is also a time for each of us to determine our own authenticity as professionals. The degree to which we can maintain faith in our profession and still strive to improve it by our own acts, the degree to which we can maintain faith in our clients while becoming involved in the process of helping them will determine the future authenticity of our practice. We are ever becoming.

Rainer Marie Rilke wrote:

"Out of infinite yearnings rise
finite deeds like feeble fountains,
that early and trembling droop.
But those, else silent within us,
Our happy strengths—reveal themselves
in these dancing tears." (14)

ACKNOWLEDGMENT

The author wishes to express her appreciation for the thoughts and support contributed by the following persons: Lois Barber, O.T.R., Jerry Johnson, O.T.R., Janet Stone, O.T.R., Doris Kroulek, O.T.R. and the staff and students of the occupational therapy department at Rancho Los Amigos Hospital.

BIBLIOGRAPHY

1. Brandenburg, Earnest, "Building Toward Professionalism," *Proceedings of Workshop on Graduate Education in Occupational Therapy*, April, 1963.
2. Yutang, Lin, (ed.), "The Manifestations of Tao," *The Wisdom of China and India*, Random House, 1942.
3. Meyer, Rose, "Dependency as an Asset in the Rehabilitation Process," *Rehab Lit*, October, 1964, Vol. XXV, No. 10.
4. Clemence, Sister Madeline, "Existentialism: A Philosophy of Commitment," *Amer J Nurs*, March, 1966.
5. Smith, Karl U., *Perception and Motion*, W.B. Saunders, 1962.
6. Ayres, A. Jean, "Occupational Therapy for Motor Disorders Resulting from Impairment of the Central Nervous System," *Rehab Lit*, October, 1960.
7. Colbert, James, "A Study Establishing the Disabled as a Minority Group," unpublished paper, UCLA.
8. Psalm VIII, verse 4, *The Bible*.
9. Roberts, David E., *Existentialism and Religious Belief*, Oxford University Press, 1960.
10. Richardson, Stephen A., "Some Unintended Consequences of Current Rehabilitation Practices," *Staff Reprint*, Association for the Aid of Crippled Children, 1959.
11. Buber, Martin, *I and Thou*, Charles Scribner's Sons, New York, 1958.
12. Barrett, William, *Irrational Man*, Doubleday Anchor Books, 1962.
13. Becker, Stephen, "On Being a Patient," *The Atlantic*, July, 1966.
14. Norton, M.D. Herter, *Translations from the Poetry of Rainer Maria Rilke*, The Norton Library, 1938.

Professional Responsibility in Times of Change

Wilma L. West, M

Abstract

Changing patterns in the organization and delivery of health services demand parallel changes in roles and responsibilities of occupational therapists. There is increasing need to identify with the field of health, thus broadening our traditional, more limited identification with medicine; to enlarge our concept from that of being a therapist to one of functioning as a health agent with responsibility to help insure normal growth and development; to think more about roles in prevention as well as in treatment and rehabilitation, about socioeconomic and cultural as well as biological causes of disease and dysfunction, and about serving health needs of people in many other settings than the hospital. We must recognize the responsibility of the profession to change with changing demands for its services, to adapt via new approaches, to assume different roles, to develop the preparation for them, and to recruit in a new mold rather than by recasting the prototype of an earlier time.

We are now convened for the final day of a conference in celebration of the 50th anniversary of our professional life. Behind us lie five decades of individual and group endeavor—endeavor to develop a profession, to define and refine a service, to improve an image and extend its acceptance, to recruit others to our ranks and train them

Reprinted from *The Americal Journal of Occupational Therapy*, Vol. XXII, No. 1, 1968.

for perpetuation of our ideals, to research new and better ways of accomplishing our goals.

At this milestone in our history, one could be tempted to look back through the years and analyze the functional relationship between endeavors and accomplishments. Such stock-taking would surely yield an inventory of assets in many areas of effort in which we might feel mutual pride. It would also, however, show liabilities for which we remain collectively responsible. Still other accounts might appear as outstanding or receivable, thus implying the necessity for continued effort in the commitment to further·progress. Depending on the perspective and purpose of the individual doing the analysis, this measure of our first fifty years might be impressive, discouraging or inconclusive with respect to net accomplishment.

Santayana has warned that "He who neglects history will be condemned to repeat it." However, awareness and understanding of effort input with reference to success or failure of outcome are most functional when new approaches are being brought to the solution of old problems. If, on the other hand, changing or new conditions prevail and hence a different set of problems is presented, there is diminishing value in more than brief review of the methods of other people and times. The example of the inadequacy of conventional defenses in a nuclear age is the obvious one, but professional personnel in medical and educational fields today face a dilemma equal to that of the military in recognizing that old ways of solving problems are no longer adequate.

Let us turn, then, from any comfortable reflection on our past to the infinitely more exciting exercise of projecting our future. Wisely approached, this can be as scientific as a retrospective analysis and surely it is a more dynamic course if we wish to have a part in determining our future rather than merely accepting one on assignment or default of others.

One cannot be in the practice of any of the health professions today without being keenly aware of the many forces shaping his future roles and responsibilities. Nor can he neglect his duty to examine the implications of these forces in three dimensions: for himself as a professional person, for the profession of which he is a member, and for the professional organization which represents and promotes his individual and group interests. In brief, the questions currently confronting us are: What is happening in both our immediate and larger worlds? and, What does this mean to us?

The general stage for this discussion may be set by an analogy from another field that is strikingly similar to that of medicine. Francis Keppel, former commissioner of the Office of Education, Department of Health, Education, and Welfare, says that America is entering a third revolution in education. In the first revolution, education of the masses was achieved by the establishment of the public school system. Later, equality of education for all people became the rallying cry for school reform. Now the astounding advances in technology demand specialized and high-quality education for all regardless of race, creed, or social class. (1)

Today this country is well into a similar multistaged reorganization of health and medical care in which equal availability and high quality of health services are sought for all people. The bipartisan endorsement of providing services to meet two of man's most fundamental needs—for education and health care—has removed the question from the arena of welfare and politics and placed it in the larger domain of basic human development.

Whether one agrees with these trends wholly, partially, reluctantly, or not at all, one fact is virtually undeniable today: comprehensive health care, among others of man's needs, is beyond individual attainment for far too many people. If we accept this fact, we can accept the organization of increasingly costly and complex programs designed to reduce disease and disability among victims of economic disparity and to raise the health standards of our country as a whole.

"Governmental involvement (then) in the financing and organization of health services is here to stay and there is every indication that it will increase." (2) I submit, however, that governmental participation and individual responsibility are neither incompatible nor mutually exclusive. In fact, we must go even further in pursuit of a rationale that is in tune with both our changing times and a high standard of personal and professional integrity. I therefore tend to agree with another commentator on this subject who has said that "placing health in the category of the rights of man involves the transformation of a social desire into a moral imperative." (3) This imperative has been stated as follows by the New York Academy of

Medicine: "That *all people* should have . . . *equal opportunity* to obtain a *high quality* of *comprehensive health care.*"

It is difficult to see how anyone could mount an argument against the humanitarian elements of this high goal. In the sense that the primary orientation of the professions is to the community interest, there *must* be concern for all people on the basis of equal opportunity and with a standard of the highest possible quality that it is within our ability to provide. Implications of most of the key phrases in this all-encompassing objective are clear. However, the last dimension—comprehensive health care—bears elaboration because it is with reference to this focus that we will examine how our profession can best adapt its philosophy and practice to future requirements.

At our annual conference in Minneapolis last year, the theme was "Dimensions of Change." Many of us, I am sure, recall the message of several thoughtful speakers who helped us read signs among today's maze of medical plans and programs that are as complex and confusing as the newest multistory interchange of highways around our large cities. I hope we also recall the repeated emphasis on *health,* as well as illness, on *prevention* of disease and disability, in addition to seeking the cures not yet discovered, on *maintenance and promotion of well-being,* not just being satisfied that there is an "absence of infirmity," (4) on *continuity of care,* in lieu of only episodic attention to emergency conditions, and on *comprehensive health services* that must replace the diagnostic or categorical approach of conventional medicine.

The trends in these directions are unmistakable. They are also irreversible. To recognize them, however, is only the first step. We must also interpret their meaning for each of our specialty areas and aggressively adapt or redesign our roles to provide a more viable future service.

No one person can or should do this for all facets of his profession. Each must, however, do it for his own focus of interest and with all the professional outlook and insight he can muster. I can best relate these changing trends and their implications to the field of pediatrics, with which I have been most closely involved in recent years. I shall attempt to do so in the general framework of comprehensive health care for children and, more specifically, with reference to selected groups which present us with some very challenging opportunities to develop a preventive role for our profession. I shall conclude with some thoughts on the implications of these and other changes for the profession as a whole.

Comprehensive Health Care for Children

What is meant by comprehensive health care for children? This is a term that is variously defined, but on the conceptual level, I prefer the following statement to all others that I have read: "By comprehensive, we mean a constellation of health services that focuses on the patient as an individual human being rather than as a collection of assorted organ systems, some of which are diseased." (5) On the practical level, we believe this ideal must be translated into programs which include health supervision in the various parameters of growth and development and the regular use of specific devices for screening deficits and dysfunctions. Comprehensive health care for children, we feel, is committed to enhancing normal development as insurance against disease or, failing that objective, to the earliest possible casefinding of those conditions which have their origin in prenatal causes or in the disabling illnesses of infancy and the preschool years.

Both the number and scope of programs designed to provide health care for children are greater today than ever before. The idea behind them, however, is hardly a new one. For it was in 1890 in France that the first nursing conferences and milk stations were established to provide preventive health services for lower socio-economic segments of the child population. At that time the motive was to reduce the enormously high infant and preschool child mortality, but from these early beginnings, clinic services of similar types have developed throughout the world. In the United States, the milk stations of the World War I era subsequently became known as well-baby clinics and today, in many areas, are called child health conferences.

It is interesting to trace the broadening philosophy of these forerunners of modern comprehensive health care for children. Since such enterprises were designed to provide health supervision of well children, one of their primary functions was to screen children for evidence of abnormality or illness that might warrant referral for care.

A classic text on preventive medicine and public health (6) tells us that the child health conference was originally necessary because a large segment of the population was unable to pay for health supervision. However, it also goes on to point out that even today such services cannot be transferred to the private practitioner. The reason, the authors state, is that education and training of medical students is still largely oriented to the patient with cellular pathology, with the result that many practitioners today have limited interest in and knowledge of the principles and techniques of health supervision of growing children. Furthermore, child health personnel even in recent years have been largely preoccupied with the development of treatment and training programs for handicapped children.

And so, it seems, have occupational therapists in pediatrics. Thus we, too, have been slow to develop a role in prevention that might greatly enhance our total professional contribution to health care. Although our traditional commitment to medicine and our orientation to illness and treatment are understandable, our greater development of a preventive role, which is "an integral part of all medical practice, wherever it may be and under whatever auspices" (7) is long overdue.

There is even a sense of urgency to the situation that cannot be escaped. Consider for example the number and diversity of settings in which new health care programs for children are constantly being developed. The well-child clinics or child health conferences that have already been mentioned are standard services of state and local health departments, but they are only one of several locales where continuing health supervision of children is assuming ever greater importance.

Probably the best known among others that I will discuss here are the Head Start programs that have received extensive publicity in the brief two years since their inception. Although the initial focus of these efforts was on enrichment of experience in preparation for school, a spin-off benefit of major importance has been identification and treatment of health deficits. It is of significance to us that the range of these deficits goes far beyond the dental and nutritional problems inevitable in the target populations and includes a high incidence of retarded or deviant physical and psychosocial development. As we well know, the chances for remediation of many such problems are infinitely better at age three or four than at beginning school age which, until now, has provided our earliest large-scale screening opportunity.

Another very new program of the Office of Economic Opportunity which was launched late this past summer could provide an even richer locus for occupational therapy in a preventive role. This is the development of Parent and Child Centers that is currently taking place in thirty-six American communities to provide services for disadvantaged families who have preschool children. A prime objective of these centers will be the use of techniques and processes both to prevent deviations and deficits and to stimulate development to the maximum potential. Among the skills and experience sought for staff are the ability to recognize and understand the developmental stages of young children and prescribe a plan for progress to meet each child's individual needs. (8)

To pediatric occupational therapists who have been concerned with the larger objective of optimal child growth and development as well as with restoration of impaired function, the possibilities inherent in these new centers must indeed be exciting. Think, for example, of the broad range of activities that could be used to provide multisensory input directed to the development of intellectual, emotional, social and physical skills. The graded and guided use of activities for such purposes is so integral a part of occupational therapy that this would seem to be a most fitting application of our skills to plan, elicit, interpret and modify both performance and behavior.

There are other groups of children for whom health surveillance could provide either prevention or earlier treatment. Sparked by the increasing prevalence of daytime employment of both parents or the absence of one parent and employment of the other, day care facilities have become a way of life for thousands of young American children. The larger of these, the day care centers, are units with seven to seventy-five or more children, a staff of one or more persons, and an organized program. In these settings today, ages of children usually range upwards from two and a half years, this being the minimum age for most children to participate in group play or other organized activities. What an opportunity there is here to prevent, restrict or retard development of problems we now see only when they are entrenched and disabling, often to a severe degree.

A final example is a group of children which has received special attention during the past year and is already providing the occupational therapist with a role in screening, evaluation and programming as well as in treatment. This is the group served by the Children and Youth projects sponsored by the Children's Bureau.

Organized in areas of economic and social disruption, these projects are designed to provide comprehensive health care for large numbers of children who, under existing circumstances, have only marginal opportunity to develop a healthy mind and body. Now, however, a broad range of health professionals is being assembled to provide services which should greatly improve their future outlook.

Included in the authorized core staff for children and youth projects is an occupational therapist whose job description reads quite differently from the specifications for other pediatric roles. If a few of these promising new positions can be filled by therapists with vision as well as skill, there are few limits on the extent to which they will be permitted to develop a broader role. For example: in New York City, two pediatric neurologists on a children and youth project added an occupational therapist to assist them in screening for neurological deficits; in Dallas and in Denver, pediatricians directing diagnostics clinics use their therapists to evaluate motor performance and behavior adjustment and to participate in programming based on team findings and recommendations; and in several other areas of the country, therapists are involving children in activities which permit assessment in numerous areas of function and providing selected experiences to promote development of neuromuscular, emotional and intellectual competencies of children.

These, then, are some of the programs made possible by the federal-state alliance to extend and improve health services for increasing numbers of people. They require of all professions a careful appraisal of changes that may be necessary as we jointly seek creative and workable solutions to both old and new problems. Although we have centered attention on one specialty of our profession, it is intriguing to think about how the number and kinds of changes in pediatrics today will inevitably, in time, affect every other age group and specialty field of occupational therapy.

Furthermore, there are equally radical changes occurring simultaneously in patterns of delivering health and medical services to all people. Witness, for example, the burgeoning community mental health programs and consider the implications of trends in that specialty of our profession. Are there not elements here, paralleling the new kinds of community-based services in pediatrics, which are dictating programs concerned with the maintenance and promotion of health as well as the treatment of illness? And hence, are there not here, too, strong indications for increased emphasis on the preventive role of occupational therapy?

Of course there are, and many progressive occupational therapists in both these and other specialties of our profession have already taken steps to keep pace with trends that require new or expanded roles. Furthermore, they have done so with such effectiveness that they have created roles and functions that greatly improve the image of our profession. In a sense, therefore, my commentary only reflects what I consider to be the best abroad in practice today, with a few thoughts on where, how and why it seems particularly urgent that we intensify our efforts in these directions and at this time.

I fear, however, that there are yet too many among us who do not sufficiently appreciate current trends and who therefore are not lending their efforts to hasten and make credible more functional roles throughout the profession. The platform at a general session of our Annual Conference and assured publication in our professional journal lend temptation to speak frankly to one's colleagues. And, the occasion of a golden anniversary provides a good point at which to cross the treacherous terrain of prophecy and hazard a glimpse of where our best future directions may lie. He who does so will always run the chance of suggesting some wrong turns, but he who does not has missed both an opportunity and a responsibility to share with others his views on areas of mutual concern.

We Are Committed to Our Profession as a Whole

I would like, now, to discuss some ramifications of these thoughts in terms of the profession as a whole rather than in the framework of any one or more specialty areas of practice. For, regardless of our individual concerns with separate fields, it is to the whole profession that we are jointly committed and for which we must cooperatively work. My remaining remarks will explore some of the reasons why it seems important that this be so.

What is the relevance to us as a professional group of the changes I have discussed, of other changes that are taking place in patterns of providing health services, and of the implications these have for traditional and transitional roles in our profession? Is it enough that there is a growing number of clinicians in each of our specialty fields who are continually sharpening conventional skills and also developing new ones? Can we rely on the work of a small but increasing number of researchers among us to confirm the scientific basis of our practice? Does the greater sophistication of today's authors sufficiently raise the level of our professional literature? Will the growing number of our members who are obtaining graduate degrees insure a higher quality of performance in the future? Are changes that are being effected by the more progressive among our educators adequate to the preparation of tomorrow's therapists? In short, will the leadership of these and other significantly contributing individuals suffice? Indeed, should it have to?

Decidedly not. What is absent from this kind of thinking is the concept of group responsibility—responsibility for awareness and interpretation of those changes which affect any part of our profession, and responsibility for whatever group action is appropriate to facilitate or hasten adjustment to change. Thus, although we clearly recognize that "All occupations are dependent on the individual contributions" of those who practice them, we must also realize that "the effectiveness of an occupation is not gauged by individual efforts alone; the total efforts of occupational members working together with some degree of cooperation must also be considered. The public image of an occupation, then, is in part individual and in part collective. . . . Moreover, the goals of an occupation are only in a limited sense individual, for the individual responsibility of practitioners and a consciousness of the aims of the occupation are very much a function of collective action." (9)

There are, of course, many terms for the kind of collective action here referred to. Among them is what I shall call professional consciousness and responsibility. This is an attribute that we in occupational therapy have to a quite considerable degree. It has served us well in the fifty years of our professional development to date, primarily, I believe, because we have used it more in the sense of professional responsiveness to public interest and need than for purposes of protecting or promoting our constituent individuals and groups. These two major purposes of a profession—meeting external obligations to society on the one hand, and internal loyalties to members on the other—may often be in conflict. That they have not created serious problems or dichotomies for us up to this time may be viewed as a mixed blessing, for readings in the sociology of development of the professions make it clear that it is only a matter of time until they do. Factors which may have delayed this apparently inevitable process include our extremely small size and the relative homogeneity of a profession with only incompletely developed specialties.

Trend Toward Decreased Professional Unity

With the passage of time, however, we are experiencing both an increase in size and a proliferation of special skills among our members. As these two dimensions grow, we become increasingly subject to the influence of factors which will tend to decrease professional unity and promote segmentation in accordance with divergent interests and strengths as they develop among us. Although it will undoubtedly create some problems, this trend is by no means undesirable. On the contrary, it usually brings with it both an improved service, which results from increased knowledge and skill of specialists, and a growing professional influence which can be used to improve the status of those who provide that service.

There are signs that the era of segmentation is already upon us; witness for example, the increasing number of special interest meetings and concurrent sessions scheduled at this year's Annual Conference. While neither deploring the problems nor lauding the advantages an increase in this trend will bring, I hope that we will retain an attitude of general professional consciousness and concern for as long as we exist. Conviction of the need for this lies in the belief that "the chief factor . . . . in the accomplishments of any profession is the unified, aggressive efforts of its members." (10)

Numerous theories have been put forth to explain why persons pursuing an occupation come together and associate in a formal manner. These include everything from the likely initial motivation for exchange with those doing the same work, to such presently accepted objectives as raising standards of competence, formulating codes of ethics, improving education, undertaking protective and promotional activities, and many others. The activities of associations as major interest groups which participate in planning and policy decisions on matters of concern to them are generally thought of as a development of recent years undertaken to counter the influence of governmental regulations on professional activities; in fact, however, these date back at least three centuries when, as one writer says, "it was characteristic of the times that powers and duties of so extensive a nature were granted to vocational associations that they may be regarded as organs of the state." (11) Thus they are illustrative of the influence a well-organized profession can have on public decisions and policies.

I make no case for our professional association to aspire to this degree of power. I do, however, believe that both as individuals and as a professional group we should be assuming a far more frequent and contributing part in the planning of health services. It will, in fact, be mandatory that we do so if, as I said earlier, we are to have a part in shaping our own development.

Izutsu believes that "it is not too late to achieve positions of leadership that will determine the future" of our profession. (12) However, he also lists several steps that we must take if we are to remain equal to changing patterns in the organization and delivery of health services. Among these are the development of leaders not only to plan for therapy but to think in the broad spectrum of social planning; training of therapists in public health principles and procedures; and exposure, in our training, to community-oriented settings and other health team members in lieu of training primarily in hospital settings.

Professionally, We Often Resist Change

I do not suppose any of us knows, with any degree of certainty, the ideal future course for our profession. We do, however, see many signs that it must keep changing if it is to stay abreast of the larger world of which it is a part. Change is seldom easy or comfortable. Yet there is little about the world in which we live today that is more characteristic of it than the continual and fast-moving changes which transcend every aspect of our lives.

Although each of us makes the necessary adaptation to these changes as they affect our personal concerns and activities, we are slower as a group to adjust our professional directions and developments to that which is new. We are often, in fact, resistant to the suggested need for change and all that it implies in the necessity for new learning and the establishment of new roles and functions. We are also reluctant to explore new potentials, to experiment, to take an occasional risk.

From Therapist to Health Agent

Increasingly, today, I believe we should identify with the field of health services, thus broadening our traditional, more limited identification with medicine. We should enlarge our concept from that of being a therapist to one of functioning as a health agent with responsibility to help insure normal growth and development. We should think more about roles in prevention as well as in treatment and rehabilitation, about socioeconomic and cultural as well as biological causes of disease and dysfunction, and about serving health needs of people in many other settings than the hospital.

One occasion on which this was expressed in a very effective way by a number of our colleagues was the conference on research in occupational and physical therapy held last February in Puerto Rico. In one of the discussion groups there was studied avoidance of the term "patient," which many felt limited their concern to illness, and a plea for consideration of health as only one aspect of the developmental process of man which should not be isolated from other factors impinging on life. This kind of thinking and discussion culminated in the group's consideration of its topic in the framework of what they called "the continuum of health services which reflect the needs of man in his environment." (13)

A broad frame of reference? Admittedly, but it is also entirely in keeping with our traditional philosophy of concern for the person rather than just his disability. For us, therefore, the idea possesses what might be called "instant validity." It now needs rapid if not instant implementation.

We are living today in a world that is vastly different from that when occupational therapy began. It matters not so much that it has taken fifty years to reach this day, as that the next fifty see more, and more rapid, progress than the last. It matters less that we are still struggling to define our profession than that we build a broader base for the better definition that will one day be written. It matters most of all that we recognize the responsibility of the profession to change with changing demands for its services, to adapt via new approaches, to assume different roles, to develop the preparation for them and to recruit in a new mold rather than by recasting the prototype of an earlier time.

On the eve of her retirement from active work in our national organization, Eleanor Clarke Slagle was paid the following tribute:

> Those of us who have been privileged to follow the winding trail of those years know of struggles, of courage in facing criticism, of disappointments and rewards, of patient waiting, persistent faith and devoted work. The questing youth of our profession accepts both with commendation and condemnation what has been so painstakingly accomplished through this quarter century. But when they too can look back over an equal span of service in this field, they, and occupational therapy, will still be moving to the measure of the thought of Eleanor Clarke Slagle. (14)

That "equal span of service" has now passed so we, too, are looking back over the second quarter of a century which immediately precedes the present day. It seemed fitting that we do so in the context of both our practice to which she gave so much, and our professional association which she helped to organize, served as an officer in four capacities, and directed as its executive for many years. I, for one, hold to much that she obviously held high among her goals for the profession. Among those goals, I feel sure, was one related to the need for professional responsibility at all times. In times of change such as these, that need and our response to it will be of great importance in determining the next fifty years of our professional life. At the turn of the 21st century, when yet another generation looks back on these times, may they see that ours was a dynamic posture of professional consciousness and responsibility.

REFERENCES

1. Keppel, Francis, *The Necessary Revolution in American Education.* New York: Harper and Row (1966).
2. Burns, Evalina, "Policy Decisions Facing the United States in Financing and Organizing Health Care," *Public Health Reports,* 81, No. 8 (August 1966).
3. Dearing, W.P., "Prepaid Group Practice Medical Care Plans," *Public Health Reports,* 77, No. 10 (October 1962).
4. Preamble to the Constitution of the World Health Organization.

5. Kissick, William L., "Trends in the Utilization of Rehabilitation Manpower," *Manpower Utilization in Rehabilitation in New York City*, New York: New York City Regional Interdepartmental Rehabilitation Committee (September 1966).

6. Sartwell, P.E., Ed., *Maxcy-Rosenau Preventive Medicine and Public Health*, 9th ed. New York: Meredith Publishing Co. (1965).

7. Freeman, Ruth B., "Impact of Public Health on Society," *Public Health Reports, 76*, No. 4 (April 1961).

8. *Criteria for Parent and Child Centers*, Washington, D.C.: Office of Economic Opportunity (July 19, 1967).

9. Vollmer, Howard M. and Mills, Donald L., *Professionalization*, Englewood Cliffs, New Jersey: Prentice-Hall, Inc. (1966).

10. Stinnett, T.M., "Accomplishments of the Organized Teaching Profession," *The Teacher and Professional Organizations*, Washington, D.C.: The National Education Association (1956).

11. Carr-Saunders, A.M. and Wilson, P.A., "The Rise and Aims of Professional Associations," *The Professions*, Oxford: The Clarendon Press (1933).

12. Izutsu, Satoru, "The Changing Patterns of Patient Care" (A Position Paper) *Research Conference in Occupational Therapy and Physical Therapy*, New York: American Physical Therapy Association (1967).

13. Group Report, "Research in Patient Care," *Proceedings of the Research Conference in Occupational Therapy and Physical Therapy*, New York: American Physical Therapy Association (To be published).

14. "In the Past, Pride—In the Future, Faith," A Documentary of the Heritage, Growth and Outlook of the American Occupational Therapy Association. Produced by the Association for its Forty-First Annual Conference, New York, New York (October 21, 1958).

Facilitating Growth and Development: The Promise of Occupational Therapy

Lela A. Llorens

A theory of occupational therapy based on a human development rationale is presented. Occupational therapy is discussed as it relates to the enhancement of neurophysiological, physical, psychosocial and psychodynamic growth as well as social language, daily living skills and sociocultural development as the human organism strives to achieve expected developmental tasks and ego adaptive behavior. The role and skills of the occupational therapist with particular attention to the function of occupational therapy within the conceptual framework of horizontal and longitudinal development are described.

Preamble

To be the recipient of the Eleanor Clarke Slagle Lectureship is indeed an awesome honor. Preparing for this moment has been an arduous task. Many of my colleagues and friends have checked periodically on my progress during the year and the answer most often given was, "We're living with it." We, including my family, have literally lived with the "Lecture" this year and the breakthrough that I was struggling for did not come until late summer during our trip to West Africa. When it did, it came in the form of ten premises which express a developmental theory of occupational therapy.

Reprinted from *The American Journal of Occupational Therapy,* Vol. XXIV, No. 1, 1970.

The theory which I am presenting has been an outgrowth of my experience and research in the field of psychiatry, both pediatric and adult, and more recently in pediatric general medicine and community health. In order to do justice to the formulation, however, I have spent considerable time in consultation with my colleagues in physical medicine and rehabilitation and with their patients. These experiences as well as the fortunate opportunities I have had to participate in a number of seminars and workshops over the past several years have stimulated my desire to think through the function and purpose of occupational therapy as I have experienced it.

Introduction

In this paper, a conceptual model for understanding the knowledge that presently supports the practice of occupational therapy is presented with a discussion of how and where occupational therapy fits into the scheme of human development.

My thesis is simply this: that occupational therapy is a facilitation process which assists the individual in achieving mastery of life tasks and the ability to cope as efficiently as possible with the life expectations made of him through the mechanisms of selected input stimuli, and availability of practice in a suitable environment. The occupational therapist serves as the enculturation agent for the conditions of physical, social and psychological health in which the developmental level being experienced by the individual in any one of a number of parameters of development is unequal to the age-related demands made of that organism as a result of natural or traumatic incident.

Developmental Theory of Occupational Therapy

The theory is based on these premises:

1. That the human organism develops horizontally in the areas of neurophysiological, physical, psychosocial and psychodynamic growth and in the development of social language, daily living and sociocultural skills at specific periods of time;
2. That the human organism develops longitudinally in each of these areas in a continuous process as he ages;

3. That mastery of particular skills, abilities and relationships in each of the areas of neurophysiological, physical, psychosocial and psychodynamic development, social language, daily living and sociocultural skills, both horizontally and longitudinally is necessary to the successful achievement of satisfactory coping behavior and adaptive relationships;

4. That such mastery is usually achieved naturally in the course of development;

5. That the fundamental endowment of the individual and the stimulation of experiences received within the environment of the family come together to interact in such a way as to promote positive early growth and development in both the horizontal and longitudinal planes;

6. That later the influences of extended family, community, social and civic groups assist in the growth process;

7. That physical or psychological trauma related to disease, injury, environmental insufficiencies or intrapersonal vulnerability can interrupt the growth and development process;

8. That such growth interruption will cause a gap in the developmental cycle resulting in a disparity between expected coping behavior and adaptive facility and the necessary skills and abilities to achieve same;

9. That occupational therapy through the skilled application of activities and relationships can provide growth and development links to assist in closing the gap between expectation and ability by increasing skills, abilities and relationships in the neurophysiological, physical, psychosocial, psychodynamic, social language, daily living and sociocultural spheres of development as indicated both horizontally and longitudinally;

10. That occupational therapy through the skilled application of activities and relationships can provide growth experiences to prevent the development of potential maladaptation related to insufficient nurturance in neurophysiological, physical, psychosocial, psychodynamic, social language, daily living and sociocultural spheres of development both horizontally and longitudinally.

This in my opinion is the promise of occupational therapy. In order to pursue this theory further, let us look at the various areas of knowledge which support the continuum of human development including behavior and ability expectation.

Current Knowledge of Human Development

The life span of the individual encompasses several phases of physical growth, neurophysiological, psychological, social and emotional development as well as a gradual decline in many of these life processes, particularly physical development, as the individual ages requiring continued growth in the adaptive abilities of the organism. Ayres has contributed greatly to our knowledge of neurophysiological development from infancy to adolescence. (1) Gesell has contributed specifically to our knowledge of the physical development of children through this same age span, as well as to our knowledge of the development of social language, sociocultural and daily living skills in this age group. (2) At the present time, however, such specific details of the physical development of adults is not easily available for either the young or the aging. Erikson has given us in his 'Eight Ages of Man' some insight into the psychosocial development of the individual in terms of his behavior both at the time of initial emotional experience and at the time of reexperience of early development in adult life. (3) He spans the life cycle from infancy to old age and emphasizes the continual growth conflicts which are inherent in living. He cautions against believing that any level of developmental achievement, once achieved, becomes a permanent part of the psychological makeup of the individual as the individual is a dynamic, changing, developing organism. Freud has provided us with an understanding of child development as it relates to personality in its organization and dynamics. (4,5)

In the process of development the human organism expects and is expected to achieve specific adaptive behaviors which equip him to cope with life. These specific behaviors assist him in the larger task of getting on in the world. In his *Developmental Tasks and Education*, Havighurst presents us with a concept of developmental tasks as being midway between an individual need and a societal demand. (6) Meeting societal demands requires adaptive skills and mastery of self and the environment. The adaptive skills correlative to this formulation have been developed from the work of Pearce and Newton and the work of Mosey. Pearce and Newton give us some insight into how residuals of early patterns of development become a part of the personality structure as an adult as well as how early patterns of development contribute to adaptation, the ability for and style of coping with life demands. (7) Mosey has defined for us specific adaptive skills required by the individual to adjust to his internal needs as well as to the external demands. (8) These are the areas that constitute horizontal and longitudinal development.

At any point in time, the human organism experiences simultaneous growth (horizontally) in the areas of physical, neurophysiological, psychosocial, psychodynamic, sociocultural development, and in the skills of daily life and social language. As he matures, he experiences longitudinal growth in each of these areas. In order for the individual to achieve in the adaptive areas of functioning it is necessary for him to experience satisfaction and mastery both horizontally and longitudinally in the developmental spectrum.

For emotional growth to proceed in a natural and spontaneous way, it must be nurtured with affection, understanding, security and discipline, and be stimulated by achievement and social acceptance. It is necessary, too, that children gain satisfaction in their relationships with others so that they may develop the feeling that they are lovable, that their individuality is respected and that they can have confidence in their own strength and capability as a person. As the child develops he explores his environment, establishes relationships and acquires knowledge and skills which enable him to successfully adapt to his world. (9)

In adolescence the activities of the period expand into social, intellectual, literary and artistic interests. Intense relationships as with a chum are particularly important to this period. Physical changes occur which must be incorporated into the self-image. It is necessary for the adolescent to have the support and understanding of his family as he reaches for adulthood.

"The primary conditions for growth for the adult are crucially different from the conditions of growth of the developmental eras of pre-adulthood. These differences relate to the adults' responsibility to initiate and consolidate experience, and also to the new significance of sharing." (10)

Middle age requires reorganization of several factors of one's life. Emotional responsibilities of parents become less demanding as children leave home and ongoing financial responsibility becomes finite and predictable. Physical and physiological changes occur which must figure in the adaptation of the individual.

Not enough information has been documented concerning physical growth and development in old age. Cultural cliches hold that growth does not take place in the aging years, that the quality of life in those years tends to be strongly determined by the nature of the outcome of the middle-aged crises.

Each stage of development in this longitudinal process is dependent upon the successful resolution of the developmental "crises" related to each growth stage. Physical or psychological trauma experienced in any one of the horizontal parameters at any particular time in the longitudinal process can interrupt the developmental cycle.

Facilitating growth and development during and following traumatic experiences is the task of occupational therapy. Understanding the needs of the individual as they relate to the determination of function and dysfunction and the choice of activities and relationships to ameliorate or modify dysfunction, to enhance remaining function and to facilitate continued growth consistent with the individual's developmental stage are the tasks of the occupational therapist.

There are sensorimotor activities, developmental play activities, symbolic activities and interpersonal relationships which are specifically significant to particular age ranges in the longitudinal process. There may be specific reason to emphasize one or another of this range of activities as well as relationships at any one given point in time depending on the horizontal area of development most affected by trauma. I wish to stress that although emphasis may be placed on the facilitation of growth in one particular parameter, simultaneous though perhaps less attention must be given to all of the other areas of growth as well in order for an integrating growth experience to take place.

Developmental Theory Illustrated

In an effort to illustrate this concept in graphic form Sections I and III of Figure 1 have been developed to show the areas of developmental growth as described by Ayres, Gesell, Erikson and Freud and the areas of expectation and adaptation as described by Havighurst, Mosey, Pearce and Newton. In order to demonstrate relevance to age, age ranges have been imposed. Caution must be observed in interpreting the age ranges as they are suggestive rather than absolute. The imposition of age ranges is particularly useful in correlating development horizontally as well as longitudinally but has its limitations in application which must be considered.

Section II of Figure 1 illustrates the tools of occupational therapy which are utilized in the process of facilitating growth and development. The age ranges are suggested by position also in a correlative fashion.

Let us look at the implications of Section I. During the first two years of life the human organism is developing sensory perception of the tactile, vestibular, visual, auditory, olfactory and gustatory functions; physical-motor behavior and body integration; is developing a balanced sense between "trust and mistrust" through these same functional areas which manifests itself in ease of feeding, depth of sleep and relaxation in elimination and is nurtured by consistency, continuity and sameness. At the same time that these areas are developing, the oral "stage" related to dynamic development as seen in dependency, initial aggression and oral erotic activity is evident. Sociocultural development at this age is centered first around the individual mothering relationship and later extends to the immediate family group. Social language is beginning first with small sounds, then coos, vocalization, listening, speaking words and responding to simple verbal directions. Activities of daily living, including early recognition of the source of food, beginning to hold feeding objects and, later, controlling elimination, are developing.

We see that there is overlap in these stages, that development does not occur in neat segments. As the infant learns to motor plan which encompasses the first four years of life beginning with the discovery of the hands and feet, he progresses to all fours then to walking, climbing, balancing, developing hand preference and coordination of eyes and hands and eyes and feet. The development of the body scheme, knowledge of body parts, development of a sense of two integrated sides with a front and back can be seen. During this period a balance between "autonomy and shame and doubt" are being developed and manifested in conflictual behavior between emotionally "holding on" and "letting go." The anal "stage" is evident in independent, resistive, self-assertive, narcissistic and ambiv-

SECTION I
DEVELOPMENTAL EXPECTATIONS, BEHAVIORS & NEEDS
(Selected for illustrative purposes)

NEUROPHYSIOLOGICAL-SENSORIMOTOR Ayres	PHYSICAL-MOTOR Gesell	PSYCHOSOCIAL Erikson	PSYCHODYNAMIC Grant/Freud	SOCIO-CULTURAL Gesell	
0-2 Sensorimotor Tactile functions Vestib. functions Visual, Auditory, Olfactory, Gustatory	0-2 Head sags Fisting Gross motion Walking Climbing	Basic Trust vs. Mistrust/Oral Sensory Ease of feeding Depth of sleep Relax. of bowels	1-4 Oral Dependency Init. aggres. Oral erotic activity	Individual mothering person most important Immediate family group important	
1-4 Integration of Body Sides Gross motor plan. Form & space perc. Equil. resp. Post. flex. Body sch. dev.	2-3 Runs Balances Hand pref. established Coordination	Autonomy vs. Shame & Doubt/ Muscular-Anal Conflict between holding on & letting go	1-4 Anal Independence Resistiveness Self-assertive- ness Narcissism Ambivalence	Parallel play Often alone Recognizes extended family	
3-7 Discrimination Refined tactile Kinesth., Visual, Auditory, Olfact., Gustatory funct.	3-6 Coordination more graceful Muscles devel. Skills develop	Initiative vs. Guilt/Locomotor- Genital Aggressiveness Manipulation Coercion	3-6 Genital-Oedipal Genital interest Poss. of opp. parent Antag. to same parent Castration fears	Seeks compan- ionship Makes decisions Plays with other children Takes turns	
3- Abstract Thinking Conceptualization Complex relat. Read, write, numbers	6-11 Energy develop- ment Skill practice to attain proficiency	Industry vs. In- feriority/Latency Wins recognition thru productivity Learns skills & tools	6-11 Latency Prim. struggles quiescent Init. in mastery of skills Strong defenses	Group play & team activities Independence of adults Gang interests	
	11-13 Rapid growth Poor posture Awkwardness	Identity vs. Role Confusion/Puberty & Adolescence Identification Social roles	11- Adolescence Emancip. from parents Occup. decisions Role experiment Re-exam. values	Team games Org. important Interest in opposite sex	
		Intimacy vs. Isolation/Young Adulthood Commitments Body & Ego mastery			
		Generativity vs. Stagnation/ Adulthood Guiding next generation Creat., pro- ductive			
		Ego Integrity vs. Despair/Maturity Acceptance of own life cycle			

Figure 1. Schematic representation of facilitating growth and development.

		SECTION II FACILITATING ACTIVITIES & RELATIONSHIPS (Selected)				SECTION III BEHAVIOR EXPECTATIONS & ADAPTIVE SKILLS	
SOCIAL-LANGUAGE Gesell	ACTIVITY OF DAILY LIVING Gesell	SENSORI-MOTOR ACT.	DEV. PLAY ACT.	SYMBOLIC ACT.	INTER-PERS. RELAT.	DEVELOPMENTAL TASKS Havighurst	EGO-ADAPTIVE SKILLS Mosey, Pearce & Newton
Small sounds Coos Vocalizes Listens Speaks	Recognizes bottle Holds spoon Holds glass Controls bowel	Tact. stim. Ident. body parts Sounds Objects	Dolls Animals Sand Water Excursions	Biting Chewing Eating Blowing Cuddling	Individual Interaction	Learning to Walk Talk Take solids Elimination	Ability to respond to mothering Mastering of gross motor responses
Identifies objects verb. Asks "why?" Short sentences	Feeds self Helps undress Recog. simple tunes No longer wets at night	Phys. exer. Balancing Motor planning	Pull toys Play grnd. Clay Crayons Chalk	Throwing Dropping Messing Collecting Destroying	Individual Interaction Parallel play	Sex difference To form concepts of soc. & phys. reality To relate emotionally to others Right Wrong	Ability to respond to routines of daily living Mastery of 3 dimen. space Sense of body image
Comb. talking and eating Complete sent. Imaginative Dramatic	Laces shoes Cuts with scissors Toilets indep. Helps set table	Listening Learning Skilled tasks & games	Being read to Coloring Drawing Painting	Destroying Exhibiting	Individual Interaction Play small groups	To devel. a conscience	Ability to Follow directions Tol. frustrations Sit still Del. gratification
	Enjoys dressing up Learns value of money Responsible for grooming	Reading Writing Numbers	Scooters Wagons Collections Puppets Bldg.	Controling Mastery	Individual Interaction Groups Teams Clubs	Learn phys. skills Getting along Reading, writing Values Soc. attitudes	Ability to perceive, sort, org. & utilize stimuli Work in groups Mas. of inanimate obj.
	Interest in earning money		Weaving Machinery tasks Carving Modeling		Individual Interaction Groups Teams	More mature rel. Social roles Sel. occupation Achieving emot. independence	Ability to accept & discharge resp. Capacity for love
						Selecting a mate Starting family Marriage, home Congenial social group	Ability to function indep. Control drives Plan & execute
			Arts Crafts Sports Club & interest groups Work		Individual Interaction Groups	Civic & social responsibility Econ. standard of living Dev. adult leisure act. Adj. to aging parents	Purposeful motion Obtain, org. & use knowledge Part. in primary group Part. in variety of relationships Exp. self as accept.
						Adj. to decr. phys. health, retire., death Age group affil. Meeting social obligations	Part. in mutually satis. heterosex. relations

The vertical letters between the ADL and Sensori-Motor columns spell: E V A L U A T I O N alent behavior. Magical thinking and anal preoccupation are also characteristic of this stage. Sociocultural development during this period centers around parallel relationships in play, isolated play and the importance of extended family. Social language is expanding into the verbal identification of objects, asking "why" and putting words together in short sentences. Feeding himself, helping to undress, recognizing simple tunes and controlling nighttime wetting become important activities of everyday life.

Between the ages of three and seven the sensory functions are refined, coordination becomes more graceful, muscles become stronger, skills are developed. At the same time a balance is being developed between "initiative and guilt" manifest in aggressiveness, manipulation and coercion.

The genito-oedipal stage is evident in the interest the child shows in his own genitals and those of the opposite sex, his possessiveness of the opposite sex parent, antagonism to the same sex parent and in castration fears or disappointment. Sociocultural development during this period centers around the companionship of others, learning to make decisions, learning to play successfully with other children, learning to play alone, taking turns and sharing. Social language development sees the child combining talking and eating, using complete sentences, expressing his imagination and creativity. His activities of daily living include shoe lacing, cutting with scissors, toileting independently and helping with chores such as setting the table and making his bed.

Beginning at about three years of age, becoming more refined around five and six and continuing on throughout life, the functions of abstract thinking, conceptualization, reasoning, the development of complex relationships and the ability to read, write, count and figure numbers develops. Physically around six the child becomes more energetic and proficient in the mastery of skills through practice. The balance between "industry and inferiority" is developing and is manifest in attempts to win recognition through productivity and learning skills and tools. The "latency" stage is evident as the primitive struggles quiet, the interest in mastery of skills becomes predominant, toleration of competitiveness, identification and acceptance of reality become important and strong defenses develop. Sociocultural development during this period centers on group play and team activities, developing independence of adults and interest in "gang" activities. Activities of daily living include joy in dressing up, learning the value of money and developing responsibility for personal grooming.

Physically, rapid growth takes place between eleven and thirteen accompanied by poor posture and awkwardness. During the adult years some physical growth, though less rapid, continues. Around eleven the balance between "identity and role confusion" is developing, manifest in identification with social roles. The "stage" of adolescence in dynamic terms is evident in the emancipation from parental control, the making of occupational decisions, role experimentation, difficulty with compromise, intensification of feelings and the reexamination of societal values. The sociocultural development of this period is centered around organized team activities and interest in the opposite sex. Activities of daily living include interest in earning money.

Adult development as described by Erikson places the struggle for balance between "intimacy and isolation" in young adulthood. This period is characterized by the capacity to commit oneself to concrete affiliations and partnerships and to abide by such commitments. Ego and body mastery must predominate. Adulthood is characterized by the struggle to maintain balance between "generativity and stagnation" which is manifest in behavior directed toward guiding the next generation, one's own creativity and productivity. Maturity is characterized by the balance between "ego integrity and despair" and manifest by the acceptance of one's own life cycle as "something that had to be."

These developmental expectations, behaviors and needs characterize the cycle of human development. Successful growth and mastery in all of these areas is the basis on which the developmental tasks of life are achieved as found in Section III of Figure 1. The developmental tasks as described by Havighurst and ascribed to the first six years of life include learning to walk, talk, take solids, control elimination, understand sex differences, form adequate concepts of social and physical reality, relate to others at an emotional level, distinguish right from wrong and develop a conscience.

The ego-adaptive skills developing simultaneously during this period are the abilities to respond to mothering, to respond to routines of daily living, to follow directions, tolerate reasonable amounts of frustration, sit still, delay gratification, share and take turns. As with longitudinal development, there are also overlaps in the horizontal plane. In this discussion the developmental tasks and adaptive behavior delineations serve to summarize the human growth continuum.

Beginning at about six years of age, learning physical skills, building wholesome attitudes towards oneself, getting along with others, learning appropriate masculine and feminine social roles, achieving personal independence, reading, writing, developing values and acceptable social attitudes are important developmental tasks. The correlative adaptive skills include the ability to accurately perceive, sort, organize and utilize stimuli and the ability to work cooperatively in groups and individually.

Adolescent developmental tasks include achieving more mature relationships with others, developing appropriate social roles, selecting an occupation, achieving emotional independence of adults while the adaptive skill most predominant is the ability to accept and discharge a certain amount of responsibility.

Young adulthood developmental tasks may include selection of a mate, starting a family, learning to manage a home and developing a congenial social group. The tasks of adulthood include the expansion into accepting responsibility for civic and social conditions, developing and maintaining an economic standard of living, developing adult leisure activities and adjusting to the reality of aging parents. The developmental tasks of maturity require adjustment to decreasing physical health, retirement and death; developing appropriate age group affiliations and meeting appropriate social obligations.

The adaptive skills correlative with this period from young adulthood through maturity are the abilities to function independently; control drives and select appropriate objects; plan and execute purposeful motion; obtain, organize and use knowledge; participate in a primary group; participate in a variety of relationships; experience self as acceptable; and participate in mutually satisfying heterosexual relationships.

In the course of human development, should the individual experience physical or psychological trauma related to disease, injury, environmental insufficiences or manifest intrapersonal vulnerability which interrupts the natural process, a gap thereby develops resulting in a disparity between expected coping behavior and adaptive facility as illustrated in Section III of Figure 1 and the necessary basic skills in growth and development as illustrated in Section I. Occupational therapy through the skilled application of activities and relationships can provide the necessary links to assist in closing the gap by facilitating basic growth and development, increasing skills, abilities and relationships in the neurophysiological, physical, psychosocial, psychodynamic, social language, daily living and sociocultural areas of development both horizontally and longitudinally.

Let us now look at Section II of Figure 1 which illustrates selected activities and relationships which are the tools of occupational therapy utilized in facilitating the growth process. Evaluation is the first step in the process of intervention, the process by which a determination is made relative to the need for as well as the primary objectives for occupational therapy intervention. Evaluation including testing, interviewing, record review, and systematic clinical observation should take into account the areas of basic growth and development represented in Section I and the expected behaviors and adaptive skills represented in Section III.

The activities and relationships available to the occupational therapist have been categorized as sensorimotor activities; developmental "play" activities, symbolic activities and interpersonal relationships and have been assigned an age relationship correlative to the basic developmental functions and adaptive behaviors by position. These positions, however, as with development, cannot be considered absolute.

During the first two years of life, activities which facilitate development of sensorimotor functions include touching; being touched, cuddled, hugged; moving, exploring, looking, hearing, tasting, smelling, identifying, sounds and objects. Developmental play media which incorporate these stimuli include blankets, dolls, animals, sand, water, books, blocks, food, and trips of various kinds. Symbolic activities of this age require biting, chewing, eating, blowing and cuddling. All of these "activities" must be practiced in an individual "mothering" relationship, the relationship of choice, to be maximally useful to the individual.

Beginning in the first year and extending through the third, the sensorimotor activities include physical exercise, balancing and motor planning; the developmental play materials include gross movement toys, pull toys, "play ground" type equipment, clay, crayons and chalk; symbolic activities of the period include throwing, dropping, messing, collecting, and destroying; and the interpersonal relationships of choice are individual interaction and parallel "play."

Between the three- and six-year span, the sensorimotor activities include listening, learning, practicing skilled tasks and games; the developmental play activities include being read to, coloring, drawing and painting; symbolic activities include destroying and exhibiting; and the interpersonal relationships of choice are individual interaction and parallel "play" in small groups. During the six- to eleven-year span, sensorimotor activities include the high level cognitive tasks of reading, writing and numbers; developmental play activities include scooters, wagons, collections, puppets, and building tasks; symbolic activities of the age are characterized by control and mastery and the interpersonal relationships of choice include individual interaction, groups, teams and clubs. Adolescent developmental "play" activities include weaving and other home crafts, machinery tasks, carving and modeling and the interpersonal relationships of choice are individual interaction, group and team relationships.

Practice and continued development of competence in sensorimotor functions is assumed to take place until the organism begins to decline in neurophysiological function, the exact time of which will vary from individual to individual. The activities engaged in leisure as well as in work from adulthood through maturity facilitate this continued development. Affective growth continues with the availability and responsiveness of the individual to interpersonal relationships as well as his ability to receive gratification through symbolic processes which continue to reactivate as the organism grows and develops.

Implications for Practice

This theory states that physical or psychological trauma related to disease, injury, environmental insufficiencies or intrapersonal vulnerability can interrupt the natural process of growth and development and that such growth interruption will cause a gap in the developmental cycle resulting in a disparity between the development of expected coping behavior and adaptive skills and the necessary basic skills and abilities to achieve such growth. It implies that the incongruence in developmental functioning evident in illness and disability is similar to conditions experienced by the individual at an earlier level of developmental functioning which requires relearning of skills, working through of emotional conflicts and redevelopment of many functions which may have been previously mastered. Further than that it is the task of the occupational therapist to determine at what level the individual is functioning in the various aspects along the developmental continuum and to program for facilitating growth and development in each of these areas in accordance with the needs of the individual and the demands of his age. The use of selected relevant activities and relationships appropriate to his level of functioning would be indicated.

In order to assist the individual in his movement toward the development of a comfortable adaptive relationship to life it is necessary to meet his needs at his developmental level as a beginning. Through careful monitoring of the treatment process and careful attention to clues that signify movement to a higher level and therefore readiness for change in programming needs of the patient, we can move toward providing an integrating treatment experience. My experience suggests that to provide activity and relationship processes for a level higher than the individual's ability to cope is to heap stress on an already overwhelmed system and to do relatively more harm than service. The permissive school of treatment within occupational therapy practice has had on its side the natural instincts of the individual to seek his level of need and therefore lead the therapist into appropriate interaction at a point of toleration for the patient provided this level could also be tolerated by the therapist. The symptom-oriented school of thought has also had some success in that symtomatology often points to needs which may indicate a level of development at which the individual is functioning provided the leads are accurate and the therapist is "listening." The disability-oriented school of treatment has had some measure of success in restoring function, however, may fail in having the restored function integrated for use if careful attention is not paid to other related levels of development.

The implications of this theory for the preservation of health and the prevention of potential maladaptation related to insufficient nurturance in the various aspects of growth and development are related to the belief that intervention at a stage that can be identified before trauma becomes overwhelming will allow the individual to continue his growth process with a minimum of interruption and continue toward the achievement of ego-adaptive skills. In cases of permanent residual or chronic physical or psychological disability, achievement of developmental tasks and ego-adaptive skills must be guided within the individual's limitations and geared to a realistically attainable level.

This formulation does not provide a recipe for practicing occupational therapy. It simply orders some of the factors relevant to a developmental theory for practice that must be validated. It provides a framework in which to understand the contribution of the various testing, systematic observation and other evaluation tools that are available to us in relationship to occupational therapy intervention, a framework in which to understand our selective use of activities and relationships and a system which speaks both to horizontal and longitudinal growth.

Within the practice of our profession, there are predictable aspects relative to cause and effect in the use of activities and the application of relationships which must be identified, applied repeatedly in a systematic manner, analyzed and documented in order to establish their validity. There are also measurable phenomena related to change relative to occupational therapy intervention which must be studied and documented as well.

Looking at our profession from a developmental point of view, one might say that we have mastered the sensorimotor levels of development and have achieved body integration, learned to walk and talk, have worked through our needs for dependency, although there may be remaining conflicts between holding on and letting go. We recognize the need for reading and writing and are developing our skills accordingly. We appear to be on the threshold of abstraction and conceptualization and working toward mastery of the understanding of the essence of our profession. This is my impression by observation; more careful evaluation would be necessary to determine the truth of these observations as well as to elicit others. In order to move us toward mastery, selected relevant activities and relationships will be needed to nurture our continued growth and development.

In closing, I would like to share with you a rather startling discovery that I made some time ago. It was, that "they," whoever "they" were, who I felt should be doing something to objectify our knowledge and raise the level of our practice included "me." I, herewith, challenge each of you to join me in that task so that "we" can move toward facilitating growth and development and fulfilling the promise of occupational therapy.

This study was made possible under Children and Youth Health Service Grant #640, Children's Bureau, Department of Health, Education and Welfare.

REFERENCES

1. Ayres, A. Jean. "Perceptual-Motor Training for Children." Lecture given during 1962 WFOT Study Course VI—*Approaches to Treatment of Patients with Neuromuscular Dysfunction.*
2. Gesell, Arnold, and Armatruda, Catherine. *Developmental Diagnosis.* New York: Harper and Row, Inc., 1967.
3. Erikson, Eric. *Childhood and Society.* New York: W.W. Norton and Co., 1963.
4. Hall, Calvin S. *A Primer of Freudian Psychology.* New York: The New American Library, 1964.
5. Grant, Quentin R. Unpublished lecture notes.
6. Havighurst, Robert J. *Developmental Tasks and Education.* New York: David McKay Co., Inc., 1967.
7. Pearce, J., and Newton, S. *Conditions of Human Growth.* New York: Citadel Press, 1963.
8. Mosey, Anne C. *Occupational Therapy: Theory and Practice.* Medford, Mass.: Pothier Brothers, 1968.
9. Llorens, Lela A. and Rubin, Eli Z. *Developing Ego Functions in Disturbed Children.* Wayne State University Press, 1967.
10. Pearce, J. and Newton, S., p. 119.

The 1971 Eleanor Clarke Slagle Lecture

The Occupational Therapist in Prevention Programs

Geraldine L. Finn

In order for a profession to maintain its relevancy it must be responsive to the trends of the times. The trend today in health services is toward the prevention of disability. Occupational therapists are being asked to move beyond the role of therapist to that of health agent. This expansion in role identity will require a reinterpretation of current knowledge, the addition of new knowledge and skills, and the revision of the educational process. Nine issues are discussed that were extracted from the process data collected during the development of prevention programs in an occupational therapy department.

Social Change

In order for a profession to maintain its relevancy it must be aware of the times, interpreting its contribution to mankind in accordance with the needs of the times. When social change was slower it was possible for a profession to make this transition gradually; to proceed in a process of evolution, with new ideas and methods slowly replacing formerly held concepts and practices. However, in our era in history, this process of adjustment has had to be accelerated in order to keep pace with the rapidity with which our society is changing. In today's world, the demand to act is often presented to us before we have had sufficient time to understand and assimilate

Reprinted from *The American Journal of Occupational Therapy,* Vol. XXVI, No. 2, 1972.

the meaning and significance behind the demanded actions. This is a tenuous position in which to be placed. One is presented with the need and the pressure to respond to that need but without the time to reflect on the knowledge and skills required to respond effectively. Reality, today, is continually outdistancing our preparation to respond to it.

Until the twentieth century, the pace of change allowed the average person the opportunity to incorporate change while feeling a sense of stability. But during this century the scope, the scale, and above all the pace of change, have been accelerated. Change in our society has developed a visibility it did not possess in former times. C.P. Snow comments, "Until this century social change was so slow that it could pass unnoticed in one person's lifetime." (1) Such is no longer the case. Alvin Toffler in his book, *Future Shock,* addresses himself to the current phenomenon of accelerated change and its impact on man's ability to adapt. Toffler reflects on the exhaustion which can engulf the individual as he reaches an overload in his capacity to adjust to the new. (2)

Occupational Therapy and Social Change

This concern about modern change is particularly applicable to the profession of occupational therapy in 1971. For at this moment in our professional history we are being asked to expand our role identity from that of therapist to health agent. Because of the change in emphasis on the delivery of health services we are being asked to move beyond the treatment of patients into the arena of health planning and the development of prevention programs: "to broaden our traditional, more limited identification with medicine... to enlarge our concept from that of being a therapist to one of functioning as a health agent with responsibility to help insure normal growth and development" (3) within the lives of all the people in a community.

This is a demand that needs to be acted on immediately if we are to take our place with others involved in the health problems of our day. Yet it is a demand that will require extensive reorganization of our current practices; changes we have not had the time to explore fully. To expand our services beyond the clinic into health planning for the community requires changes in the interpretation of our current knowledge, the addition of new knowledge and skills, the abdication of learned behavior patterns, and the revision of our educational process.

This expansion of role identity will require us to give up something we know for something new and unknown. Our education has trained us to work with the disabled person, usually within an institutional setting. Our knowledge, our training, our experience have all formed us to function within a clinical model-evaluating, treating, and rehabilitating the disabled person. We know the problems of today's society as they are reflected in the life of a particular patient but that is quite different from dealing with the problem at a community level. Yet we are faced with the request to change. Not to change gradually over a period of years but to change now; to be relevant to the needs of the times in which we live we must change our model of practice.

We find ourselves in the position of having to act while simultaneously trying to gain the knowledge necessary to act within our new role identity. The printed words in the books written about change in today's society have come alive for us. In our professional life we are actually *experiencing* the words. In today's world the demand to act is often presented to us before we have had sufficient time to understand and assimilate the meaning and significance behind the demanded action. We are living in a professional reality that is outdistancing our preparation to respond to it.

Faced with the drama of this situation we have a choice as individual occupational therapists. We can deny the urgency of the need to become involved in health planning and prevention programs and go on with our everyday activities; we can accept the importance of the mandate but feel that we can contribute more to the service of mankind by remaining in our present role as clinician; we can admit the concept of role identity change and ponder its significance in isolation away from the daily realities of practice; or we can accept the challenge and begin to change the emphasis of our practice, implementing new programs as increased knowledge and understanding are achieved.

As a clinician and administrator I chose the route of expanding my own identity to incorporate the role of health agent, and assumed the responsibility of reorganizing an occupational therapy department according to the new emphasis in health services. This reorganization has now been in progress for two years. In preparation for this lecture I attempted to study this process of change; not to report to you an autobiographical journey but rather to share with you some of the issues that became evident during this experience—issues we need to understand if we are to develop comprehensive prevention programs and revise our curricula to prepare the future occupational therapist in the role of health agent.

Practice of Occupational Therapy—1960 to 1970

In order to understand these issues as they relate to the process of expanding services into the community, it is necessary to relate these issues to the practice of occupational therapy and the changes within the health services.

To understand the position of occupational therapy practice at this particular moment when changes are being demanded of it, we need to consider the developments within our practice during the past decade. The mandate for expansion of our services into health planning comes at a time when we are just beginning to develop our full identity as a profession within a therapy role. We have progressed from technician receiving a prescription from the physician to our present position as principle agent in the treatment of patients who require an intervention process employing the therapeutic use of activities.

After years of intuitive service to the sick and disabled we have now begun to define our practice and validate our clinical impressions through research studies. During the decade of the 1960's we began, in earnest, to study the process of normal growth and development and to interpret this knowledge as it applied to the patient with developmental deviations or fixations. We studied the theorists in cognition and began to refine our understanding of the role which specific activities and experiences play in the development of perceptual-motor-cognitive skills. (4) We probed deeper into the psychological aspects of activities. We increased our knowledge of group process and the use of task-oriented groups in developing one's interpersonal skills. (5) We began to communicate to others the debilitating effects of disability on the satisfaction of these basic needs. We no longer had to apologize for our association with the practical activities of daily life because we had reached the level of awareness that it was through these activities that the disabled person was able to maintain his sense of human identity: to keep that sense of self-dignity and independence that can be so quickly lost in an institutional setting. We took our new understanding of human functioning and started to develop evaluation and treatment methods to correct specific deficits impeding the ability of the patient to fulfill these basic human needs. We responded to the permanently disabled person's need to maintain a normal way of life within the limitations of his disability, and helped him develop his social, vocational, and avocational interests.

The 1960's were productive years in the maturation of occupational therapy and the advent of the 1970's could be looked upon as the time for greater refinement in our clinical practice. At last we were beginning to define clearly the contribution of activities to the treatment of the sick and disabled. We had grown beyond the need to seek our identity by simulating the services or appearances of another profession. Therefore, as we entered the 1970's, there stretched out before us an array of avenues to follow in analyzing activities, in refining our evaluation procedures, and in developing more effective treatment techniques.

Change in Delivery of Health Services

But the needs of a particular period in history do not wait upon a timetable of priorities. Emphasis was being placed on developing prevention programs in the fields of mental health and pediatrics. Starting in the 1960's concern was centered on the importance of preventing disorders in children through the implementation of special programs. Well-baby clinics were established in local communities, Head Start for the preschool child was introduced, and more attention was given to the child with learning disabilities. (6) In the field of mental health the trend away from large state institutions and the establishment of community mental health centers was developing. Although these centers provided clinical services to people in a particular geographical area, specific attention was directed toward the establishment of collaborative relationships with other institutions in the community as a means of developing primary prevention and early intervention programs. In the field of public health there was growing concern for the increased numbers of people suffering from long-term chronic conditions such as arthritis, diabetes, mental retardation, and alcoholism. (7)

Fully recognizing the continuing need of many people for direct clinical and treatment services, there was the growing realization that many of the problems dealt with daily in the clinic could be prevented or modified if only earlier intervention had been available. Those within our society who had studied the health demands of today were saying that, for both human and economic reasons, we must expand our efforts to create an environment that would prevent serious illness and disability. The time had come to recognize that unless we began to refocus our attention on keeping people well, we would never be able to stem the tide of human suffering in our country.

The era of maintaining the health of a community through the control of communicable and infectious diseases was behind us. We had the knowledge to conquer these destroyers of human life and we must now move on to those chronic and disabling conditions that do not cause immediate death but, rather, years of human suffering and waste of human potential. In public health we had passed the time when all our energies had to be focused on the most basic physical health needs of the people. We were now able to devote our attention to the social disorders which not only affect the physical life of the individual but also have social, psychological, and economic ramifications for the individual, his family, and the society at large. Sudden illness and death have been replaced by disorders spanning an extended period of disability. Many chronic conditions limit the individual's ability to function for years. It is the length of time involved in these chronic disorders, the variety of services required, and the large numbers of people affected by them which have made chronic disorders such a major health problem today. (8)

Realizing, therefore, the need to counteract the amount of disability in our society, and recognizing that the most viable way to stop this amount of disability was through preventing it from occurring, emphasis was placed on prevention. In addition to this desire to prevent disability was the desire to provide an environment in which each person would be free to reach his fullest potential of human development. The achievement of this supportive environment was seen as an extremely complex task but it was felt that the effort made to reach this goal would be worthwhile. The need to improve the quality of all aspects of life was seen as part of the responsibility of health planning because health problems are interrelated with all the other aspects of life. It is not possible to consider the solution of health problems without being aware of the influence of other social factors, such as, economics, housing, and family life, on one's state of health.

The interrelationship of health issues and the other social forces in the community is illustrated graphically by the current problem of the elderly in our society. The control of communicable disease and the advance of medical science have combined to allow the individual of today a longer life span. This extension of life has presented complications when considered in relationship to other forces in our society. The technological advances have created a trend toward urban living, with smaller houses, constant mobility, and the separation of the nuclear family from its extended members. As a result of this life pattern there is usually no room for the aging parent in the home of the child. Housing, therefore, becomes a major concern for the elderly. Even if the elderly remain in their own homes, neighbors change so often that the sense of security among friends is often missing. Further, the cost of living continues to rise in our society. Financial retirement plans made twenty or thirty years ago are no longer sufficient to sustain the older person. Although many elderly people are still capable of working, the retirement policies of business and industry force inactivity on the older individual. Unable to work, concerned about finances, and often alone, the older person begins to withdraw from life experiences. Depression, poor eating habits, and inactivity often result. Then again protection from disease has not completely eliminated the degenerative conditions that often result from the aging process—conditions that require the older person to receive assistance with his daily life. Too often, however, the needed services which would allow the person to remain in his own home are not available. As a result, the older person must be placed in an institution. Here care is available but the expense is great. Institutions, no matter how comfortable, can never replace one's own home, and the elderly person begins to develop a sense of hopelessness. Often the children are concerned but are so caught up in coping with our rapidly changing environment that feelings of resentment begin to develop against the parent. Financial assistance beyond the family is usually needed and the care and expense of the older person becomes society's responsibility. The problem of aging becomes, therefore, not simply a health problem but a complex social problem. (9)

Issues to Consider in Prevention Programs

Supported by a growing body of knowledge in occupational therapy clinical practice and aware of the need and priority of health prevention service, it is now necessary to begin the examination of the kinds of issues to be considered by occupational therapists, as we accept the mandate to move beyond the role of therapist and become health agents and progress along the continuum from hospital and clinical services to the community and health programs.

Issue One. The first issue relates to the environment in which one carries out his practice. Prevention programs are carried out in the community, with the primary institutions—such units as the family, the school, the law, places of business, the health center, and the church. Each of these institutions makes a contribution to a person's life to one degree or another. They provide each person with the opportunities to gain the "increments of ego strength and personality robustness" (10) which enable him to cope with the demands and pressures of daily life. To maintain the sense of well-being of the people in the community and to allow them the opportunity to develop their human potential, these primary institutions must respond adequately to the needs of the people. If they do respond in effective ways then the environment provides the nurturing elements needed for human growth and happiness. Unfortunately, the perfection of these institutions has not been attained and one of the responsibilities of those engaged in prevention work is the development of programs and services that will contribute to the perfection of these institutions.

Included in the list of primary institutions are ones which have usually been outside the professional interests of the occupational therapist. Little concern has been given, for example, to the functioning of local industries, or the overall administration and policies of the school system. Until the present time the occupational therapist has limited himself primarily to the health center. Even here, though, the occupational therapist has related more to the internal functioning of the health center rather than concerning himself with the health center's role and responsibility in the community. The occupational therapist is familiar with what goes on within the walls of the health center, but the remaining primary institutions in the community are often perceived only at the level of vague general awareness.

When moving, therefore, into community programs it is necessary for the occupational therapist to become knowledgeable about these other institutions, to understand more fully their functions, their goals, their policies, and their methods of operation. It is only in this way that the occupational therapist can begin to develop appropriate communications with the primary institutions. In collaborative efforts with these primary institutions the occupational therapist must discern those areas in which he can make his contribution.

Issue Two. Consideration of this factor of collaboration introduces us to a second issue. Before the occupational therapist reaches out to the primary institutions he must have a clear understanding of the services he has to offer. Although the occupational therapist has been responsible for delineating the kinds of services he has to offer to the patients within a clinical setting, treatment programs have had the advantage of years of experience in relating specific treatment services to a particular disability. Prevention programs are new for occupational therapists and there are no traditions upon which to base one's actions. It is possible to try to reinterpret clinical programs so that they fit the particular needs of a community but it must be remembered that the clinical programs were developed for the person with a specific pathology. The programs in the community have to relate to the maintaining of a person's health. Therefore, in considering community programs the occupational therapist must have an understanding of health in order to develop appropriate prevention programs.

Dubos notes that, "solving problems of disease is not the same thing as creating health. . . the task of health demands a kind of wisdom and vision which transcends specialized knowledge of remedies and treatments and which apprehends in all their complexities and subtleties the relation between living things and their total environment." (11) Health is far more than just the absence of disease. The word *health* is an abstract term that has been given to a highly complex, multivariable condition of man. Those who have attempted to define health have come up with a series of characteristics.

Gordon Allport suggests six principle characteristics of the healthy personality. First, he considers the capacity of the individual to extend himself to interests outside his own body and material possessions. The second characteristic Allport attributes to the healthy personality is self-objectification. This is the capacity of the individual to achieve a spatial and temporal quality in his orientation to life. The third attribute is a unifying philosophy of life. Allport states that his philosophy of life may, or may not, be religious, but in any event it has to be a frame of meaning and responsibility into which life's major activities fit. Fourth, Allport sees a healthy person as one who is capable of relating to other human beings in a warm and profound manner. Fifth, Allport attributes an importance to the possession of realistic skills, abilities, and perceptions with which to cope with the practical problems of life. And sixth, Allport considers the capacity to possess a compassionate regard and respect for all men and the willingness to participate in common activities that will improve the human lot. (12)

Using Allport's six characteristics as a foundation, let us attempt to develop a definition of a healthy person. A healthy person is one who is accepting of himself, responsive and concerned about other people, sees meaning in his existence, and is capable of productively fulfilling the daily demands of his life. Now, no definition of health, however, completely expresses the full understanding of this concept, but such a definition as the above does provide a basis upon which to develop a more comprehensive understanding of the subject.

It is significant to note in Allport's description of the healthy personality the role played by one's involvement in active participation in his environment. The healthy person does not remain preoccupied with self-interests but extends himself to others and related to them in a productive manner within the daily events of life, accomplishing this through the use of his skills and abilities.

The healthy person is an active person, This fact has been recognized by philosophers and psychologists searching for a greater understanding of man. Aristotle stated that virtue is activity, by which he meant the exercise of the functions and capacities that are peculiar to man. Happiness to Aristotle was the result of activity and use, it was not a quiescent state of mind. (13) According to Erich Fromm, "man is not only a rational and social animal . . . he can also be defined as a producing animal, capable of transforming the materials which he finds at hand, using his reason and imagination; not only can man produce, he must produce." (14)

Issue Three. Armed with a realization of the concept of health, and particularly the aspect of human activity and man's relationship to the activities in his environment maintaining his sense of health, the occupational therapist must begin to reinterpret his body of knowledge. He must begin to relate his understanding of the ways in which man, throughout the stages of his life and in his active interactions with his environment, develops the characteristics that define health. He must begin to consider ways in which he can apply this knowledge within the primary institutions within the community. One example would be the association of play experiences in the cognitive and emotional development of the preschool child, and the application of this knowledge to the education of child-care workers in a community day care center.

Issue Four. This reinterpretation of the occupational therapist's body of knowledge and skills brings us to the next issue—the importance of thinking creatively. In order to meet the challenge of developing effective prevention programs we must begin to exercise our imaginations. The imagination is a mental process which, all too often in our technological society, has been dulled. We have been trained to take facts and put them together logically without the benefit of our own mental images. In our educational process the imagination has too often been relegated to a creative writing course, or a literature course, and omitted from our more scientifically-oriented courses. Yet how do people begin to see associations that have not been perceived before if they do not use their imaginations.

We are often amazed at the way a poet seems to see inside a situation and extract from it the richness of its essence. One reason for this skill rests on the development of his imagination; on his capacity to think in mental images. One poet I know refers to the specialization process in education as training people to put their knowledge into boxes. If one gets a thought that does not fit the criteria of the box, then it is discarded. A poet instead has transcended the box mentality and is open to all aspects of reality, manipulating them mentally into new images and associations.

It is this process of creative thinking which is required of us, as occupational therapists, in order to interpret our knowledge about human performance, growth and development, work, play, and human relations so that it becomes functional material for developing prevention programs in the service of maintaining the health of a community. It is necessary for us to begin to think creatively about our particular understanding of man's needs and to start to build new images around this knowledge.

Issue Five. Once we have begun the process of recombining our knowledge it is necessary to consider ways in which this knowledge can be translated into actual programs. This brings us to another issue—the development of a method to translate one's plan into action. Over a period of years we have broken down our units of knowledge and applied them in the treatment situation. For most of us in our professional careers, we entered practice with associations already established between a plan and the act. In our educational process we have studied man physically and psychologically, learned the various ways in which his functioning may be pathological because of a disease or disability, and have practiced the methods employed to treat the problem. Therefore, in our clinical practice the process of proceeding from a plan to an act has centered on the particular patient coming to us for service. We have adapted our general knowledge to translating a plan into an act for a particular patient. The situation in the community, however, is quite different. Instead of working with a single patient, we are working with a primary institution or several primary institutions possessing a litany of complexities far beyond the problems of a single person. The primary institution does not have a single, well-defined problem which is seeking solution. The primary institutions are coping with a wide variety of factors impinging on the health of people in the community. The task that is presented to us is the establishment of a method of processing the needs of the primary institutions and the services the occupational therapist has to offer.

A method which has proved satisfactory consists of conceptualizing ideas and plans into progressively more specific conceptual units until one is able to express his thoughts in action-oriented terms. This process requires the mental discipline to continue to breakdown a thought until it can be translated into a specific action relating directly to the initial idea. When dealing with such broad concepts as human performance, health, and social systems there is a tendency to forget that these words represent a complex association of facts that must be analyzed carefully if the particular components of these concepts are to be combined so that a definite plan can be carried out. Without breaking down these concepts, a chasm which cannot be crossed exists between the thought and the act. Everyone sometime in his life has had the experience, I am sure, of being able to speak knowledgeably and at length about a particular concept, but finds that he is totally lost when asked to express this concept in a concrete act. In this situation the person has not conceptualized his knowledge in action terms. But once he has broken down the concept into units of action he is able to act.

Issue Six. Once we have broken down our concepts it is possible to act—to begin to take our knowledge of activities and their significance to man and develop new programs. The implementation of new programs brings with it a recognition of risk-taking, which is the next issue to be discussed. We are most comfortable when we know the route and the expected outcome of our actions. In the process of developing new programs within a new environment it is not possible to know fully the route which the program will take nor the specific details of the final outcome of the plan. Over the years we have become familiar with the expected behaviors of those working within a medical institution and have been able to transfer this information to new staff and students. Health planning, however, requires us to relate to people from nonmedical settings and from different organizational structures. Often one is involved with people from various settings simultaneously. Without the comfort of knowing the behavioral responses to expect, anxiety and apprehension can become overwhelming feelings. To cope with the need to become comfortable in unfamiliar situations we must begin to develop new skills in interpersonal relationships; to become more acutely sensitive to the behavioral cues of others as well as more conscious of our own patterns of relating.

Issue Seven. Of particular importance in dealing with new situations is a deeper understanding of the communication process. Through our professional education we have embraced a style of relating technical information comprehensible only to others trained in medically-oriented fields. We have developed a way of thinking about certain information and often assume that everyone else thinks in the same frame of orientation. When we speak, for example, about the stages of development we are thinking about the process of development—the particular process by which a person progresses along the developmental continuum. Many teachers, however, see stages of development from a static frame of orientation. They think about the child at age five, or age six, or age seven but not about the process by which the child grows from age to age.

In order to communicate with parents, teachers, Golden Age directors, clergymen, and the like we must be able to communicate our ideas in language that is understandable to the other person. This requirement forces us to admit those areas of our knowledge which remain vague and ill-defined under the mantle of the professional term. For example, unless one fully understands the psychosexual stage of orality it is very difficult to help a neighborhood recreation leader realize the particular needs of a boy in his sports group fixated at this stage of emotional development.

Issue Eight. Clear communication provides an important step in the introduction of new ideas or programs. The introduction of new ideas, new programs, or new ways of thinking and acting in a primary institution represents the core issue in prevention work. As clinicians we are used to having patients come to us for help. The person is in need and seeks our assistance. In prevention work the occupational therapist goes to the people in the primary institutions. The significance of this reversal of roles must be fully understood. It is necessary to demonstrate to the other person or group of people the feasibility of accepting the plan, the idea, the program, or the service offered by the occupational therapist. Unless the occupational therapist fully understands the service he has to offer, believes in the value of the service, and can explain how that service will benefit the other person, the desired collaboration will not occur. In order to present appropriate programs and communicate clearly about them, therefore, a great deal of thought and planning must go into the preparatory work for prevention programming.

Because the other people sometime do not see the worth of the proposed plan, or are hesitant to accept the plan because of internal organizational factors, the element of frustration accompanies the implementation of prevention programming. Most clinicians have had the experience of a patient refusing to attend occupational therapy and know the feelings of frustration and futility that such an experience can arouse. In developing prevention programs these feelings are magnified because of the amount of preliminary work that has had to go into each plan and the endless variations in the problems and obstacles encountered. As Leonard Duhl says, "The input of information constantly redefines the situation, the problem, and the possible range of solutions." (15) Therefore, a well-defined, well-planned program may have to be revised a dozen different ways before there is agreement on the details of the plan.

Issue Nine. Because of the complexity of factors involved in developing prevention programs the morale of the staff becomes our final issue. Effective prevention work is carried out at the grass-roots level of the community. If change is to take place within the primary institutions in a community it is not sufficient that the person at the head of the institution, such as the school superintendent for example, be in agreement with the ideas. The people who actually carry out the daily action plans are the ones who must be enthusiastic. In order to maintain this kind of willingness to change on the part of others the occupational therapist must be able to maintain his sense of objectivity and interest in the project. To do this the occupational therapist must have the opportunity to look at his own feelings and also see the personal growth opportunities in the experience. To accomplish these things the occupational therapist must be receiving assistance in sorting out his own feelings and obtaining guidance in continuing his own personality development. It is for these reasons that staff supervision becomes a crucial part of any prevention-oriented program. The supervision must relate to the individual needs of each staff member for specific knowledge and skills, for the ability to deal with one's feelings, and for the development of a professional identity as an occupational therapist in the role of health agent. Because of the need for the development of a supportive system for staff involved in the pioneering work in health planning and prevention programming, a hierarchy of supervision can be developed where each staff member receives supervision from a more experienced therapist while in turn supervising a less experienced therapist. This method provides for the development of a network of support, and through this process the individual occupational therapist begins to learn ways in which he can find support for his efforts within himself, and is able in time to relinquish the great need for external support.

Summary of Issues

We have now concluded the discussion of the specific issues which began to crystallize as we proceeded through the process of expanding an occupational therapy department from an inpatient service to include prevention programs. Nine separate issues were extracted from the process data gathered over the past two years of developing prevention programs. To restate them again, they include (1) the function of primary institutions in maintaining the health of the people of a community and the need for occupational therapists to understand the functions, goals, and policies of these primary institutions; (2) the planning of appropriate programs and services based on man's need to engage in interaction with the objects in his environment in order to maintain his health throughout his life; (3) the need to reinterpret the body of knowledge available within the profession of occupational therapy in order to apply it in the service of keeping people healthy rather than in helping people minimize their disabilities; (4) the creation of new associations of our available knowledge in order to respond more accurately to the pressing reality needs of today; (5) the establishment of an organizational model which will allow translation of abstract plans about activities, human action, and the delivery of health services into concrete actions; (6) the presence of risk-taking and its ramifications on one's ability to function and perservere when faced with an unfamiliar environment; (7) the necessity of reexamining communication patterns to insure real communications among people; (8) the need to create a climate of acceptance for a planned program and the development of the skills needed to assist others in seeing the value of these programs; and (9) the role of supervision in maintaining the performance and professional growth of the staff members.

Community Programs

Before proceeding to the concluding section of my presentation I would like to share with you the kinds of programs that provided the process material from which these issues were extracted. These programs include early intervention programs for children, ages 4 to 12 years, who are beginning to present the first indications of behavioral and learning problems; a consultation service to teachers; an inservice education program in developmental screening and program planning for teachers in day care centers; an outreach program to community agencies assisting the elderly; a workshop for mothers and preschool children in early childhood development and parent-child relationships; an inservice education program on perceptual-motor development for mental health workers; development of new models of parent education and counseling; and the introduction of knowledge about developmental levels in human performance in a community drug program.

Curriculum Changes

Having localized some of the issues arising out of prevention programming we are now faced with their significance in the mandate to occupational therapists to move beyond the role of therapist to health agent. In discussion of each of these issues I have alluded to the change that must occur in the education of occupational therapists both at the level of academic professional education and at the level of continuing education for practicing occupational therapists.

In order to expand into the areas of health planning and prevention programs, occupational therapists must possess a comprehensive knowledge and understanding of the meaning and significance of activities in the development of man's fullest potential. It is natural for man to be active; to interact with the objects in his environment, to develop his physical, cognitive, and psychosocial abilities.

Man must exist in an environment which provides him with the opportunities to grow and develop as a total human being through his interaction with people and with the activities and objects in the environment if he is to remain healthy. The study of activities and the application of this knowledge to provide man with a better way of life are the essences of the profession of occupational therapy. Therefore, as the profession with this charge, we must move beyond the confines of focusing our attention on the value of a specific activity to achieve a specific result and include a more comprehensive understanding of activities and human action. It is only with such an understanding that we will be able to respond to the needs of the primary institutions in our communities and develop the kinds of particular services these institutions require in order to maintain the health of the people in the community. We must not give up the knowledge we now possess in activity analysis as it applies to the physically and psychologically disabled person, but rather we must expand this knowledge.

Secondly, we must develop our ability to become leaders; to move with confidence into the community and collaborate in the creation of a healthier environment, contributing our knowledge of activities and human action. We need, therefore, to be able to problem-solve, to understand the factors involved in complex systems and define the problems where we can make a contribution.

And thirdly, we must increase our knowledge about the society in which we live. We must understand the effect of technology on man's way of life today, to realize the reasons behind the young people's push to return to a more human-oriented life style, to understand the economic, political, and social forces that predominate in today's society.

Summary

The trend, today, in health services is toward the prevention of disability. We are a profession possessing knowledge that is particularly necessary to maintain the health of people. To move from therapist to health agent demands us to change but to change in a forward, positive way. We do not have to give up what we know, rather, we must instead be willing to know more.

For years we have been concerned with the disabled person's right to maintain his dignity and self-worth by reaching his maximum level in human functioning. The needs of our times are now asking us to contribute to the preservation of each person's right to achieve his highest level of human functioning.

References

1. Toffler A: Future Shock, New York, Random House, 1970.
2. Ibid.
3. West WL: Professional responsibility in times of change. Am J Occup Ther 22: 231-249, 1968.
4. Llorens LA: facilitating growth and development: the promise of occupational therapy. Am J Occup Ther 24: 93-101, 1970.
5. Fidler GS: The task-oriented group as a context for treatment. Am J Occup Ther 23: 43-48, 1969.
6. West WL: The growing importance of prevention. Am J Occup Ther 23: 226-231, 1969.

7. Smolensky J, Haar FB: Principles of Community Health, Philadelphia, WB Saunders Company, 1967.
8. Ibid.
9. Berezin AB, Stotsky BA: The geriatric patient. The Practice of Community Mental Health, Boston, Little Brown Company, 1970.
10. Bower EM: Primary prevention of mental and emotional disorders: a conceptual framework and action possibilities. Perspectives in Community Mental Health, Chicago, Aldine Publishing Company, 1969.
11. Ibid.
12. Allport GW: Personality and Social Encounter, Boston, Beacon Press, 1960.
13. Fromm E: Man for Himself, New York, Rinehart and Company Inc., 1947.
14. Ibid.
15. Duhl LJ: Planning and predicting: or what to do when you don't know the names of the variables. General Systems Theory and Psychiatry, Boston, Little Brown Company, 1969.

Occupational Therapy: A Model for the Future

Jerry A. Johnson

The success and perhaps survival of occupational therapy may well depend upon our ability to clearly identify our product and services, to determine where we can best provide these services, to obtain adequate sources of support for occupational therapy services, and to insure that we have experienced competent personnel to provide these services. This paper draws on concepts from business and biology to assist occupational therapists in the development of models to facilitate successful adaptation and negotiation which will enable us to provide occupational therapy services where there is need for them and in a manner consistent with our professional standards of quality care.

Introduction

Occupational therapists repeatedly throughout our history have demonstrated concern for the individual and a strong belief that through involvement in the occupational therapy process, those individuals who cannot contribute to, or fully participate in society's marketplace can determine the quality and style of life they seek and can thereby influence their health. Mrs. Eleanor Clarke Slagle associated such concern and belief with occupational therapy when she refused an offer to go to France in 1918 to head a hospital for "shell-shock cases." Instead, she elected to remain in Chicago where she had started courses in occupational therapy as she felt her efforts

Reprinted from *The American Journal of Occupational Therapy*, Vol. XXVII, No. 1, 1973.

could best be devoted to meeting the needs of wounded veterans in that fashion. (1)

While concern for the individual has been demonstrated consistently, our knowledge of individual behavior and social behavior has expanded so that our efforts to promote and support man's desire for health through the occupational therapy process have shifted from sole focus on the individual to recognition that equal focus must center on helping man learn to achieve a satisfying interaction with his social system or environment.

Defining the occupational therapy process has been difficult. Early in our development we found success when we employed the concepts of "moral treatment" with psychiatric patients. (2) Within this framework we were concerned with the whole man, and we attempted to provide wide-based, health oriented services to individuals which were consistent with and responsive to society's needs. At the same time we were able to retain our belief in the individual and to demonstrate the value of his involvement in occupation to restore function and promote healing.

At other times we have lost sight of man as a whole and have concentrated on mechanics, media, or techniques, usually in an effort to influence pathological processes. (3) When we put aside our strong orientation toward health, we seem to be less successful and to harbor more doubts about the viability of occupational therapy.

At this point in time, we, as a profession, are faced with the challenge of making critical decisions which may well determine not only our success—but our survival—as a profession in the future.

This presentation will attempt to delineate a model to serve as a guide in our decision-making process as we develop a strategy for the future. I will discuss five elements, all interrelated as part of our decision-making process. I will also raise questions for our mutual consideration as we move toward decision-making.

The five elements in the decision-making process are: organizational behavior and societal change; the occupational therapy product; the marketplace for occupational therapy; the marketing process; personnel requirements.

The terminology and concepts utilized herein are derived primarily from business and biology, rather than from medicine, because we must examine many models before we can select those which are most appropriate for our professions.

Organizational Behavior and Societal Change

History reveals that our desire to provide services of professional status and quality have prompted us to accept and seek to fulfill the criteria of professionalism defined by medicine and also accepted as "the authority" by other professions, who also view the physician as the "professional par excellence." (4)

Fidler (5) and Yerxa (6) in their respective Eleanor Clarke Slagle lectures identified and examined our progress in fulfilling these professional criteria in our educational and practice systems. Among the criteria they examined were the following:

Acceptance by the profession of a body of knowledge, supported and substantiated by research;

Establishment and enforcement of ethical standards for membership behavior;

Acceptance of responsibility for making independent judgments and for operating autonomously;

Establishment of and control over educational standards for admission of members into the professional association; and

Identification of services associated by the public with occupational therapy.

Our desire to move from competence to excellence has been equated with fulfilling the above criteria of professionalism. This has led us to direct our primary attention to internal matters over which we could exert some degree of control. This behavior was demonstrated in an era in which professions were distinct and often isolated entities. Lawrence and Lorsch, in their studies of organizational behavior, found that this was a generally accepted pattern of organizational behavior and that it represented a method whereby organizations could find "the one best way to organize." (7)

While we and other professions have spent most of our efforts and energy focusing on internal change and revision, and have erected organizational structures reflective of the past, the very foundations which govern all aspects of our lives have shifted. Drucker, among others, writes that in a very short period of time society has emerged from an era of experience into an era of knowledge. One of the most dramatic changes resulting from this societal transition is that the requirement for every job—skilled or unskilled—

will be knowledge-based. Schooling, rather than apprenticeships, will provide job foundations because the worker's productivity will depend upon his ability to employ concepts, ideas, and theories. (8)

The moon shots exemplify this point for we had no previous experience upon which to build as we sent men to the moon. Rather, we had knowledge and technology which enabled us to anticipate and approximate experience and consequences of decisions.

A side effect, or consequence, of the emerging era of knowledge is the decreasing amount of isolationism and the increasing interrelatedness and interdependence which is found in all areas of life today. Individuals, as well as professions and organizations, are equally affected.

A case in point is that of the alcoholic whose life typifies complexity and interrelatedness in that his drinking affects his life, the lives of his family, and society at large. His behavior can endanger the lives of others. His children demonstrate more pathology than do children from nonalcoholic homes. His family as a whole seems to feel a greater sense of guilt than do other families. Ultimately, society may have to assume responsibility for both the alcoholic and his family.

Similar examples of increasing complexity, interrelatedness, and interdependence, are found in the areas of health, ecology, conservation, and pollution, for we are learning that our behavior and actions may have consequences extending far beyond any which could have been conceivable in earlier times.

For example, the October 1, 1972 issue of the Washington, D.C., *Sunday Star and Daily News* reported that "thousands of men and women who worked in shipyards during World War II are threatened by a rare form of cancer stemming from exposure to asbestos . . . The disease, a tumor affecting the lining of the chest or abdomen—has only recently begun to appear, 30 years after exposure . . . until the last decade mesothelioma was so rare that it did not warrant separate classification as a cause of death . . . Now it is possible that 32,500 to 225,000 of the 3.25 million World War II shipyard workers still living could be killed by the disease . . . which is invariably fatal."

As demonstrated by the above examples, our lives are becoming more complex, more interrelated, and more interdependent. With the rapid advancement of technology and the availability of increasing amounts of knowledge, the importance of experience diminishes as we move into areas in which man has had no experience. It becomes necessary to rely upon knowledge to help us anticipate the future and predict more accurately the consequences of our decisions and behavior.

There are two direct and immediate implications for occupational therapy which emanate from the knowledge era. The first implication relates to an expansion of the populations which we can service. The second implication relates to our need to expand our concept of professionalism to meet criteria we establish and to develop an organizational strategy which enables us to relate to and interact with other professions and disciplines in positive, constructive ways, without sacrificing the concepts in which we believe.

Drucker supplies evidence upon which we can predict an expansion of the populations we serve when he says that our present manpower shortage will increase because marginal and unemployed individuals frequently lack, and perhaps cannot acquire through the educational system, the habits, tools, and skills which are prerequisites for employment today. (9)

If we believe Reilly's hypothesis as proposed in her Eleanor Clarke Slagle lecture, "that man, through the use of his hands as they are energized by mind and will, can influence the state of his own health," (10) we have a responsibility to expand our service base. Dubos provides substantiative support for Reilly's hypothesis in that he proposes the distance of a direct relationship between meaningful occupation and health. (11) We as occupational therapists, can offer valuable services to those individuals who are cut off from the mainstream of society because they cannot effectively utilize our educational channels or compete in life's marketplace. These individuals need opportunities for experience, which are no longer readily available to them, to learn and to help them find an outlet for their skills and abilities.

The occupational therapist's knowledge of individual behavior, social behavior and occupational (or experiential) behavior as these components influence health leads to an understanding of the contribution of the occupational therapy process as it is relevant to present-day individual and societal needs.

The second implication emerging from the knowledge era is that it is not sufficient to attend to standards for the development of

individual professional occupational therapists, as we have traditionally done. Now we must go beyond concern for the individual
therapist to develop a strategy for the profession of occupational
therapy as a whole. This strategy will need to be concerned with the
interrelationships and interrelatedness between occupational therapy
and other professions. It may also require that, as Lawrence and
Lorsch suggest, we develop several different organizational characteristics and behavioral patterns, responsive to differing external conditions, if we are to be a successful organization in the context of
societal change. (12) Finally, it may require us to develop our own
criteria for professionalism and excellence.

In summary, we can utilize knowledge to anticipate and predict
change in the larger social context and to identify the implications of
those changes for occupational therapy as they affect our service
functions and our organizational behavior. Examination of the social
system thus enables one to take a fresh look at the product of
occupational therapy.

The Product

Occupational therapists share a common goal in their desire to
influence occupational performance in the knowledge that the individual's involvement in occupation bears direct relationship to the
state of his health. Occupation is defined as any goal-directed activity
meaningful to the individual and providing feedback to him about his
worth and value as an individual and about his interrelatedness to
others. Occupational performance consists of components of emotional, biological, cognitive, and social behavior. Each of these behavioral elements can be viewed separately, but to fulfill the goals of
occupational therapy the components must ultimately be viewed in
terms of their interrelatedness. Dubos lends his support to this approach by saying that the most pressing problems of humanity can
be resolved only as we study "systems as a whole in all of the
complexity of their interactions." He also challenges science to move
from an atomistic, reductionist approach to one which deals with the
responses of the "total organism to the total environment." (13)

Because occupational therapists have traditionally viewed man
as a total organism seeking to influence his state of health through
occupational pursuits, we have also been able to see the need for the

occupational therapy process to be concerned with individuals, their social systems, and their occupations. The client and the therapist participate in a collaborative process or transaction whereby the therapist provides an experiential learning environment in which the client can initiate or participate in occupational performance meaningful to him. As a result of this learning experience, the individual should develop a sense of competence and mastery as he learns to cope with, adapt to, and conduct negotiations and transactions with his social system, thereby facilitating mutual change.

The crucial test comes when the individual is required to perform in his own social system. If we have fulfilled our responsibilities adequately, the individual should succeed for it will be possible for him and the social system to produce changes and adaptations necessary for compatible coexistence. In summary, through this process man learns to make decisions about the quality and style of life he seeks to achieve and to influence his health.

Viewed in this light, occupational therapy is an applied social science, eclectically drawing upon the biological, social, and behavioral disciplines for our basic understanding of man, occupation, and social-organizational systems.

In summary, our product is basically a service, emanating from the following knowledge:

> That each individual has some capacity to be involved in meaningful occupational performance;
>
> That occupational performance provides feedback, conveying a sense of dignity, worth, and competence to the individual; and
>
> That through the use of occupations and his attitude toward them, the individual can determine his life style and influence his state of health.

The opportunity for individuals in our society to learn from experience is diminishing and may be gone. Through the services provided by occupational therapists, those individuals who require experience to acquire and utilize knowledge can continue to have opportunities which enable them to make decisions about their lives, and to cope with, adapt to, and negotiate with their social environments.

The above description of our product is broad and purposefully aimed at the commonalities in our professional activities. This was done in the belief that attitudes about roles and functions should be built upon a professional foundation rather than predicating the profession's future upon the role of the therapist in any given marketplace.

The Marketplace

Given the fact that our product is a service, where should we market it?

Traditionally, the hospital has been our marketplace. Should we continue, in light of the changing social context and the product as it may be defined, continue to be hospital-based and medically related?

Will the changing structure of hospitals permit us to remain there even if we wish to do so? Will our own professional goals permit us to retain our primary affiliation with medicine?

Two particular changes occurring within the spectrum of health care prompt me to question the retention of our primary ties with medicine. In the first instance, there is increasing discrepancy in health needs and expectations as identified by the public and in the needs identified by medicine. Until recently, the scope of medical care (with the exception of public health) was limited by the "germ theory." Theoretically, this theory suggested that the cause of illness or disease was a germ. If the germ could be identified, a cure could then be effected through medication, surgery, or some other prescribed regime. (14)

In contrast, the concept of illness now extends to include persons with social or behavioral problems. These problems, once considered to be of a legal or moral nature, were handled by judges or ministers who prescribed punishment or forgiveness. Now persons with such problems are candidates for health care.

The second change occurring within health care is the emergence of a new relationship between the "patient" and health professionals. The relationship involves (1) a difference in degree of patient involvement in the treatment process; (2) a movement away from the dependence and compliance required earlier of patients; and (3) a desire on the part of the patient to know more about the rationale for and consequences of the treatment program. Perhaps this change results from the greater incidence of chronic conditions and the different approaches required to change behavior.

In many instances, the cure, eradication, or control of health problems becomes a function of the contract and relationship negotiated between the health professional and the individual participating in the service program. Many of these individuals do no require hospitalization, nor will the regimented schedules and dependency states fostered of necessity by hospitals produce the desired behavioral changes necessary to enable the individual to live in relative harmony with himself and his social system.

If we are to successfully provide our services to patients, we need time which is a commodity not readily available in most hospitals. Thus, we either have to seek to change the hospital system or move into other environments. There are many other changes in medical care which cause me to question whether we can even realistically see ourselves as desiring to retain a primary affiliation with medicine and hospitals, but these instances highlight my concern.

With the changing social context, the product as I have defined it, the needs of our potential service population, and the time required to produce behavioral change, occupational therapy's greatest contribution may be other than hospital settings. We might be located in sheltered environments where opportunities for experiential learning are provided or in the individual's own social system, whereby he learns to cope with its demands, adapt to its requirements, and enter into a transactional arrangement with it.

Thus, the most ideal marketplace for occupational therapy may be in community health centers, school systems, day care centers, early child-care facilities, institutions for the chronically ill or for persons requiring long-term care as a result of either biological, social, cognitive, or behavioral problems, industrial settings, environments designed to reverse the cycles of poverty and welfare, vocational settings, or in specified medical settings where medicine and occupational therapy share or jointly seek common goals.

The decision or decisions related to the most appropriate marketplace have yet to be made, but we must explore, and evaluate all possible alternatives in order to determine whether our product can be effectively marketed in any of the marketplaces identified above.

Product Marketing

As we consider a change in the marketplace, one of our first orders of business will be to identify sources of financial support. Examination of the medical profession reveals that any movement toward a new service delivery system is accompanied by plans which insure a solid base of support for physicians. The interest in prepaid medical plans, as a means of insuring financial security, is so great that lawyers, dentists, and insurance companies are exploring the feasibility of utilizing this approach on a widespread basis.

Occupational therapy faces a more difficult problem than does medicine, dentistry, or law in that our name is not yet associated by the public with the services we provide. In reality many of the needs and problems identified by society are those for which we maintain that we can provide services. Yet a gap exists between our perception of our services and the public's ability to recognize those services as being provided by occupational therapy. Evidence also suggests that we are identified by our media, rather than by our goals and functions, and we seem to perpetuate this image by many of the advertisements which appear in our professional literature and at our professional conferences.

One of our greatest challenges is to clearly identify our product or services for ourselves and the public, particularly if we wish to achieve success in marketing them.

The inadequate solution to this challenge utilized by therapists moving into new environments has been to relinquish their professional identity to obtain jobs. It is only after they have succeeded in their jobs that they may admit that they were successful because their education and experience prepared them to contribute to the solution of certain problems. If we persist in this pattern, we run the risk of losing many excellent therapists. This is a loss we can not afford.

We have made some inroads into marketing our product through our increased reliance upon public information systems, public relations, and development of educational brochures and materials, and our efforts to influence and utilize the legislative process. These have been tentative, hesitant steps, and we must find a way to more directly and more forcefully close the gap between our perception of our services and the public's perceptions of our services.

Drucker, in addressing the issue of marketing as business views it, defines it as the systematic purposeful organization of work to sell a product, deliver it to the customer, and receive pay for it. The purpose of marketing is to translate knowledge or technology into products or services which are economically productive. Questions he raises are: (1) What are the needs, satisfactions, and expectations of the customer? (2) What can the customer afford? and (3) Who is the customer? (15) The purchaser of the service and the consumer of the service may be different and the distinction is an important one. It certainly has relevance for occupational therapy because we have traditionally been paid by hospitals to provide services to patients—and the implications of this method of financing upon our professional behavior may not yet be clear to us. I tend to believe however that financial dependency does little to help therapists become either advocates or activists.

In essence, as we think of marketing our product, the questions proposed by Drucker may be important ones for us to consider.

Personnel Requirements

As we consider a reorganization of the delivery of occupational therapy services, the personnel required to market the occupational product becomes a primary focus of consideration. We must decide how to provide, maintain, and retain experienced practitioners who provide service, and we must decide whether we will attempt to provide manpower to fill all of the positions or first try to identify and fill critical positions.

Our profession has been slow to recognize the true value of our practitioners, and while we establish standards to improve the level of practice, we have done little to increase the prestige, status, financial rewards, or opportunities for advancement within the clinical field of our experienced therapists. Our competent practitioners have to leave clinical practice to advance or to fulfill the goals of occupational therapy. Our most distinguished researchers have difficulty obtaining grants and financial support to conduct the studies to substantiate professional knowledge. If this trend continues, the most vital component of our profession—the practice of occupational therapy—may be left in the hands of young, inexperienced, or unknowledgeable therapists, of assistants and aides, and of therapists who may be complacent with competence but who do not aspire to excellence.

This is a critical problem for which we must find resolutions quickly. We must create opportunities within areas of clinical practice so that clinicians can move up in terms of professional responsibility, financial reward, and prestige without having to "move out to move up." Part of the solution to this problem may well relate to the identification of our marketplace and our ability to find sources of economic support and financial security for occupational therapists.

If clinical practice is to be assured of its rightful place within our profession, our educators have special responsibilities. We need to overcome "town-gown" attitudes of medicine for we do ourselves and our profession a serious disservice when we indulge in such negative attitudes. These attitudes are reflected in the form of criticism, frequently without apparent recognition of the fact that clinicians are the product of our educational institutions. If our clinicians fail to meet our expectations, we must examine the criteria against which we are judging their performance. We must ask why, in view of the knowledge we have imparted to them, they do not meet our expectations. Perhaps we fail to help students learn to identify for themselves, the external forces to which they must be responsive, the occupational therapy product, the marketplace in which services can be delivered, and ways of seeking financial support for our product of service.

We may fail as educators, just as therapists fail with their patients, when we focus on the product and forget the market. The patient must be able to survive in his social system. He must find a sense of satisfaction, a sense of achievement, a sense of mastery and competence—much of which is fed back to him through his occupational performance. The clinical therapist (as well as the administrator, the researcher, or the educator) must also find these satisfactions in his social system through occupational performance, and thus it behooves us to help them learn how to transact the necessary negotiations with the system in which they live and/or work in order to provide the full benefit of our services to patients.

The second way in which we demonstrate negative attitudes toward clinical therapists is perhaps most evident but not limited to university teaching hospitals. We utilized two sets of standards in hiring academic and clinical faculty and the salaries may reflect a considerable differential between academic and clinical faculty members. There is frequently reluctance on the part of academic faculty members to include the clinical faculty members in the decision-making process concerning the curriculum and the educational process. There are differing recognition and reward systems for academic and clinical faculty members. I appreciate the fact that funding for these two groups of faculty members frequently comes from different sources, but that does not relieve us of the responsibility for attempting to find alternatives and resolutions.

Clinical occupational therapists are the core of our profession—they provide the services which we value and in which we believe. It is to educate clinical therapists that our educational system exists. Research becomes necessary to improve the quality, content, and direction of practice and education, and administrators provide the facilities and other resources needed by our practitioner.

We must find ways to enable our most experienced clinical therapists to remain in the field and this is a challenge for the whole profession.

Other personnel-related issues to be anticipated as change occurs in our product, our marketplace, and our marketing process include change in professional behavior and increased conflict as we come to grips with the occupational therapist as generalist or the occupational therapist as specialist. Freidson, in studies of the medical profession, found that the nature of practice determines physician behavior. More specifically, he identified "client-dependent" and "colleague-dependent" practices. In the "client-dependent" relationship, the physician must be responsive to patient needs and expectations if he wishes to retain his patients and his income. In the latter instance, the "colleague-dependent" physician (the radiologist, pathologist, etc.) receives patients by referral from other physicians and so he is primarily responsive to their expectations, rather than the expectations of the patient. (16) This concept has relevance for occupational therapists in that we are just recognizing the implications for our behavior that are inherent in the constraints imposed by the marketplace in which we work and the source of financial support for our services. Certainly movement into new areas, often with loose or few affiliations to medicine, may be reflective of the fact that it is necessary to be employed by, or in, an environment in which there is a shared philosophy and a shared goal—or in which there is opportunity to create with others the goals which are to be shared. To be employed, without an opportunity to influence or negotiate with one's social system, is seldom satisfying. Thus, as we seek new marketplaces we may anticipate change in professional behavior, reflected by our determination to define for ourselves the standards of professionalism we wish to attain, change in our professional behavior will also reflect our growing ability to exert force, influence, or political power to see that our clients have access to adequate services. Increased conflict as an anticipated issue, may arise in response to the argument to prepare generalists versus specialists. This issue has plagued occupational therapy for years, and the prospect of expanding our horizons into new service areas may intensify the conflict.

One alternative to a discussion of the merits of the generalist versus the specialist is suggested by Lawrence and Lorsch, and Dubos, respectively, as differentiation and integration or universality and diversity. Drawing from systems theory, we know that as organizations grow, they differentiate into parts which must be integrated if the entire system is to be viable. In biology, the human body follows a similar process through its differentiation into various organs, all of which are integrated through the nervous system and brain. Each system, whether in business or biology, is concerned with differentiation, integration, and adaptation to the outside world in order to survive. Both differentiation and integration are necessary for successful interaction with and achievement in any given environment, but the unavoidable consequence is conflict. According to organizational researchers, the organization's success ultimately depends upon how well it tolerates and resolves conflict so that integration is facilitated without sacrificing the need for differentiation.

For us, as occupational therapists, it will be necessary to think of our common goals as our point of integration. While specialization may be centered upon the behavioral components (biological, social, emotional, or cognitive) of occupational performance—or related to the areas in which to work. Again, our own future success may well depend upon our ability to tolerate and resolve conflict in order to facilitate integration without sacrificing needed differentiation within occupational therapy.

These issues—retention of experienced practitioners in the service areas, changes in professional behavior, and conflict resolution—

demand attention now and will continue to occupy our time and energy, particularly as changes occur in our product, marketplace, and marketing process until we can find appropriate solutions to them.

Summary

In summary, I have raised several challenges to which I believe our profession must respond:

1. How can we utilize knowledge, rather than rely solely upon experience, to help us predict social change and anticipate the consequences of such change for occupational therapy?
2. Can we develop a strategy and organize ourselves, as a profession, so that we can conduct negotiations and transactions with the larger social system in which we exist, thereby insuring the provision of our services to those who have need of them?
3. Can we identify clearly—for ourselves and for the public—the product, or services, we can provide? Can we identify the purchasers of our services, and can we, in actuality, provide those services?
4. Can we decide where our product should be marketed and can we anticipate and plan for the changes which might occur as we move into new environments? In relation to this, can we define for ourselves the criteria for professionalism we seek to fulfill?
5. Finally, can we insure the necessary support for clinical therapists who represent our larger corporate body?

The challenges I have identified are ones for which I have no ready answers—but recognition and awareness often precede problem-solving. I cannot help but believe that the wider our base of operations, the more responsive we will be to social needs, and the more responsible and accountable we will become. Furthermore, if we can identify our services as meeting identified public health needs, support may be forthcoming from many sources: from school systems, industry, proprietary as well as voluntary agencies providing a wide variety of human health services. Possibly even physicians and insurance companies will contract with us to deliver specific services to their patients. I feel that economic independence may not only facilitate but promote the move toward professional growth if we can identify how we wish to market our product. I also believe that the answers for a profession come not so much from individuals as from collective attempts and wisdom to identify problems, to resolve the conflict inherent in them, and to consider and select the alternatives which offer the most appropriate solutions.

In conclusion, I feel comfortable leaving these challenges unanswered because I believe in the ability of occupational therapists, based on demonstrated convictions about the worth of occupational therapy to clients, to help in the process of finding answers to these challenges.

ACKNOWLEDGMENT

The author wishes to express appreciation and gratitude for the contributions and assistance given by my colleagues, students and secretarial staff at Boston University, by Anne Henderson, O.T.R., Lela Llorens, O.T.R., and Elizabeth Yerxa, O.T.R., and by my mother.

REFERENCES

1. Dunton WR: National society for the promotion of occupational therapy. Maryland Psychiatr Q 8: 55-56, 1918.
2. Bockoven JS: Legacy of moral treatment: 1800's to 1910. Am J Occup Ther 25: 223-225, 1971.
3. Mosey AC: Involvement in the rehabilitation movement—1942-1960. Am J Occup Ther 25: 234-236, 1971.
4. Freidson E: Professional Dominance, New York, Atherton Press Inc, 1970, p 51.
5. Fidler GS: Learning as a growth process: a conceptual framework for professional education. Am J Occup Ther 20: 1-8, 1966.
6. Yerxa EJ: Authentic occupational therapy. Am J Occup Ther 21: 1-9, 1967.
7. Lawrence PR, Lorsch JW: Organization and Environment, Homewood, Illinois, RD Irvin Inc, 1969, p 3.
8. Drucker PF: The Age of Discontinuity, New York, Harper and Row, 1969, p 41.
9. Ibid, p 15.
10. Reilly M: Occupational therapy can be one of the great ideas of 20th century medicine. Am J Occup Ther 16: 1-9, 1962.
11. Dubos R: The Mirage of Health, New York, Harper, 1959.
12. Lawrence PR, Lorsch JW: Organization and Environment, p 14.
13. Dubos R: So Human an Animal, New York, Charles Scribners Sons, 1968, p 27.
14. Freidson E: Professional Dominance, pp 5-6.
15. Drucker PF: The Age of Discontinuity, pp 52-53.
16. Freidson E: Professional Dominance, pp 91-93.

Academic Occupational Therapy: A Career Specialty

Alice C. Jantzen

I would like to express my appreciation to you as colleagues for the accolade of being selected as the sixteenth recipient of the Eleanor Clarke Slagle Lecture Award of our Association. In particular, I would like to thank the therapists who nominated me and also the many therapists with whom I have been associated during my professional life in occupational therapy education.

Having free choice in the selection of a topic for the lecture and one year to work on the assignment does create some dilemmas, as I am sure any student would understand. Throughout this past year I remained convinced that I should talk with you today about the area of occupational therapy of prime concern to me and the one that I know best—that of occupational therapy education.

The booklet, "Chicago . . . Occupational Therapy Beginnings," by Beatrice Wade and Barbara Loomis, came to my attention recently, and I am pleased that they provided me with some ideas that make my presentation on this topic especially appropriate for a conference in Chicago. To quote, "a significant portion of occupational therapy education history occurred here, in Chicago, with the pioneer efforts of Eleanor Clarke Slagle." Further, "the . . . Lectureship was established in 1955 by AOTA to honor the contributions of Mrs. Slagle to occupational therapy education, to the profession and to the professional organization." (1)

Some of my Slagle predecessors have expressed their concerns about education. Ruth Brunyate Wiemer talked about clinical education; Mary

Reprinted from *The American Journal of Occupational Therapy*, Vol. 28, No. 2, 1974

Reilly presented "A Theoretical Basis for Planned Change in Professional Education"; Gail Fidler spoke about the teaching-learning process involved in education for professions; while Wilma West has written on graduate education, and in the 1960s, under her leadership, our Association carried out an ambitious curriculum study project (2–6). I plan to talk about occupational therapy education from a somewhat different point of view. I would like to have you consider academic occupational therapy as a career specialty in our field, grounded in the basic bodies of knowledge required of clinical specialties, but requiring additional knowledge for competent performance in the academic setting.

Perhaps before I launch into the topic of academic occupational therapy it might be well to present my concept of what is meant by the term specialization.

The practice of occupational therapy is the heart of our field— the delivery of our particular kind of health care services to patients or clients is the reason for the existence of occupational therapy. In the practice setting, the different types of patients we work with demand that we become specialized in the knowledge required to provide effective service—psychiatric, physical disabilities, developmental— thus, we become clinical specialists. But there is another concept of specialization that needs to be clearly acknowledged. This is that the knowledge gained in clinical specialty areas is implemented in different types of career roles. These career roles—all of them essential to occupational therapy—include expert practitioner, program supervisor, researcher, and educator. And the last three require a second set of specialized competencies in addition to clinical expertise. Thus, to return to my topic of academic occupational therapy, I propose that the educational component is both a necessary and essential part of our total field of endeavor and that competent performance as a university faculty member requires both clinical knowledge and additional knowledge and skills specific to this career role. The recent upheavals throughout higher education and the many and diverse changes occurring at this time demand that we give consideration to our educational activities. Since I feel qualified to talk from my own experience, some of my presentation will be autobiographical. However, I believe that the concerns I shall express are not unique to me, but are shared by all of us in this area of our field.

Establishment of a Program

Fifteen years ago I accepted a position at the University of Florida with the responsibility to initiate an undergraduate curriculum and, simultaneously, to establish an occupational therapy service program in the yet-to-be-opened teaching hospital. There were pluses and minuses in the situation, as is true of most situations. On the minus side there was no student awareness of the field; thus, prospective students were nonexistent. Persons in the Health Center and university professed almost no knowledge as to what role occupational therapy played in health care services. At the time there were only about 25 occupational therapists working in Florida, most of them located in the central and southern parts of the state, and there was thus little opportunity to provide reference points for understanding of our field. There were no clinical training centers within an 800-mile radius of the university, and most of the therapists in the southeastern region had never been involved in training students. In essence, I found myself moving into a community in which it would be necessary to carve out and establish the role of occupational therapy in health care delivery, thereby justifying the validity of establishing the educational program.

In some ways no knowledge turned out to be a plus, since I was not confronted with a traditional mind-set about occupational therapy, but largely with lack of information. To be on board in a new venture was also on the plus side—a newly established Health Center complex, designed to house all medical and health-related disciplines, in a state that had not previously trained its own health professionals. The administrative structure was such that we were housed, along with six other academic programs, in a separate College of Health Related Professions. A further plus was the inclusion of the teaching hospital as an integral part of the Health Center. In order for the academic and service programs to be in concert with each other, the chairman of each academic department was appointed as the director of the corollary service in the hospital. Another plus was the fact that the Health Center was located on the main campus of the University of Florida, a large university composed of 15 colleges with a multiplicity of departments and course offerings.

Thus, 15 years ago I saw the setting as having much to offer occupational therapy education. Further, I was most fortunate in being able to recruit five occupational therapists—Genevieve Jonas Widmoyer,

Miriam Thralls, Grace Straw, Reba Anderson, Karen Rasmussen Rusnak—who were willing to join in a pioneering adventure of starting a curriculum and a clinical service program simultaneously.

The essentials for an accredited curriculum tend to foster the idea that our programs should preferably be based in universities with medical schools attached. Such universities usually also have many doctoral level programs, as illustrated by the fact that the University of Florida offers 255 possible majors for a doctoral degree. While there are certain advantages to such a setting, over the years I have learned that in the present stage of development of occupational therapy education, these settings are not without concurrent penalty for us. University administrations tend to reward post-baccalaureate professional programs, such as medicine and law, and those departments which offer Ph.D. programs. In fact, the cost accounting for teaching at the different levels varies, and not in our favor. Furthermore, our programs are inclined to be considered very small operations. For example, while our enrollment figures seem reasonable to us, in terms of numbers we are working with only three-tenths of 1% of the total number of students in our university. Thus the visibility of our program is difficult to achieve; and visibility is the determinant in the long run of staffing and funding for the program. Programs in colleges and universities where the primary emphasis is on undergraduate students are frequently in a far better position than ours to be recognized and rewarded for their endeavors.

Also, I have recently learned that the advantages which led to the decision that all university academic operations be on the same campus resulted in the University of Florida being today one of the three most complex university administrative structures in the nation.

While the heart of the activity of a university occurs at the academic departmental level, there are usually many layers and levels of administrative activities which affect departmental operation, ranging on our campus from academic affairs, to finance and accounting, sponsored research, contracts and grants, and the registrar's office. On the other side, a university has numerous supportive services and resources which can be very helpful in our activities. These include the computer center, teaching resources laboratories, testing and counseling bureaus, student health services, and the financial aid office. A multiuniversity also has a multiplicity of elective course offerings available to our students. At the same time the numerous faculties in such a university provide a major challenge to us when we seek to make course and curriculum changes. In the same way, graduate programs, such as ours, which must work through the graduate school of a university, can have a more difficult time than those in colleges and universities that do not set this requirement.

When I accepted the position as chairman, I was quite naive about the complexities of university administration, but I must admit that today I enjoy the challenge of making us both visible and academically respectable as an educational program. However, the job is not easy, and each year the pressure seems to increase rather than diminish. Further, with changes in the demands for membership in the university community, changes in the university administrative thinking in terms of accountability, time-shortened curricula, and the like, changes in the life demands made on students, as well as increased knowledge of the learning process and of methods of education, the task of providing quality education for occupational therapy students has become increasingly complex.

In order to clarify my views about academic occupational therapy, I shall talk further about faculty, about students, and about our common point of reference, the curriculum.

Faculty Responsibilities

First, some thoughts about occupational therapy faculty, our specialized job demands, and the resultant need for specialized credentials to meet these responsibilities. On our campus, faculty activity is cost accounted into eight categories. I intend to talk about three of these—teaching, service, and research.

Let me talk first about our teaching responsibilities. "That *some* kind of preparation for college teaching is helpful there can be little doubt. But what kind?"(7) The Commission on Undergraduate Education in the Biological Sciences has issued a series of helpful monographs. One, concerned with the preparation of college teachers, categorized the activities and competencies of teachers under six headings. The dimensions are "content mastery," which includes the generally held idea "that one must know something in order to teach it, and that the teacher's information should be up to date"; "the ability to organize a domain of knowledge, to design and plan a course, to establish instructional objectives; effective presentation skills—the 'management of learning'; personal interaction with students," which includes four paramount characteristics—accessibility, authenticity, possession of useful knowledge, such as how to register for next term, and the ability to relate to students; "ability to rigorously evaluate one's own teaching effectiveness; and professionalism" . . . those qualities that differentiate a scholar from an instructor (7).

While in my view the above six dimensions should apply for both academic and clinical teachers, the locus of our work—the university, the classroom, and the laboratory—makes different demands upon our teaching skills. We even have a different jargon, as was pointed out recently by a new faculty member, an experienced clinical teacher, who remarked after attending her first departmental faculty meeting that she hardly understood a thing we were talking about. Just as we, early in our occupational therapy education, received some orientation to medical technology, so, too, faculty members need an orientation to academic terminology.

In occupational therapy education, our faculty activity reports frequently look all right in terms of classroom teaching—student credit hours generated or time devoted to classroom contact. However, our faculty efforts at clinical teaching, a concept well accepted in medical and dental schools, have not yet really been recognized by university administrators. Occupational therapy education programs have been part of colleges and universities since World War II, but our clinical practice requirement seems to be a long way from being accepted as a university responsibility. The one program that led the way in implementing a plan for solving this was the University of Illinois under the leadership of Beatrice Wade. Yet, when deans and administrators seek to find how many faculty are necessary for an academic program, they continue to look to the average number, four or five, needed just for classroom teaching, and to ignore the educational staff of about 17 persons at Illinois.

Next, let me talk about faculty responsibilities for service. This component of a faculty member's role includes the university expectation that we serve on a variety of university committees and not just focus on departmental or college committees. In addition, we are expected to be active in service to the community outside the university confines, be it local, state, regional, or national community. At times I have heard people grumble in AOTA that educators seem to be over-represented in state and national organizations. This is not merely for self-seeking aggrandizement as some might perceive; it is viewed by the university as one of our inherent responsibilities as faculty members. So too, we are expected to be active in a wide variety of local community service organizations and to serve as consultants to various groups and facilities. In other words, we are expected to communicate our portion of the university's storehouse of knowledge.

Next, let me discuss the research responsibilities of faculty. We tend to think the time spent for research is limited to undertaking a formal research project and following it through to conclusion. This is an erroneous assumption. As Van der Kloot says, "Time allocated for research almost invariably also includes time spent in the library, at seminars, talking with colleagues, and at scientific meetings. If I were to stop research tomorrow, all the activities mentioned must still be done, or else I would soon lose touch with my field and all effectiveness as a teacher." (8) So, faculty must devote research time to simply keeping up with their areas of knowledge.

According to Van der Kloot, "The view that the university is solely responsible for teaching, merely as an extension of the high school, is one of the most potentially disastrous ideas circulating in our society. The university has traditionally been responsible for teaching, for research, and for the preservation of knowledge. The tradition evolved because each activity feeds on the others. Any attempt to evaluate how well the job is being done by measuring only one parameter is bound to be incredibly misleading." (8)

To further clarify faculty activity, a final comment is worth making. The university is rightly considered a storehouse of knowledge, but the storehouse is not the libraries as some might think. The storehouse in each university is in the heads of a few hundred professors who constantly keep up-to-date on their areas of specialized interests and who share this knowledge with colleagues and consumers. The university "can be understood only when the role of professor in processing, ordering, and storing information is taken into account and when we realize that the pressure for increasing faculty size comes from the exploding supply of information." (8)

When we consider that the field of occupational therapy reaches out in so many directions and that we present ourselves, in totality, as a field dealing with a myriad of problems, of people ranging in age from infants to elderly, it is apparent that our curricula are grossly understaffed to accomplish the true dimensions of responsibility of university faculty members. In essence, in terms of accountability for faculty time, some of us have been too naive in our knowledge of a university, how it functions, and what it considers important in terms of faculty effort. We, I believe, have therefore been unnecessarily penalizing ourselves and, in fact, the field of occupational therapy, by not paying sufficient attention to university concerns not only for teaching, but also for service, research, and the preservation and expansion of knowledge.

Faculty Credentials

An understanding of the multiple responsibilities of a faculty member in a university leads to identification of the credentials required for faculty status. Since ours is an applied field with the aim of education to prepare practitioners, we ourselves generally require that candidates have a period of work experience as practitioners. When seeking faculty members, we, in addition, usually look for persons with competence in specialized areas of practice, such as pediatric or psychiatric occupational therapy.

Whether we support the idea or not, universities no longer consider competence in the doing, as demonstrated by performance as practitioners, as sufficient for faculty status. We are expected to be more than clinicians and teachers. We are expected to be scholars, and to contribute to knowledge. Thus, universities generally require that faculty candidates have earned the highest degree available in their particular discipline. For us presently that is a master's degree. The fact that most of us with graduate degrees have them in other fields points to the realization that in terms of knowledge areas we do not yet provide the necessary spectrum of options for our own field. Faculty members, in addition, need specialized skills for college teaching and knowledge of how to design strategies for implementing research activities compatible with their interests. They also, as scholars, need to write for publication since the only way, other than by casual conversation, that they can be judged as to their development of specialized knowledge is by having the opportunity to read the results of their explorations. Thus, today we must pay realistic attention to university demands for specialized credentials for faculty.

Students

Now for some comments about today's students. I shall discuss the explosion in numbers of students seeking admission to programs, some of the developmental issues that today's students face as individuals, their potential for becoming helping professionals, and the interaction inherent in communications between students and faculty.

Fifteen years ago we were looking for students, and in 1959 found three willing persons and started our academic program. For several years we had essentially open enrollment, accepting all students who met the admission requirements of the university. It shortly became apparent that many students were interested in majoring in occupational therapy, but 10 years ago it was somewhat like a voice crying in the wilderness to suggest that at a national level we should focus not on student recruitment but on expanding consumer awareness of the services occupational therapy offers.

Today, academic programs are flooded with applicants. Why are so many of today's students selecting occupational therapy as a major? I wish I had a ready answer. Some of it is undoubtedly due to society's shift from a technological imagination to a social imagination; some due to the recent so-called glut of persons prepared in other fields who cannot find jobs. In any event, we as faculty and clinicians are communicating some positive and rewarding behaviors and attitudes which cause students to wish to join our ranks. Having talked with several thousands of prospective students over the years, what I find especially encouraging is their lively concern for the ills of man and of society and their wish to bring about some improvement in the human condition.

In terms of providing a quality education, programs that are able to limit enrollment on the basis of available resources are fortunate. For the past few years we have had three to four academically qualified applicants for each place in the class, a situation which results in our being confronted with a process of selecting which students to admit. Some attempts have been made to find criteria for selection in addition to placement scores and grade point averages. Unfortunately, we as yet do not have other measures which have been proven valid, reliable, and defensible, and the knowledge that seemingly all other helping professions are having the same difficulty is small comfort. The fact is today we must justify the exclusion of many qualified students from the program. How to handle pressure from parents, politicians, administrators, and other health professionals has therefore become an important element of an occupational therapy educator's role.

Next I shall comment about what today's students are like. I shall limit my remarks to those of typical undergraduate age—late teens and early twenties. I do this not only because it is the age group with which

I am most familiar, but also because nationally most of our students are enrolled in undergraduate programs.

Today's college students are dealing with many shifts in values and standards in our society. Need we remind ourselves that this includes occupational therapy students? In our day we were guided by the indoctrination of an established set of values, moral, social and religious, that were geared to the premise that, although changes might occur, they would not be substantial, radical, or continuing. We expected the world we faced upon graduation to represent a milieu perpetuating the best of the past, and the stable endurance of the present. How wrong we were. College students of the 70s are facing the crucial need of a hierarchy of new values to guide them through the turmoil and crises of continuing changes (9). On campuses many of the rules and regulations for student conduct have been eliminated, and a wide range of situations requiring personal decisions now confront today's undergraduates. Even as recently as five or six years ago such choices were largely deferred because of university strictures or were even nonexistent. Situations range from how to live in coed dormitories, to communal living arrangements, the drug scene, the "pill," and abortion. We as faculty need to be aware that our students are dealing with such concerns in their personal lives. Fortunately, most of today's occupational therapy students have lively and healthy character structures and seem able to handle decision making in terms of their personal lives in an effective and mature fashion.

In considering the potential for professional development of today's undergraduate students, we find them to be a very bright and questioning group of young people. While they are ready to learn the necessary skills and techniques, they, along with their fellow students in the university, are ready to question the relevancy of what we teach in terms of both present and future performance demands. In essence, they wish to know not only "how to do," but "why" it is done that way. Fortunately, they are also generally effective in interpersonal relationships, and for us not only a challenge, but fun to work with.

In our roles as faculty some of the learning that took us so long to achieve we can shorten for them by communicating our present knowledge, pointing out uncharted areas demanding solutions, and directing them toward other areas of knowledge that may provide some of the answers they seek. We depend on them to keep the field alive and lively and, by their performance as practitioners, to realize some of our dreams, hopes, and visions for the field. They depend on our experience, the knowledge we have gained, to guide them into becoming competent and confident occupational therapists. So far as I am concerned, that is what the role of educator is all about.

All effective educators fully expect some students to outdistance them in their performance and accomplishments. As educators we derive satisfaction from this. While grades are an important measure of competence, especially for undergraduate students, students need and merit positive reinforcement in still other ways which will indicate to them that they are on the right track toward achieving excellence. Frequently, I am afraid, we tend to focus on the student with problems and neglect to consider that the competent and capable student deserves equal, if not more, attention. Student-faculty interaction is, fortunately, a two-way street, and we as faculty do receive some measure of positive reinforcement from students and graduates. Some we get from teacher evaluations at the end of each quarter. Some from reports on the calibre of performance of our graduates at clinical affiliation centers. We derive satisfaction from a view of the accomplishments of graduates and also from incidental remarks, such as "Whatever you're doing, keep it up!" Such feedback makes it possible for faculty each year to pick themselves up off the floor of exhaustion after working with the presently enrolled classes and to have the courage to start all over again each September with a new class of beginning students.

Curriculum

I would like now to talk some about curriculum both at the basic professional level and also as advanced education. While I shall not discuss assistant-level education, I believe that some of my remarks could reasonably apply to such curricula.

In 1958 I had some ideas that I attempted to incorporate into the curriculum. These were a balance in course offerings between human biology and behavioral sciences, a design of so-called occupational therapy theory courses to emphasize evaluation and treatment principles in the two broad areas of physical and psychological dysfunction, and the inclusion as early as possible of clinical experience concurrent with didactic courses—which we term practicum. When the accreditation team arrived in 1960, we were informed that we met the essentials, but in a rather different pattern than was then usual. As one survey team member said, the plan was too revolutionary and probably would not work.

When one is responsible for another person's education, such a remark can be rather upsetting, but we derived comfort from the knowledge that the same kinds of remarks had been made to the College of Medicine faculty by their survey team. In retrospect, I am happy to say that the curriculum has worked, and very well when judged in terms of the performance of Florida graduates.

During the past 15 years, my ideas about curriculum design have evolved so that today I see curriculum in the following context. A curriculum is more than just a listing of general education courses, prerequisite courses, and required courses in a major. A curriculum should have both an underlying philosophy and a specific identifiable design of the sequencing and patterning of course offerings.

I see two primary factors as determinants of the design. The first is an awareness that the educational objectives of an occupational therapy program include all three components in the taxonomy of objectives: the cognitive domain, the affective domain, and the psychomotor domain. The second major determinant of curriculum design is the awareness that the curriculum needs to be planned in a developmental frame of reference. This developmental focus determines both the sequencing and patterning of courses and also creates a necessary awareness of the developmental process occurring in the students themselves.

Let me first talk further about the three domains in the taxonomy of educational objectives. A group of college examiners interested in achievement testing developed a system of classifying the goals of the educational process by the types of responses specified as desired outcomes of education. They found that most objectives could be placed into one of three major classifications or domains: cognitive objectives, emphasizing recall of knowledge and the development of intellectual abilities and skills; affective objectives, which include interests, attitudes, appreciations, values, and emotional sets of biases; and psychomotor objectives which emphasize motor skill, manipulation of material and objects, or acts which require neuromuscular coordination (10,11).

The practice of occupational therapy clearly emphasizes all three areas. When one reviews the essentials of an accredited curriculum it is evident that all three domains of educational objectives are included. It appears that occupational therapy is a prime example of an academic program whose goal is the development of learning in all three areas. I submit that the entire curriculum should be carefully planned and thoughtfully designed to meet the goals of cognitive, affective, and psychomotor learning required for occupational therapy practice.

In considering the developmental frame of a curriculum, just as Lela Llorens presents occupational therapy practice as facilitating growth and development of patients in seven defined areas necessary for effective performance, so too, we as faculty propose education as facilitating growth and development of students in the cognitive, affective, and motor skill areas of learning necessary for professional performance. "The development of a professional self-conception" according to Lortie, "involves a complicated chain of perceptions, skills, values and interactions. In this process, a professional identity is forged which is believable both to the individual and to others."(12) Vollmer and Mills state that, "You ... have to go through an extended period of socialization ... until you finally develop a psychological and social commitment to a professional career," and further, that "this period of socialization certainly includes formal training."(13) It seems essential, then, in designing academic programs that we keep clearly in mind that this time span is the beginning set in the development of the professional self-concept of an occupational therapist. To have education truly serve as a facilitating process in the growth and development of a professional occupational therapist requires that we consider not only students from a developmental frame of reference, but also all curricular components, the learning experiences, from a developmental frame of reference. This latter requires that we look cross-sectionally at all course offerings— what learning experiences should be offered concurrently; and that we should also look longitudinally to determine the sequencing of learning experiences.

Let me now attempt, by some illustrations, to clarify for you what I mean by curriculum design. When we accept a new class of juniors each fall, we know that in general they are about 20 years of age and that for most of them their major activity since about age 5, three-fourths of their life span, has been to go to school. Most of their formal education to date has focused on the cognitive domain of learning, ranging from the three R's through English, physical science, humanities, biology, and the like. As occupational therapy faculty we seek to continue their cognitive learning in content areas germane to our field. We strive to have them be well-grounded in selected basic areas of human biology; in behavioral science; in the pathology, deviations and disorders to which human beings are subject. We also seek to ensure that they acquire sufficient motor skill in some of the tools of occupational therapy, those environmental things that we use in the treatment process.

Simultaneously, we wish to encourage affective learning in order that students become competent, helping health professionals. The affective domain is not only the hardest to communicate, but it is the area that students most resist. We seek to have them know who they are—to understand themselves, to know how others affect them, including patients who "look very different," fellow students, authority figures, and of equal importance—to help them understand how they affect others. How does one communicate to a student whose own reward system almost exclusively emphasizes high academic achievement that more is needed both as a clinician and a staff member than proof of A's in anatomy, neurology, skills, and the like? I am suggesting that it both can and has been done successfully and that we do it in our roles as educators working with students. Topics such as interpersonal and interprofessional relationships, group dynamics, and the like are built into the program and accomplished by how each course is structured and scheduled. We also seek to have students explore these affective dimensions through the kinds of questions asked on tests, by the reports—written and oral—we require, by term paper assignments, and by how we structure discussion groups.

Now for some examples of the developmental approach to curriculum design. We start off where students are and expand their knowledge of what is normal in the human condition, thus, courses in anatomy and growth and development. They also learn to observe normal social behavior among a wide range of the population; in community day-care centers, nursery schools, boys' clubs, girl scout troops, the hamburger joints and pizza parlors adolescents frequent, adults at work and at play in a variety of settings, and the healthy elderly in their struggles and pleasures found in this business of living in today's society. Simultaneously, other components of the curriculum begin—that of learning necessary skills of occupational therapists—ranging from such content as weaving, woodworking, and leathercraft, to activity analysis, chart reading and reporting, and use of a medical library.

From these bases we move into providing students with knowledge of the abnormal—pathology, neurology, delayed development, with some emphasis given to the sociocultural overlay as an essential factor of concern in identifying physical or behavioral pathology and its effect upon possible remediation of a disorder. In subsequent terms we move to their learning the specific evaluation and treatment procedures which we use in working with people with physical or psychosocial problems. It has been our experience, using a developmental frame, that some topics which might come first in the ordering of chapters in a textbook or in a course outline, can be better presented with meaning to the students at the end of the course or of the program. It is not that we arbitrarily turn programs topsy-turvy, but the sequencing of topics needs to be planned thoughtfully in order to achieve the best learning.

Throughout the entire program students participate in part-time fieldwork, ranging from observations in the normal workaday settings, as described earlier, to practicum assignments in the available clinical settings which surround the program. As they move along and gain knowledge in the content areas of the courses they are taking, they are concurrently expected to become participants in the activities of a clinician to whom they are assigned. Since we wish students to establish a professional identity, for practicum assignments we consider it essential that this in-process occupational therapist—one still learning to become a professional—must have a qualified occupational therapist to serve as role model in the assigned setting. We are also interested in students' learning all the facets of the practitioners' jobs, so it is not necessary that the supervising therapist always be with a patient, as students are, we hope, not learning to become patients. Thus, our felt need for faculty, knowledgeable about the total curriculum, who can serve primarily as clinical educators, role-modeling for students as occupational therapists do in our familiar settings. Furthermore, we consider that the student, still attempting to determine what occupational therapy is all about, cannot realistically assess the role of occupational therapy in locations where none exist. Thus, we feel the need for additional faculty to explore, while at the same time sharing this experience with students, our potential roles in school programs for high-risk first graders, in camps for diabetic children, in crisis intervention centers, health programs for migrant workers, or in a work evaluation unit for hard-core unemployed.

Students themselves consistently tell us that the practicum, this part-time clinical experience component of the program, is one of the most meaningful experiences for them in the curriculum. It provides a "try-out" opportunity to help them determine if the role of occupational therapist suits their personal frames of reference, and also provides them with the reasons to concentrate on learning the content of the standard type courses.

Up to now I have focused my remarks about curriculum design on the undergraduate basic professional level of occupational therapy education. I think, however, that these same considerations need to be given to advanced education in occupational therapy. The cognitive, affective, and motor-skill areas of learning and their interweaving, need to be considered as does the developmental frame of the course offerings and of the students enrolled. At this point it also seems important to reiterate some of my earlier comments as to how I perceive specialization in occupational therapy, since it directly affects my concept of advanced, graduate education for our field. Occupational therapy clinical specialties are grounded in the specialized problems of the different types of patients with whom we work. Career specialties in occupational therapy define the settings and types of positions in which we apply this specialized competence—teacher, practitioner, or administrator.

Ten or 15 years ago, and when I did my several stints in graduate school, I saw the rationale for us in occupational therapy to earn graduate degrees as primarily that of education for competence in career specialty areas of teacher or administrator. After conversations with colleagues in charge of doctoral-level programs, I have become more recently aware that our graduate programs in occupational therapy can be designed to evolve the body of knowledge needed for our field. Graduate education should, therefore, primarily focus on expanded knowledge in the clinical areas of occupational therapy. These areas can be classified developmentally, such as problems of children, adolescents, adults, or the aged; or according to type of insult to the persons we seek to help, biological or psychological. The information needed as administrator, consultant, teacher, or researcher can be gained by means of electives in the program and integrated with the expanded occupational therapy content.

Colleagues in clinical psychology, speech pathology, and medical anthropology have made clear for me that faculty and adventuresome graduate students in their disciplines started together in search of new insights and a clear-cut identification and expansion of the body of knowledge specific to their fields. As time passed, much was learned. Old shibboleths were disproved and dropped, new directions were charted, and today these fields have achieved a status and are making contributions that far outdistance their original roles. Occupational therapy needs to be infused with the same adventuresome spirit, as has occurred in other fields.

According to Ethridge and McSweeney, "the acquisition of knowledge through research, and the subsequent dissemination of this knowledge through publication . . . establishes the basic literature so necessary for the acceptance of occupational therapy as a profession."(14) Since research is an inherent job responsibility of university faculty members, I suggest that occupational therapy faculty take leadership in the research activities for our profession. Further, I suggest that we who are university faculty members begin to demand that university administration support us in these endeavors. Although our graduate program is just beginning its second year, I can guarantee that there is an excitement in working with enthusiastic colleagues and graduate students, each seeking to achieve excellence in a particular specialized area of occupational therapy. Parenthetically, I am sure that our present shortage of qualified faculty could be readily alleviated if clinicians were to perceive that this is the type of interaction in which we are engaged.

It is here that we must begin to think of academic occupational therapy as a career specialty area in the field, no less than academic medicine, academic sociology, psychology, and the like. A combination of the clinician's insight and the academician's discipline, as demanded by his environment, can serve to move the field to take its rightful place among others in the university setting. And this academic status will result in an enhancement of our contributions in the practice setting.

In summary, I have talked with you about occupational therapy education. First off, I identified my own frame of reference in order that you might understand the points of view I have about this phase of occupational therapy. I discussed briefly universities and colleges, their complexities and differences and how these affect an occupational therapy curriculum. Next I gave some information on what are considered by universities to be inherent responsibilities of faculty and some of the consequent qualifications that are considered necessary today for faculty status. I then provided some perceptions about today's students; pressures that they are dealing with, the qualifications of those presently entering the field, as well as dilemmas surrounding the explosion in numbers of prospective students. Following that, I gave some of my views concerning curriculum design—the necessity for considered sequencing and patterning of courses in terms of areas of learning, and in terms of the developmental process of both the students and of the educational objectives. Finally, I discussed advanced education in occupational therapy, a definition of what such education means to me, and suggestions as to how we can foster and develop this phase of the field.

I trust that my remarks will point out for you that, while I consider, as I said earlier, that the heart of occupational therapy is the practice of our field, the educational component, those of us who work in this career role, and our endeavors, are both necessary and essential to the totality of occupational therapy.

REFERENCES

1. Loomis B, Wade BD: Chicago . . . Occupational Therapy Beginnings: Hull House, The Henry B Favill School of Occupations and Eleanor Clarke Slagle, Chicago: Curriculum in Occup Ther, Univ of Ill, 1973
2. Brunyate RW: Powerful levers in little common things. In *The Eleanor Clarke Slagle Lectures 1955-1972*, AOTA, Publisher, Dubuque, IA: Kendall-Hunt, pp 29-48, 1973
3. Reilly M: A Theoretical Basis for Planned Change in Professional Education, University of California at Los Angeles, unpublished doctoral dissertation, 1959
4. Fidler GS: Learning as a growth process: A conceptual framework for professional education. In *The Eleanor Clarke Slagle Lectures 1955-1972*, AOTA, Publisher, Dubuque, IA: Kendall Hunt, pp 137-153, 1973
5. West WL: The present status of graduate education in occupational therapy. *Am J Occup Ther* 12: 291-292, 299, 1958
6. AOTA: Curriculum Study, 16 volumes, New York, AOTA, 1963, mimeographed
7. Dean DS: Preservice Preparation of College Biology Teachers: A Search for a Better Way, Washington, Commission on Undergraduate Education in the Biological Sciences, pp 16, 17, 20, 22, 1970
8. Van der Kloot WG: Comments on financing education. In Anlyan WG et al: *The Future of Medical Education*, Durham: Duke Univ Press, pp 191-192, 1973
9. Bowes N: The development of human values for the college graduate of the '70's, Bedford: June 1973, unpublished college commencement address
10. Bloom BS et al: Taxonomy of Educational Objectives, The Classification of Educational Goals, Handbook I: Cognitive Domain, New York: David McKay, pp 4, 7, 1956
11. Krathwohl DR, Bloom BS, Masia BB: *Taxonomy of Educational Objectives*, The Classification of Educational Goals, Handbook II: Affective Domain, New York, David McKay, p 7, 1964
12. Lortie DC: Laymen to lawmen: Law school, careers and professional socialization. In Vollmer HM, Mills DL (eds): *Professionalization*, Englewood Cliffs: Prentice-Hall, 1966, p 98
13. Vollmer HM, Mills DL (eds): *Professionalization*, Englewood Cliffs: Prentice-Hall, 1966, pp 88, 98
14. Ethridge DA, McSweeney M: *Research in Occupational Therapy*, Dubuque, IA: Kendall-Hunt, 1971, p 1

Occupational Therapy: Realization to Activation

Mary R. Fiorentino

Today I find myself standing before you in this honorable position feeling humble, yet privileged. It is with the deepest appreciation that I acknowledge all those who gave me the support, the assistance, and the contribution to my knowledge, to enable me to be in this position this afternoon.

It was very difficult to select a topic I felt could contribute to the ongoing growth of the profession as it relates to service in the habilitation and rehabilitation of children. In doing so I knew it was necessary to go back in time and return to the lower levels of my own professional development, and to proceed with the sequential maturation that eventually brought me to this "standing position."

In narrowing down the broad spectrum of topics, a review of previous Eleanor Clarke Slagle Lectures revealed that both Lela Llorens and our President Jerry Johnson very aptly expressed two of my major concerns. Lela Llorens presented "a conceptual model for understanding the knowledge that presently supports the practice of occupational therapy with a discussion of how and where occupational therapy fits into the scheme of human development."(1) Jerry Johnson presented "the success and perhaps survival of occupational therapy may well depend upon our ability to clearly identify our product and services, to determine where we can best provide these services, to obtain adequate sources of support for occupational therapy services, and to ensure that we have experienced, competent personnel to provide these services."(2)

Reprinted from *The American Journal of Occupational Therapy*, Vol. 29, No. 1, 1975

In the global overview of occupational therapy, these concerns continue to be of major importance. Does the occupational therapist fit into a developmental scheme, beginning as a neophyte in the profession and progressing to a therapist with special skills, competence, and a secure feeling about basic knowledge? If so, what is the scheme? As a profession, are we able to identify and define this scheme from both an academic as well as a clinical viewpoint? Can we provide competent, professional therapists who are ready to provide services that will meet the demands of health care as we know it today? Are we ready to be challenged by the ongoing advances being made in medicine and research and changes in health care brought about by federal and state regulations? Finally, can we deal with the nebulous definition and role of occupational therapy as it is understood by third-party payees?

Therefore, from my vantage point, I made the decision to follow the theme: The growth and development of pediatric occupational therapy, and the pediatric developmental therapist, or occupational therapist, as they relate to the habilitation and rehabilitation of the physically handicapped child. I would like to explain how this growth and development can evolve, how it can be accomplished in a manner similar to the maturation of a child who is initially at the apedal level, who advances through the quadrupedal level, and finally reaches the highest level of control and skill, that is, the standing position, or bipedal level. I shall not delve into any fancy philosophy. I will attempt to deal with the facts as they have unfolded over the years during my own levels of development evolving from "realization to activation."

The parallel to be drawn between a child's development in all spheres and an adult's development into a highly professional, skilled, competent therapist has many striking similarities. Also, many of the axioms or principles we use from the neurosciences, or more specifically the maturation of the nervous system, have their corollary in the educational development of the occupational therapist.

Let us compare the development of the occupational therapist with the development of the young child. We know now that the infant with an intact nervous system is born with all of the primitive reflexes and reactions. These are basic and necessary in order to have higher skills occur as integration and maturation proceed. We also know that an infant begins at the lowest level of development, the apedal level. He is born with many mechanisms for survival. He has all of the basic senses, cells, and systems of a normal infant's central nervous system (CNS) plus a full potential for learning and maturing. The amount of sensory input received into this nervous system, that is, how the infant is stimulated and handled, will eventually determine his ultimate potential. It is at this early age that the infant's CNS is the most pliable and capable of learning the fastest. Researchers today believe that it takes up to 21 years before the CNS is completely myelinated and matured; however, learning does continue within this system for many years (3).

Initially, the infant relies on his mother for care, for proper or adequate stimulation, and for integration of the feedback resulting from *his* handling of the stimuli. Although he is essentially unable to sustain his own life without assistance, he learns to manipulate his environment by his behavior. The quality and quantity of these stimuli, their reinforcement, and their meaning to him as an organism will have a profound effect on his future development. As stated by Kaluger and Kolson (4), "Each child develops a neural pattern for learning, which includes organizing the cerebral functions and structures involved in the learning process to perform in sensory input, associative functions and motor output." They explain further that integrating basic reactions and reflexes through use of a complex combination of cerebral processes for input, decoding, encoding, and output functions enables the child to progress to a purposeful, responding, conceptualizing individual.

A child in the first several months of life has no mobility, cannot explore his environment and must have experiences brought to him. He is fed, bathed, dressed, loved, spoken to, played with . . . all his senses are stimulated. There is constant change occurring and, if the stimuli are purposeful and meaningful, the child learns. The constant demands placed on the nervous system through all types of stimulation create the basic learning processes necessary to meet the requirement of future development and behavior.

Correlating this concept with a person entering a school of occupational therapy reveals that this individual has many of the same potentials and needs. A student must be provided with all experiences and exposures to ensure that he or she has a base upon which to develop a future as a therapist. The climate of a university allows for assimilation of material at a more rapid pace, but only if that material is presented in a manner that is meaningful, and allows for participation of the individual. It has been proved through animal and human studies that when there is deprivation of sensory stimuli there is no learning. Only when there is active participation does the individual learn more quickly and forget less.

Just as the basic mechanisms for learning and potential are altered if the newborn infant has CNS damage, so the basic education of an occupational therapist can be compromised if the material is not meaningful because it is outdated, or it is irrelevant to clinical advances. If the material is recognized by the student as not having observable application, the result is poorly understood information and inferior application of this knowledge to other situations in a generalized manner. The student or the infant then approaches his next level of development, the affiliation or quadrupedal level, ill-prepared to respond to a new set of stimuli, those that require a greater expertise from him.

At the quadrupedal level the child is ready for mobilization. The student should be ready to synthesize academic knowledge, explore new ideas, learn independently, develop interests, and make each experience as meaningful as possible to have the learning process continue. Therapeutic output will reflect the basic input received during the academic years. If basic courses have been appropriate, if basic preparation has been sufficient, then the student will take advantage of the meaningful experiences of the clinical centers. If the basic preparation has been meaningful, but the affiliation has not given the opportunity to explore, create, problem-solve, and learn, then sensory deprivation will predominate and learning will diminish. The student will continue to need the maturation and integration gained through experience to become a competent, self-sufficient individual performing at the highest level of development.

If there is lack of sensory input into a normal system, abnormal development will be manifest as a functional deficit during the life of the organism. Research tells us that each new learning experience, if properly reinforced, may cause a change in the nervous system to such an extent that behavior can be modified or even permanently changed. Therefore, the quadrupedal individual, infant or student, begins to mobilize and explore his environment, creating new experiences, changing his behavioral patterns while continuing to build up blocks of learning so that further integration can occur. Sequentially, he begins to prepare himself for the next higher level of development.

In the ongoing process of growth and development, the young child reaches standing and walking positions by the end of the first year. Much learning and maturation has occurred during this time; however, he has only basic motor movements and perceptions. The capacities of the adult evolve to meet the requirements of his natural environment. The extent to which these capacities are developed from birth and the rate at which they mature thereafter will depend upon the demands of the postnatal environment.

We know that in the learning process and in the maturation of the nervous system, the infant "perceives" through sensory stimuli into this system. This calls for a response that, in turn, creates new sensations which are immediately fed back into the CNS. Through repetition of an act, the response is "engrammed" into the system and a pattern of behavior is developed. Not until he utilizes this pattern over and over again will the response be an ingrained or semiautomatic, learned response, well integrated into this nervous system.

Thus, the CNS of the child by one year of age has integrated many primitive reactions and has developed higher reactions which enable him to reach the bipedal level. This has occurred through the learning process of perception, then repetition, then active participation. The child has undergone the learning process in all areas of behavior. He is beginning to reach out into his environment, extending his exploration for new fields of learning. He is becoming more independent in his decision making, constantly changing and adding to the information which he has in order to develop higher cognitive skills necessary to cope with his adult environment.

In like manner, the "infant" therapist has basic knowledge at her command. She has perceived, repeated, and utilized this knowledge in preparation for achieving the higher level of development. At this point, he or she must now synthesize and act according to the dictates of this knowledge, problem-solve, make independent decisions, and continue the learning process. All of these actions require higher cognitive skills of behavior. If there has not been a "lesion" created somewhere along in the process of development, the new therapist will evolve into a competent, self-sustaining individual. He or she will be secure in the knowledge of the role of the occupational therapist and in the definition of occupational therapy as an essential discipline in the health fields. The idea of competent, skilled therapists solves the problem of establishing professionalism. Just as one cannot superimpose fine motor activities on a cerebral-palsied child who has no head or trunk control, one cannot superimpose professionalism on people ill-prepared to perform.

I would like now to discuss the role of occupational therapy in a pediatric setting as it relates to rehabilitation of the physically handicapped child. Let us go back down the road to when I started my professional career as a new therapist, full of enthusiasm and idealism about curing the ills of children. As would be expected, I felt that I had some competence and professionalism, but had no idea that, in reality, I was on the apedal level of development. Many events, problems, and frustrations have occurred over these many years to bring me to the bipedal level of development. It should not be necessary to say that, even at my age, I still have some dendritic, collateral growth left in my nervous system to continue to learn and to change according to the dictates of health care with these children. Similarly, our profession still can learn and change.

In the 1950s, when I started my career, the rehabilitative movement was predominant. As stated by Anne Mosey "During the period of 1942 to 1960, perhaps the most significant event influencing occupational therapy was the growth of the rehabilitation movement."(5) She considered the major catalyst for this growth to be the number of returning disabled World War II veterans and the failures of established institutions, the family, school, and organized medicine, to meet their needs. Together with other professional groups, occupational therapy jumped on the bandwagon first and then decided what our role would be in this rehabilitation process. We borrowed, begged, and maybe stole to supplement our armamentarium. The main therapeutic measures in the area of adult physical disabilities were activities of daily living (ADL) training, prosthetic and orthotic expertise, maybe some vocational training along with muscle strengthening and range of motion exercises accomplished mainly through the use of crafts. The latter were also used for diversional and "busy work" activities. These same treatment goals and these same craft modalities were used for children. In many instances, occupational therapy sessions were, in reality, all diversional in nature.

As an unsuspecting therapist starting her career, I had to apply these goals, methods, and modalities to all types of physical disabilities. If you will recall, I said that the therapist at this level of development does not have the expertise to generalize from her academic and brief clinical experiences. Therefore, can she really know what she is doing? Can she know where she is going? Can she know who she is, especially when she realizes that no one knows what occupational therapy is? What she hears is the label of "busy work" or "play ladies." On occasion we received a direct referral for ADL training, or to improve hand-eye coordination, or some type of order to supplement physical therapy in strengthening the upper extremities. Less frequently but more appropriately, we received referrals for upper extremity prosthetic training.

Can you remember when you received a referral requesting ADL training for a severe quadriplegic cerebral-palsied child? How successful were we? We know now that the abnormal patterns laid down during maturation of the CNS are the only patterns that can be elicited, especially on voluntary movement. Sensory input is abnormal; integration is abnormal; motor output is abnormal; sensory feedback into the CNS is abnormal. The child is still dominated by primitive reflexes and/or abnormal tone, and he can move only in these stereotyped patterns. In the realm of emotional and psychosocial areas of behavior, we were seeing adverse reactions because of the child's frustration at his inability to succeed. He knew cognitively what he wanted to do, but could not work out the concept, the process of the task. Under these circumstances, what tools did we have to determine how to cope with this problem? "None." Where did we go for assistance? "Nowhere." The only conclusion was frustration! Frustration, not only for the therapist, but also for the child and his parents who were expected to carry out the therapist's directives.

At this time, in the 1950s, therapeutic media and goals of treatment could be equated to the apedal level of development. I said previously that the infant is born with tremendous potential for development and learning, and that how he is stimulated and handled will determine the realization of this potential.

What is the quality of this stimulus when crafts are the only treatment modality? What is the meaningful experience to the child? Will it have a profound effect on his future development? Crafts were and are non-meaningful to a child's function. There was and is no scientific basis underlying their use (6). In addition, and perhaps even more damaging, the visual image created by these crafts as a treatment modality, and the inability of the therapist, many times, to give a convincing rationale for their underlying value, other than diversional, certainly was not and is not worth the cost to the professionalism of occupational therapy.

It was at this point that I "jumped" into my second stage of development, the quadrupedal level. My experience had not been a meaningful one. I had explored, tried to create, problem-solved; but sensory deprivation was setting in. It was necessary for me to mobilize if I was to provide quality treatment. Also, it was necessary for me to mobilize so that the role of occupational therapy could be accepted as a professional service to the rehabilitation of children.

Self-analysis was important at this point. I asked myself, "Who am I?" "What am I doing?" "Where am I going?"

Who am I? A qualified registered therapist with a certain body of knowledge and experience. What am I doing? Attempting to use this body of knowledge and experience to rehabilitate handicapped children in all areas of behavior to the best of my ability. Where am I going? I didn't know! Frustration and failure in accomplishing the goals of treatment pertinent to the needs of the children were obvious. Added to this frustration was an awareness of the lack of knowledge and acceptance of the profession as a necessary adjunct in the rehabilitation process.

As a consequence, it was imperative that I make a change or forego the pleasure of being an occupational therapist. The choice was clear. To make a change and mobilize into the next higher level of my development, it was necessary to deviate from the established protocol; change the working definition of occupational therapy; change the concept of occupational therapy; and, of utmost importance, alter the modalities.

One definition of the word "change" is to alter, implying the making of some partial change, as in appearance, but usually preserving the identity. Change was necessary to establish the professionalism of occupational therapy. Gross states, "As any occupation approaches professional status, there occur important internal structural changes and changes in the relation of the practitioners to society at large. A useful way of discussing these changes is by reference to the criteria of professionalization: the unstandardized product, degree of personality involvement of the professional, wide knowledge of a specialized technique, sense of obligation (to one's art), sense of group identity, and significance of the occupational service to society."(7)

Herein lies a basic professional concept for occupational therapy. If change is to occur within the organization to meet the standards of professionalism, the primary alteration must be made in the basic formation of a conceptual framework from which an individual can synthesize and then expand his knowledge. Explicit criteria that set standards of performance emanating from this basic conceptual model must be met. In this way a continuous spiral of behavior can be produced to meet and maintain these standards of ethics, group identity, personal obligation, and quality of service. In my estimation, many of these criteria were not manifested in an acceptable manner for recognition. Therefore, change had to come about secure in the knowledge that the identity must remain, that the personal characteristics of the professional must not be lost.

The next decision was to determine how to bring about this change in therapeutic modalities and goals of treatment. Therefore, I asked myself the questions, "What is important in this child's life? What does he need in his process of development to make him a functioning individual capable of coping with the problems of his environment?" Having made this decision, I then attempted to reach the professional stature of an accepted, scientifically based profession.

In his developmental process, important facets in any child's life are gross and fine motor skills, perception, and specific developmental stimulation. These are the concerns of occupational therapy. The therapist attempts to bring the child up to, or close to, his age level, with a thorough understanding of his emotional and social development.

How is he to gain these skills? I felt that the only way was to treat the problem directly and not through a diversional activity such as leather lacing, or weaving. The body of knowledge and expertise the occupational therapist has at her command are far too important in preparing a child to cope with his environment to be relegated to the realm of relaxation with craft activities. This is a basic concept that I feel is essential if we are to be considered a professional discipline.

The first step in the process of my development from apedal to quadrupedal integration went from "realization to activation" of the problems revolving around the needs of the children. The second step was to determine methods to give a child these skills. Through the process of integration of learning, higher levels were attained and I was closer to the bipedal level of development.

In the process of establishing the bipedal level, or the cognitive level of the adult, it was necessary to synthesize all the learning of the two previous levels; therefore, extended exploration into the tools and methods of treatment to professionalize the role of occupational therapy was carried out. This meant standardized evaluations, as much as possible; media which were meaningful to the needs of the child; technical expertise with a knowledgeable background; and, last but not least, the courage of my convictions to carry through these changes in spite of criticism by my peers.

In the areas of gross and fine motor development, we cannot accept, as a goal of treatment, functional use of the hands without first attaining stability of everything to which the hand is attached. Development is cephalocaudal, proximal-distal, medial-lateral, gross to fine. This is how treatment should progress if we are to give children their maximal functional potential. Also, we should place our emphasis on normal developmental sequences of CNS development; for example, learning on a subcortical basis, followed by cortical, voluntary learning, finally reaching the stage of spontaneous, automatic movements.

To reach this process in a meaningful manner, it was necessary to change to techniques of treatment that revolved around the sequential maturation of the CNS and that also emphasized the normal growth and development of the child. To give meaning to the use of these techniques and to provide the secure knowledge and competency to justify these techniques, it was necessary to learn the basic concepts of neurophysiology which were believed to underlie these methods of treatment. In this way I knew that I was not working in a vacuum; I knew that I could confront any physician and justify the "means to an end." This was not a simple task. I was told at one time that it would take 20 years to nurture and develop the "germ" of an idea, and it has taken that long.

Based upon this process of developmental learning, children, such as the cerebral palsied or others with a neuromuscular dysfunction, have benefitted from this treatment to a much greater extent than ever previously attained. Significant changes have been noted in their abilities, resulting in improved function. Many times when basic gross motor movement and then higher motor development have been attained, the child has sufficient fine motor control to begin voluntarily to function by feeding himself, removing his socks and shoes, or playing with toys. At this point, *he* is beginning to manipulate his environment, rather than allowing the environment to manipulate him.

In the process of attaining a goal of treatment, such as feeding, we cannot look at just the skilled act and feel that this is where the role of the occupational therapist begins. We know that the child cannot feed himself if he does not have at least some measure of head, trunk, and arm control. We know also that if the asymmetrical tonic neck or symmetrical tonic neck reflexes are dominating his nervous system with resulting interference of higher motor skills, he cannot perform this skilled act.

The inhibition and/or facilitation of these preparatory mechanisms are a part of the total functional skill. We, as occupational therapists, must have the knowledge, skill, confidence, and security *to treat the total child*. Why should we expect the physical therapist to "prepare" the child and then the occupational therapist merely to teach the child a given skill? First of all, we might find ourselves out of a job; with basic stability the child might function spontaneously. Second, the concept of upper extremities for the occupational therapist and lower extremities for the physical therapist is outdated. You cannot divide the child into parts, especially if you treat developmentally. It is more than the sum of all the parts which leads to the total normal organism; it is the integration of the parts. Therefore, let us break down our defenses and integrate our efforts, making the child our focus, and not permit personal prejudices and preconceived ideas to interfere with what we are all interested in, "The Child."

Two other major areas of treatment for the occupational therapist in pediatric rehabilitation should be: (1) Enhancing perceptual-motor and visual-motor integration; and (2) stimulating children who have lags in their growth and development. I will not proceed through the same process of paralleling development from apedal to bipedal, or from realization to activation, since both were similar to the development of the motor program. Suffice it to say that both of these programs are important in total functioning of any child. They must be included in any pediatric program.

Other rehabilitative goals specific to varying diagnoses are indicated in the area of pediatric-physical disabilities; however, the therapist must decide what is most important in meeting the goals set for her patients. The therapist must have the security and confidence to substantiate these goals and the competence in the methods used to reach them. It is not possible to be all things to all people. For this reason it may be necessary to select fewer major goals of treatment rather than attempting to encompass the gamut of defined goals of occupational therapy. In the judgment of this writer, the occupational therapist in a pediatric setting should utilize her expertise for the development of the child in all areas of behavior. This, we hope, should lead to an integrated functioning individual capable of reaching his maximum potential. Let us remember that a handicapped child is a child first, and then is a child with a handicap.

I should like to read a few statements from an article published in *Scientific American:*

It is obvious that the organism with fully developed and integrated sensory and motor capacities is better prepared to deal with its environment than is one who is lacking in development of these abilities. Beyond the coordination of input and output, however, additional skills are necessary for the higher organism to be successful in its world . . . the basic concepts of action and reaction, cause and effect, behavior and its consequences—which must be acquired through experience with the environment—are the building blocks upon which the organism's continuing understanding of his world will depend (8).

Once we have gained the depth of knowledge necessary to substantiate with confidence our definition of occupational therapy and the role of the occupational therapist, and once we have decided and identified the means through which we can give our services as a professional service, then and only then will we be able to say that we have reached the highest level of development. Occupational therapy has undergone the same process of learning and development as the young child; but it has not reached its fullest potential. Cognitively we realize this; but we need to activate the realizations to meet the changing world of medicine, the controls of government, the demands of professionalism, and the obligations of competency *if we are to survive.*

In summary, the process of the growth and development of occupational therapy and the occupational therapist was compared to the growth and development of the infant from apedal to bipedal levels. A similar comparison was made of the methods of treatment and the modalities used to reach the highest level of development. Neurological maturation and integration must occur in the infant if he is to reach his highest level of development and to be able to function in his environment. Similar sequential maturation must occur from the student level to that of the skilled therapist if he or she is to become a competent professional. An overview of the course of occupational therapy revealed the necessity to mobilize from "realization to activation" so that the role of occupational therapy can be accepted as a professional adjunct in the rehabilitation of the child.

ACKNOWLEDGMENTS

The author wishes to express appreciation for the contributions and assistance given by Constance Harasymiw, OTR and Karen Stonesifer, M.S., OTR, of my staff; Patrick J. Fazzari, M.D., Josephine Moore, Ph.D.,

Ann Grady, OTR, Elnora Gilfoyle, OTR, Paula Habecker, OTR; and my mother and sister.

REFERENCES

1. Llornes LA: Facilitating growth and development: the promise of occupational therapy. *The Eleanor Clarke Slagle Lectures, 1955-1972*, AOTA, Publisher, Dubuque, IA: Kendall/ Hunt Pub. Co., 1973, p 192
2. Johnson JA: Occupational Therapy: A model for the future. *The Eleanor Clarke Slagle Lectures, 1955-1972*, AOTA, Publisher, Dubuque, IA: Kendall/Hunt Pub. Co., 1973, p 229
3. Moore JC: *Neuroanatomy Simplified.* Dubuque IA: Kendall/Hunt Pub. Co., 1969. pp 89-95
4. Kaluger G, Kolson CJ: *Reading and Learning Disabilities.* Columbus: Chas. E. Merrill Pub Co, 1969, pp 29-30
5. Mosey AC: Occupational therapy—A historical perspective: Involvement in the rehabilitation movement—1942-1960. *Am J Occup Ther* 25: 234-236, 1971
6. Moore JC: Are we halfbreeds? (Editorial) *Am J Occup Ther* 17: 200, 1963
7. Gross E: *Professionalization*, Englewood: Prentice-Hall, Inc., 1906, p 9
8. The Nature and Nurture of Behavior. Readings from *Scientific American*, San Francisco: WH Freeman and Co., 1972, p 83

Behavior, Bias, and the Limbic System

Josephine C. Moore

Human and animal behavior has always fascinated me. In my early years, Freud, Adler, Jung, Erickson, and others seemed to suggest the most plausible basis for understanding human behavior. However, during the 1930s and 1940s, scientific disciplines began to study behavior from a different perspective. Biochemistry, endocrinology, and neurophysiology studied behavior in relation to biochemical individuality, the function of enzyme deficiencies, and genetic defects and stimulation studies of the brain. In psychology, a number of individuals broke away from the Freudian school of thought in order to investigate behavior in relation to group interaction and environmental manipulation. Studies were extended into such areas as architectural design, color phenomena, crowding of populations, the effects of sensory deprivation, and other areas too numerous to mention. A number of neuroanatomists began to take a renewed interest in the organism they were studying, especially in regard to the functional implications of various systems, instead of just their structural and mechanical aspects. Paralleling this upsurge of interest in behavior, another group decided to study animals in an entirely new light. These scientists, who called themselves ethologists, realized that animals living in their own environment behaved quite differently from animals confined to a laboratory or an enclosed area. Therefore, the ethologists went out into the field in order to study animals in their natural habitat. By the 1960s a great deal of new and fascinating information had been accumulated from all of these different scientific disciplines concerning animal behavior. Because of my interest in this area, I began to look at man's nervous system, and especially the limbic system, in an entirely new way. Animal research seemed to provide

Reprinted from *The American Journal of Occupational Therapy*, Vol. 30, No. 1, 1976

a great deal of insight into the complexities of the limbic system in relation to man's behavioral mechanisms. Where is the limbic system in the brain and what are the principal functions of this area?

The Location of the Limbic System

Picture a target with a gray bull's-eye and several alternating white and gray bands surrounding the central area (see Figure 1). The gray areas represent the location of specific groups of nerve cell bodies. The white areas represent the fiber connections between these gray areas. In actual numbers, the target has only three gray areas with two white ones interposed. The first gray area, or the bull's-eye, represents the diencephalon or the thalamus, the next gray area represents the basal ganglia, while the outermost area represents the cerebral cortex. These concentric circles graphically depict the basic pattern of the gray and white matter of the brain. The lower parts of the nervous system—that is, the brain stem, cerebellum, and the spinal cord—have been removed in order to use this target concept to understand the structural and functional aspects of the brain in relation to the limbic system.

Returning again to the target concept, the bull's-eye represents some of the oldest evolutionary areas of the brain. The intermediate gray band represents the younger structures, while the most recent phylogenetically evolved area is located on the periphery. The same sequential pattern, from central to peripheral, also illustrates the functional hierarchy of the brain. As the newer and more peripheral structures develop,

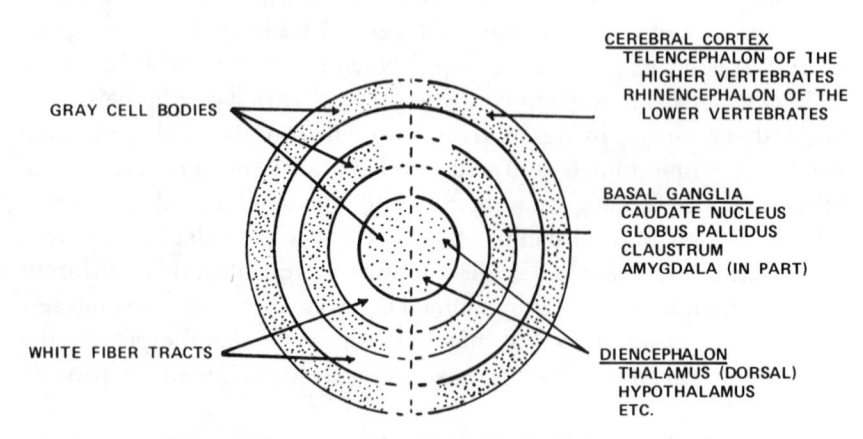

Figure 1 Target concept of the brain (brain stem removed)

there is a tendency for these areas to control and regulate, to some extent, the older centers. Yet, due to the numerous white fiber tracts interconnecting all of these centers, the entire nervous system functions as a total unit.

The target illustration also aids in understanding the names of each of these gray areas. As previously mentioned, the central gray area is called the diencephalon or the thalamus. Diencephalon means "through brain." This implies that almost all of the information received by one's senses, from any part of the body, must pass through this area. The diencephalon integrates and modifies this information before relaying it to surrounding structures. In addition, numerous components of the motor pathways of the nervous system are influenced by this area. Last, but not least, is the fact that part of this area is the master controller of the endocrine system and the autonomic nervous system. Thus the term diencephalon identifies some of the basic functions of this central gray area. But how about the other term, the thalamus? This word means a "bridal chamber." Perhaps the forefathers of anatomy chuckled when they applied this term to this centrally located part of the brain. After all, this area is hidden away in a rather secluded and relatively safe location. Maybe these anatomists were also thinking about the synapses that occur here, and the importance of this center in relation to homeostatic mechanisms in the preservation of the species. Nevertheless, the term thalamus is a rather apt word for remembering the location of this area.

The next gray circle surrounding the thalamus is known as the basal ganglia. During early development of the brain, the ganglion, meaning a mass of gray cell bodies, was located at the base of the brain, hence the term basal ganglia. As the brain matured these cells divided into several distinctive groups and migrated upward in a circular fashion to partially surround the diencephalon (see Figure 2). The basal ganglia were destined to become regulatory centers for many stereotyped reflexes, for sensorimotor functions, for some aspects of visceral behavior, and for a multitude of other functions too numerous to mention.

The outer layer of gray matter represents the cerebral cortex or the bark of the brain. However, if one examines the brain of many of the lower vertebrates, having only a minimal amount of cortex, this outer gray ring represents the rhinencephalon or smell brain (see Figure 1). The rhinencephalon is the oldest part of the cerebral cortex. As the higher vertebrates developed, this older cortical area was displaced medially and was eventually buried in a deeper location as additional cortex was added (see Figure 2). In man, the exposed surface of the brain is still called the cerebral cortex, but the rhinencephalic cortex, which lies hidden from view, is now called the limbic cortex (see Figure 2). What is the reason for this change in terminology? It is because this area of man's cortex is no longer concerned only with the sense of smell and survival mechanisms. As can be seen later, many other functions were incorporated into this area. However, the word *limbic* is a descriptive term, meaning border or the outside edge of a structure. If one examines the medial view of the human brain, the limbic cortex forms an almost complete ring or border of gray matter around all of the deeper structures of the brain (see Figure 3).

This target concept is acceptable for understanding the very basic structural relationships of the brain, but it is limited when discussing different systems of the brain. What is a system in comparison to a structure? The easiest way to explain this is to compare the word *nerve* or *neuron* with the term *nervous system*. A *nerve* is a structural entity

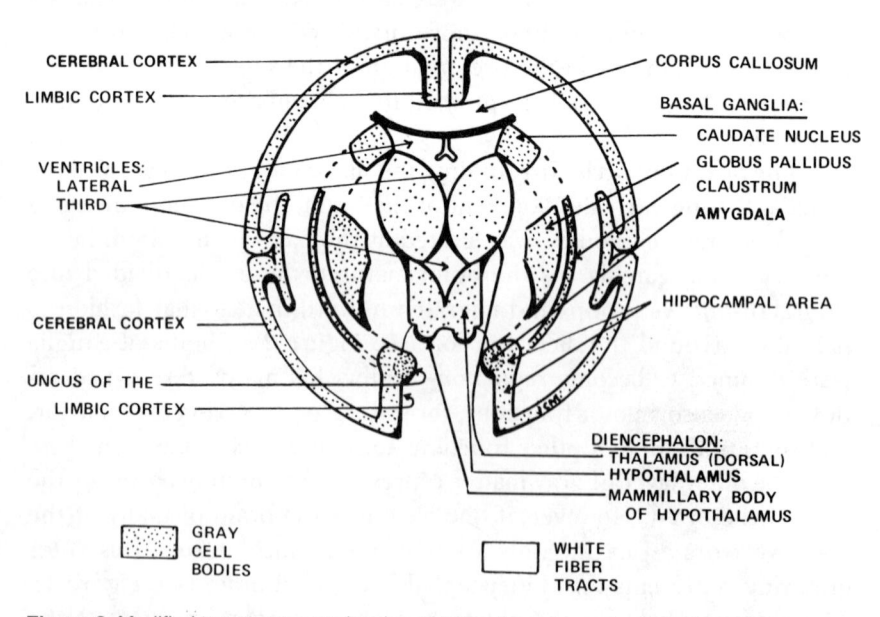

Figure 2 Modified target concept showing white and gray areas comprising the major structures of the brain

consisting of a neuronal cell body and all of the processes, whereas the term *nervous system* refers to all of the neurons and their processes, which function as a total unit and make up the entire nervous system. In other words, the term *system* denotes numerous components incorporated into one functional unit. In the same way the limbic lobe or limbic cortex is ·a limited structural area, while the limbic system comprises *parts* of the old and new cerebral cortex, as well as parts of the basal ganglia, thalamus, midbrain, reticular formation, autonomic nervous system, and on and on. It is not my intention to list in detail all of the structural and functional components of this system as volumes have been written on this subject. Rather, it is more important to understand a few concepts about this system. The *first concept* is that the limbic system ties together or integrates the newest cortical or cognitive centers of the brain with the older sensorimotor systems and the primitive visceral and reticular structures of the nervous system (1-5). The *second concept* is that several of the major structures which comprise man's limbic system evolved from the rhinencephalic cortex or the small brain of lower vertebrates (5-8).

In lower animals the smell brain is the most prominent structure of the entire nervous system. In these animals it is regarded as the area which is primarily responsible for controlling and regulating instinctual drives and survival mechanisms. As the brain of the higher vertebrates evolved, the smell brain diminished in size in comparison to the newer evolutionary structures. However, the function of this area remains as a primary means of survival for the animal kingdom. For example, the sense of smell is necessary for hunting, for locating sources of food and water, and for tracking down distant prey. It is also used to recognize members of one's own group as opposed to those of the same species belonging to another group. It is important for knowing the boundaries of one's territory, finding a den or shelter after a hunt, or for following others during migration. And naturally, smell is one of the primary senses used for procreation of the species. Smell also enables the animal to react defensively or offensively when threatened because this primitive cortical area has a direct influence upon the animal's autonomic nervous system. Thus many of the behavioral instincts of the lower and higher vertebrates are incorporated into this area of the brain (5-8). Even though man's limbic system is much more complex than the animals', man still retains many of the behavioral instincts of the other forms of animal life (5-10). One of nature's basic laws is to retain and enhance behavioral traits which have proved to be effective survival mechanisms, especially those which have assured the preservation of the species. Therefore, the basic functions of man's limbic system are similar, with some exceptions, to that of the higher vertebrates. Let us look at these functions and identify their relationship to behavioral mechanisms.

Limbic System Functions

Perhaps the simplest way to understand the functions of the limbic system is to use the mnemonic word "M-O-V-E." The limbic system is believed to "move" or drive us so that we can survive as individuals and as a species.

M . . . of the word "move" stands for **memory**.

O . . . stands for **olfaction** or the sense of smell.

V . . . refers to **visceral** or autonomic nervous system functions.

E . . . represents the **emotional** components of behavior.

First, let us look at the limbic system in relation to memory. Part of the limbic system appears to be involved with the organism's ability to have instinctual or genetic memory, as well as short- and long-term memory. This does not imply that all memory is confined to the limbic system. Rather, parts of this system appear to contain vital centers through which information must be processed or retrieved in order that the entire nervous system can utilize memory for survival (1-3,6,7).

For example, in the medial aspect of the temporal lobe there is an area, known as the hippocampal formation, which is involved in one's ability to have new memory (1,3,11) (see Figure 3). Two theories have been proposed concerning how this area functions in learning. One theory is that new information has to be processed through this center before it can be retained as memory. The other theory is that this area helps provide recall of memory, that is, this area is part of a memory retrieval system.

If this structure is destroyed on one side, the individual has a temporary loss of the ability to remember new information. Usually the person recovers and is capable of learning new facts. However, if the opposite side is subsequently lost, the individual is unable to learn anything new. Both short-term and long-term memory is permanently lost. Emotional memory, such as swearing, crying, or laughing, and basic defensive mechanisms usually remain and may, in fact, be enhanced or greatly exaggerated (1,11).

A similar lesion at the base of the diencephalon, which destroys structures known as the mammillary bodies, may also cause this same syndrome (1,11) (see Figure 2). The reason for this is that both of these centers are relay stations along a major route or pathway that is necessary for either memory storage or retrieval of information. Therefore, destruction of either area interrupts circuitry, not only within the limbic system, but also between it and the newer areas of the cerebral cortex.

There is another area of the medial temporal lobe which is located slightly anterior to the hippocampal formation (see Figure 3). This area and the surrounding tissue (the amygdala and surrounding cortex) can be destroyed unilaterally due to CVA (cerebral vascular accident) involving small branches of the middle cerebral artery. The interesting feature about the loss of this area, is that no real predictions can be made concerning the behavior of an individual who has a lesion in this center (1,11-13). One person might become docile. Another may be

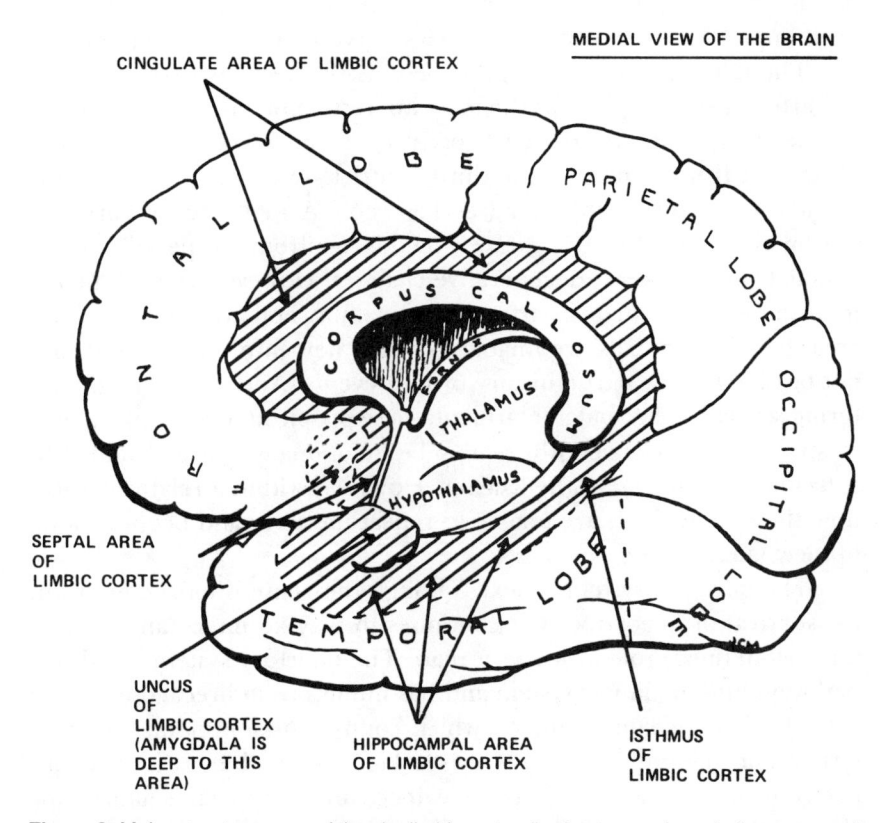

Figure 3 Major structures comprising the limbic cortex (brain stem and cerebellum removed)

overly aggressive. Some may lose the ability to visually discriminate between different objects or be unable to recognize any object at all. Probably the most common syndrome resulting from this type of lesion is the loss of the ability to recognize people. There are several reasons for the behavioral variations seen following this kind of brain damage. One is that this area of the limbic system is intricately interconnected with several different cortical and subcortical structures that are concerned with some of the more primitive behavioral mechanisms used for survival—such as fear, anger, and submissiveness, and visual and olfactory recognition (1,11). Another reason depends upon the exact location of the lesion, such as a relatively small lesion occurring in the more posterior and lateral structures of this center, as opposed to a larger lesion encompassing many adjacent structures (1,3,11). The third reason concerns individual differences, such as one's basic inherited personality, one's biochemical individuality, and the environmental influences which have been impressed upon each individual's nervous system (1,3,11,13-15).

Though there are many other lesions of the limbic system which can affect memory, perhaps the most interesting one is Korsakoff's syndrome (1,11). This syndrome can occur in chronic alcoholics, but it may also result from tumors of the third ventricle or from CVAs (cerebral vascular accidents) in this area (see Figure 2). Actually, several areas of the limbic system can be involved in this syndrome, especially if this results from long-term degenerative changes. However, the most common site is in the medial part of the thalamus. Following a loss of this area, these individuals are unable to retain new information, and may not be able to give a true history of past events. And even though suffering severe intellectual impairment, these people may retain the ability to spin fascinating tales which may be emotionally charged and thus extremely convincing to the listener. However, within a relatively short time these individuals are unable to repeat the story and begin making up new tales.

The olfactory system is next. Though this sense is more important for survival of quadrupeds, it continues to play an important, though not well-defined, role in modern man. The olfactory system has direct pathways into the limbic system and has numerous indirect connections with the hypothalamic centers, which control the autonomic nervous system and the endocrine system (see Figures 2 and 3). It is also connected with the reticular formation, which functions as a mechanism for alerting the entire cerebral cortex (1-3,11). One can understand why the smell of a sizzling steak or the scent of a freshly baked pie can cause saliva and digestive juices to be secreted and make a person feel hungry. Certain smells can also trigger emotionally charged memories which may be accompanied by visceral responses such as an increase or decrease in heart rate, respiration, sweating, or dilation of the pupils. For example, the odor of burning pine logs may remind one of pleasurable events surrounding a wonderful camping trip. This person may become relaxed and drift into a dreamy state recalling past memories. Another individual might be aroused because the pine odor reminds him of a fire which destroyed a home. Thus, odor can be an effective stimulus for bringing back rather specific memories, alerting individuals, or calming them down. It can also be used to stimulate digestion and enhance taste sensations. The reason is that the sense of taste and smell and their central connections in the nervous system are intricately associated with one another as well as with the limbic and autonomic nervous system.

Certain smells also play a very important role in man's sexuality. Many of these odors are believed to be more effective as stimulants if they are perceived on a subcortical or limbic level rather than at the level of cortical awareness. It is no wonder that the perfume and soap industries of the world have made billions of dollars a year catering to these behavioral mechanisms.

Lesions of the olfactory bulb and tract are not very common in man. When they do occur, especially if only one side is involved, they may not be noticed by the individual. However, there is one interesting area on the medial part of the anterior temporal lobe, called the uncus, which can be involved in irritative lesions and does present some rather specific symptoms having to do with olfaction (see Figures 2 and 3). This area of the limbic system helps to integrate olfactory and visual sensations with emotional memories. A tumor or irritative lesion in this area can cause an individual to smell putrid odors which are not present in the atmosphere. This sensation may be accompanied by visual hallucinations associated with the unpleasant smell. As the lesion spreads, the person may have a focal seizure or "uncinate fit" following the sensation of the odor. Fortunately, this type of seizure tends to remain localized within the limbic system—it does not spread to the cerebral cortex. Thus the person usually remains conscious, even though he may not be aware of the seizure per se (1,3,11).

The next major limbic system function concerns the visceral components of behavior. It is now known that everything we do, that is, all behavior, is colored by concurrent changes taking place within our autonomic or visceral nervous system. This in turn modifies all future behavior. Thus the limbic system is believed to help integrate and coordinate visceral responses with cognitive, emotional, and sensorimotor behavior. In this way, the normal system maintains a homeostatic balance in favor of pleasurable rewards and away from painful or nonrewarding stimuli (3-5,7-9).

However, there are occasions when this homeostatic balance goes astray. This is usually the result of excessive physical or emotional stress which is put upon a nervous system, which is unable to cope with these stresses (13,16,17). The resultant behavioral patterns which develop are many and varied and depend upon multiple factors. But usually the limbic system reacts with the most basic survival instinct known to mankind and this is fear (4,5,9,13,18-21). Once this behavioral mechanism is aroused, the entire nervous system is alerted, especially those areas of the autonomic nervous system which control our fight or flight response. If this arousal mechanism is allowed to continue for a long period of time, it may begin to dominate the other systems of the body. Homeostasis is lost, and eventually the entire nervous system can exhaust itself. Man has been trying to cope with this problem for ages. He has used a variety of methods to treat this syndrome, such as witchcraft, prefrontal lobotomies, electroshock and insulin therapy, psychotherapy, and more recently, drug therapy and biofeedback training. Unfortunately, no one method has been successful, or probably ever will be, for all individuals concerned. This is because of man's individual genetic and biochemical differences as well as his multiple and highly variable relationships with his environment (9,13-15).

In the final analysis, no two nervous systems function alike, and this is especially true in regard to each individual's limbic system. Not only has each of us inherited our behavioral traits from different genetic pools, but no two of us have experienced the same environmental stresses. Because of this we have learned to cope differently. Therefore, the behavioral mechanisms of each person are biased by one's individual emotional needs, in spite of the fact that all humans share certain basic limbic drives (4,9,10,12-17).

This brings us to "E" of the word M-O-V-E, or our emotional tone or drives. These drives have long been referred to as the "3 F's," that is, the feeding, fighting, and reproductive drives. Many believe today that these three basic drives are genetically endowed—that is, they are inherited (6-9,16).

Probably the most important of all of the limbic system mechanisms, if one can rank any facet of survival as more important than any other, is found under "E," the emotional drive. This is the feeding drive. Actually, this drive for sustenance consists of two very fundamental and slightly different components. The first and most important is simply called love or TLC (tender loving care). The second component is food. Food, of course, is rather vital for survival but it appears to be less necessary than the need for love (9).

In lower animal terminology, love is defined somewhat differently than for man. Basically, however, it consists of the same principal components, such as the need to be touched and fondled, to be communicated with and accepted. It now appears that the genetic drive for TLC must be fulfilled, to some unknown degree, in order to assure survival. Also, TLC is believed to be the primary drive of gregarious animals. It is not believed to be directly linked to the productive drive per se. Rather, reproduction results only if this first drive is adequately fulfilled (5,7,9).

Research is also showing that this drive "to love and to be loved," to belong, to be accepted, may be the very foundation upon which many higher animals, including man, strive "to be"; upon which some of their territoriality may be based; and upon which survival of normal individuals is assured or lost. Indeed, this drive may be the very reason for standards, laws or codes of behavior, and biases which are found within and among the societies of all gregarious creatures. This drive for love, if adequately met, assures survival of the individual, the family, and the society (4,5,7,9,16,18-21).

Thus the limbic system appears to be the seat of our ability to have memory, emotions, genetic drives, and pre-endowed standards of behavior. Just as important, of course, is the fact that this system is strongly influenced by the environment. Interaction with the environment continually shapes, modifies, and biases our memory, behavior, and emotional tone in relation to everything we do at any given moment.

This continual modification or change of one's behavioral mechanism is not just the result of learned behavior. A great deal of it is probably due to the fact that much of the sensory information received from the environment is handled or taken care of by the nervous system at a subliminal or subcortical level (3,9,22). In fact, much of our early learning is believed to be primarily subcortical, that is, we do not have to think about our basic actions and reactions. The nervous system functions adequately for us on the lower emotional, autonomic, and sensorimotor reflexive levels of behavior. In fact, memory circuits are formed in these lower centers long before cortical control is fully developed and integrated into the limbic and subcortical centers (1-3). Likewise, since man is an emotional animal, he continues to function on this level throughout life, especially when he encounters either positively or negatively charged situations, such as love or fear. Man's nervous system is also genetically endowed or biased to gravitate toward rewards and away from that which is threatening. Likewise, as the nervous system matures, Man, or the animal, quickly learns to reinforce or bias his drives toward pleasurable events, especially if he has received a normal amount of sensory stimuli from the environmental surroundings (3,16,22).

This biasing or reinforcement of the behavioral drives may be accomplished primarily at the limbic or emotional level of the nervous system. One of the most fascinating features of the limbic system is the complexity of the fiber connections of this area, not only with adjacent structures but within the confines of the system itself. It has long been known that electrical stimulation of the limbic system causes long-lasting afterdischarges—that is, a single stimulus can cause this system to continue to reverberate for a relatively long period of time after removal of the stimulus (11). This is not surprising if one examines the intricate connections of this system. In comparison to other areas of the nervous system, this center has a multitude of pathways which are circular in nature, that is, they feed back to themselves. Many of these are also reciprocal. Thus stimulation of any one area not only feeds to other areas of this system, but in turn these feed back both directly and indirectly into the same area which was initially stimulated. It has taken anatomists years to unravel the complexities of this reverberating circuitry, and even today many of these are not completely understood. In spite of this, man has experienced the reverberating nature of this system and has unknowingly used this circuitry for emotional learning. For example, following a stressful situation, these reverberating circuits may cause the entire episode or particular aspects of the event, to keep coming back into the mind, over and over again. The event will continue to reverberate until it is resolved or forgotten. Likewise, a few notes of a song may be heard, and throughout the day the entire tune keeps repeating itself in one's mind. Undoubtedly the reverberating nature of this system is what enables the brain to learn, and store, emotionally charged memories much more rapidly and usually more permanently than nonemotional memory. This is also believed to be one of the reasons why emotional language, such as swearing, singing, crying, and laughing, is usually preserved when a cerebral vascular accident destroys either our cortical language center or its pathways within the nervous system.

Man and the Animal

We have discussed man and the animal in relation to the limbic system and behavioral mechanisms. Man, of course, is rather different from other species. Therefore, is it fair to compare him with animals, especially since he is endowed with a generous amount of cerebral cortex and has the most complex nervous system known to mankind? After all, doesn't man need to use all of this gray matter for learning erudite things he believes he must know in order to interact with and survive in this modern world? Yes, in some respects this makes man different. He is also different in that he seems to have lost some of the ability to function at a limbic or emotional level, that is, he appears to use his intellectual pursuits to override his own needs as well as the needs of others. Could it be that man has not lost his emotional tone or ability to relate to others, but instead he is fearful of developing some kind of oral or anal complex? Perhaps he has also brainwashed himself into believing that he will be dominated by his reproductive or sex drives instead of his primary drive for love. It is my belief that man could eliminate some of his biases and fears by studying the animal, not just intellectually, but also on an emotional or on a limbic level. If he did this, he might begin to see why he behaves as he does, almost instinctively, to various situations he encounters in life. He might even learn more effective, and perhaps simpler and more direct, ways of coping with life without fearing himself or his fellow man.

It is interesting to note that man has associated himself with the animal long before the dawn of history. He has shared his home, affection, and some of his livelihood with four-footed creatures, such as the canines and the felines, down through the ages. These animals were not always used as beasts of burden, sources of food or for protection. Rather the animal as a pet probably enabled man to relate on a limbic level to a creature which readily understands and accepts him for what he is. The animal usually offers unlimited affection in return for a friendly word, a morsel of food, and perhaps some shelter. This enables man to unleash his intellectual drive and express his primary emotional need for love and understanding without the fear of being challenged, dominated, or questioned. Just as important, of course, is the fact that primitive man learned from and understood many of his own behavioral mechanisms and drives from his close association with animals. For example, according to the Indian legend of the Sioux Nation, the wolf was considered as a brother and a teacher. The Indian and the wolf lived together in harmony, sharing the same territory. It is said that they did not fear one another and even helped each other survive, especially if one were wounded, trapped, or lost. Modern man, on the contrary, somehow drifted away from having respect for and a mutual understanding of his four-footed friends. He came to consider animals as beasts of prey, unlimited sources of food or economic wealth, or as threats to his very existence. It is true that man continued to keep animals as pets, but intellectually he divorced himself from them. He denied that their behavior and drives were in any way related to his basic needs. He became so biased that he even failed to use any of his senses to recognize the similarities between himself and what he called "the lowly creatures." This may have been the time when man began to lose a great deal of his ability to comprehend himself, his environment, and especially the animals which resided in it. Fortunately, in the last several decades, man has begun to reverse his opinions. He is taking a new look at himself and his fellow creatures especially in relation to his surroundings, his evolutionary heritage, individual differences, and emotional drives. Man knows, for example, that he is not the only animal with the capability of learning a language and communicating this to his offspring or to others. He knows that he shares the ability to use tools with many of the higher vertebrates, and that this ability can be taught to others. Likewise, man is not the only beast having emotional needs such as the drive for love, touching, acceptance, communication, and understanding. His reactions are now known to be very similar to those of the animal, especially when this need is threatened or fails to be adequately provided throughout the entire life span of the animal (4,5,7,8). Likewise, man recognizes the need to form bonding pairs, family units, and social groups. He is just beginning to comprehend why he has territorial needs, and how he can cope with this kind of behavioral mechanism. He is understanding why there are and have to be natural laws which regulate societies of gregarious animals, such as rules and standards of conduct which govern the behavior of all of the members and demands that individuals accept certain responsibilities if they wish to survive as individuals, as a family unit, and as a society.

Perhaps, through an in-depth study of animal societies, man will gain additional insight and understanding concerning the differences between the emotional needs of the sexes. It is well known that the female and the male are genetically, biologically, and socially different from each other. It is theorized that, because of innate biochemical differences, the limbic or behavioral patterns of male and female are substantially different from one another throughout life (4,7,12,14,15,17). Research in many scientific fields indicates that, among gregarious animals including man, the female of the species instinctively looks to the male for protection, security, and leadership (4,7,9,10,14,16-21). This facet of behavior has never implied, either biologically, phylogenetically, or ontogenetically that the female is inferior to the male. It does say that she is different and has different needs and drives in relation to the opposite sex. This may explain why long ago the females of the human race recognized the need for and established many of the health care fields such as our own and numerous others, and why they have continued to be a major contributor and energy source behind societies which care for the needs of others. Also, it may explain why many of these "care organizations" have experienced rather turbulent histories trying to gain recognition and equality with fields that were established by and have been dominated by the opposite sex. If the male of the species does not or cannot fully recognize and understand the needs which the female recognizes, then it becomes rather difficult for the female to gain recognition, let alone equality, in those areas in which the male has less interest or limbic drive. Likewise, when intellectual beliefs are impressed upon these basic genetic differences, then it begins to look, especially from a man's point of view, and perhaps eventually the woman's, as if the female is the inferior individual. Is it not more accurate to say that the environment creates a feeling of insecurity, not inferiority, in the female of the species? It is well known that the female is neither inferior nor superior. Rather she is different, just as the male is different. Each sex has different drives in relation to one another. Likewise, each sex looks at and experiences the environment from a different biochemical and genetic perspective. This could be expressed as follows: the male drive is more concerned with the conquest of nature, while the female's is to nurture nature. However, both sexes have the same drive to be nurtured. All of these are of equal importance and are essential in the emotional preservation of the species. Animal societies recognize these differences and accept them for what they are. But the human primate has a tendency to forget or ignore them, because of his need to use his cortical gray matter for intellectual pursuits. Also, humans may be different, in that they have a built-in excuse for not understanding others on an intellectual level. It is theorized that the nervous system may not be capable of cortically comprehending that which it has not personally experienced. By the time the nervous system reaches maturity the intellectual brain is believed to be biased toward that which it can readily understand, and away from that which is different, strange, or unknown. It is no wonder then that man appears to be the only species among the higher vertebrates of the animal kingdom who sometimes fails to comprehend his fellow creatures and seems to spend a great deal of intellectual energy denying his emotional needs and forever defending his own biased views, instead of listening to the needs of others.

Conclusion

In conclusion, it is my biased belief that humans need to understand their emotional or limbic brain before they attempt to comprehend their complex intellectual brain. Humans should pause several times each day during their busy lives to observe, study, and interact with a family of canines, felines, or other gregarious animals so that they can begin to understand themselves. It is only in recent times that man has allowed himself to see the similarities which exist between humans, the higher vertebrates, and the environment. Also I feel that man can learn more from observing the animal, rather than his own complex species, because the animal presents a simplified, nonthreatening, and rather rewarding model for comprehending behavioral mechanisms.

Through this avenue of understanding behavior, we might begin to take a second look at some of the comments we hear about our profession. Perhaps one of the most common remarks is that many of our treatment techniques are successful merely because we have the ability to motivate people. The intended implication is that no matter what we do, the individual seems to improve because of the motivation factor. Is this really what is being said? If it is, then the person is admitting that he or she has never listened to us with an unbiased mind. Also, it implies that the individual has failed to read the literature that substantiates many of our treatment techniques. Another implication might be that we, along with many other professions, need additional scientific research to verify some of our techniques. Actually, this remark could mean many things, but in reality the speaker is not listening to what he or she has said. It is a well-known fact that treatment of any kind may fail unless the individual being treated is motivated and has faith in those who are helping him. Thus a person who makes this kind of remark does not realize that he or she is actually giving us one of the highest compliments known to mankind. In effect, the person is defensively saying . . . "How in blazes can you motivate a person to do something when I can't?" Little does the individual know that certain kinds of motivation—or what might be called motivation at a limbic level—is of the utmost importance when working with those who need help. The ultimate expression of all of our limbic drives is the need "to be" . . . to be loved, to be understood, to be wanted and accepted for what we are, or just the need "to be." Unfortunately, this drive is an extremely intangible entity to measure and, of course, man must measure everything he does before he can accept anything as fact. Also, it is rather difficult to measure how quickly this drive "to be" can be lost or shaken when one is confronted with disease, injury, mental illness, loneliness, fear, loss of loved ones, radical changes in life, or any factor that upsets the routine of living. Persons who are not able to perceive the feelings of individuals who have lost some of this drive "to be" may not be able to understand others who have this perceptual ability. This initial lack of insight may also prevent these individuals from being able to comprehend the techniques we utilize in patient treatment. Because of these factors, our profession and others like us may never win many accolades or be understood and recognized as equals in the health community. However, this should never deter us from utilizing treatment techniques which we feel are appropriate for the individual needs of each person. Above all, we should continue to perfect our perceptual abilities which enable us to relate to others on a limbic level instead of functioning entirely at the level of a biased intellectual.

REFERENCES

1. Barr ML: *The Human Nervous System*, 2nd Edition. New York: Harper & Row, 1974
2. Eccles JC: *The Understanding of the Brain*, New York, Mc-Graw Hill Book Co., 1973
3. Williams PL, Warwick R: *Functional Neuroanatomy of Man*, Philadelphia, WB Saunders Co., 1975
4. Smythies JR: *Brain Mechanisms and Behavior*, New York, Academic Press, 1966

5. Barnett SA: *Instinct and Intelligence, Behavior of Animals and Man*, New Jersey, Prentice-Hall, Inc., 1967
6. Beritashvili IS (JS Beritoff): *Vertebrate Memory Characteristics and Origin*, New York, Plenum Press, 1971
7. Hinde RA: *Biological Basis of Human Social Behavior*, New York, McGraw-Hill Book Co., 1974
8. Sarnet HB, Netsky MG: *Evolution of the Nervous System*, New York, Oxford University Press, 1974
9. Harlow HF: *Learning to Love*, New York, Jason Aronson, 1974
10. Goodall JVL: *In the Shadow of Man*, Boston, Houghton Mifflin Co., 1971
11. Willis Jr. WD, Grossman RG: *Medical Neurobiology*, St. Louis, CV Mosby Co., 1973
12. Valenstein ES: *Brain Control*, New York: John Wiley & Sons, 1973
13. Snyder HS: *Madness and the Brain*, New York: McGraw-Hill Book Co., 1974
14. Williams R: *Biochemical Individuality: The Basis for the Genetrotrophic Concept*, Austin: University of Texas Press, 1969
15. Levine S: Sex difference in the brain (April 1966). In *The Nature and Nurture of Behavior*. Readings from *Scientific American*. San Francisco: WH Freeman & Co., 1966
16. Dubos R: *So Human an Animal*, New York: Charles Scribner's Sons, 1968
17. Selye H: *Stress Without Distress*, Philadelphia: JB Lippincott, 1974
18. Lorenz K: *On Aggression*, New York: Harcourt, Brace & World, Inc., 1963
19. Ardrey R. *The Territorial Imperative*, New York: Dell Publishing Co., 1966
20. Mech D: *The Wolf*, New York: Natural History Press, 1970
21. Mowat F: *Never Cry Wolf*, New York: Little, Brown & Co., 1963
22. Moore JC: *Concepts from the Neurobehavioral Sciences*, Dubuque, IA: Kendall/Hunt Publishing Co., 1973

Touch With Care or a Caring Touch?

A. Joy Huss

For 18 years my career as an occupational therapist has been predicated and developed on the premise that sensory input can influence motor output if used appropriately. As I have studied the literature, worked with and observed patients, students, and colleagues, and have been a patient as well, I have come to an additional conclusion—the theme of this presentation. Since effective sensory input includes handling or touching the client, what implications does touch have in our culture, in the framework of occupational therapy, and as individuals? As I informally surveyed colleagues and students, I have been surprised to find that approximately 60% indicate that they are personally uncomfortable touching clients. Some have even expressed feelings of fear. Why? Is this necessary? If touching is therapeutic, how can we learn to be comfortable with it? What implications does this have for our educational curricula and for continuing education? Is touching applicable not only in physical dysfunction but also in psychosocial dysfunction? Are touching (handling) with care and a caring touch mutually exclusive or inclusive? Is touch to be used indiscriminately or are there some possible guidelines? What is the neurophysiological rationale?

Review of the Literature

The neurobiological literature indicates that, first, the skin and the nervous system are derived from the same germ layer, the ectoderm, which provides a critical link between the two. Second, there are basically two major avenues for reception of touch/tactile information (1-3). Various terms have been used to differentiate between the two types of information. In the strict sense, touch is described as the spinothalamic

Reprinted from *The American Journal of Occupational Therapy*, Vol. 31, No. 1, 1977

system—protopathic, primitive, or protective—and is carried primarily in the ventral half of the spinal cord. Tactile information is described as the lemniscal system—epicritic, discriminative, or exploratory—and is carried principally in the dorsal half of the spinal cord. The sense of touch is older, whereas the tactile sense is newer phylogenetically and ontogenetically. Both provide us with information regarding the environment, although each may be processed differently and have different effects on higher centers. Until the touch system is integrated within the functioning of the central nervous system, the tactile system apparently cannot function adequately (4). Tactile areas, especially the lips, index finger, and thumb, have the largest cortical representation both sensorially and motorically. Because the nervous system functions holistically, final interactions of the touch/tactile inputs have effects on the autonomic, reticular, and limbic systems, thus having a profound effect on emotional drives. Moore, in the 1975 Slagle Lectureship, spoke of the need for tender loving care (TLC) as a basic primary drive of the limbic system for survival (5). One of the important components of TLC is touch/tactile input.

Developmentally, touch is one of the first systems to myelinate and thus become functional. The fetus will begin to respond to touch at about eight weeks gestation. In utero, the skin is constantly stimulated by the amniotic fluid and the touch/pressure of the womb. There is tremendous stimulation of this sense during birth. Leboyer has been concerned with providing soothing input to tactual and other systems with his method of *Birth Without Violence* (6). After birth, the baby experiences the environment through touch: by being handled, by clothes, surfaces, objects, and by experiencing himself. It is through this system that the infant gathers information about his body and his external environmental relationships (7). Studies have shown that, without appropriate touch and handling, the infant will not thrive normally even though nourishment and other needs are attended to carefully (8). Does this not speak to the need of the nervous system for meaningful tactual input?

Does this need not stay with us throughout life? Our vocabulary reflects this need with a multitude of references to touch: "keep in touch," "handle with care," "I am touched," "I feel. . .," "how does it feel?" "it feels like. . .," and an experience is "touching." We use such expressions as "being tactful," "rubbing someone the wrong way," "we all need certain strokes," someone has a "soft touch," or "human touch," or is "touchy," and we speak of the need for "tangible" evidence. In addition, many adjectives such as rough, smooth, tender, and painful would have no meaning without previous tactual experience.

Frank (9) indicates that, because the tactual system is one of the first functional systems, the infant uses this as a primary mode of communication. As other systems (auditory, visual, and kinesthetic) mature, they gradually supercede the tactual mode, leading eventually to symbolic communication. The individual learns the taboos of tactual experience through satisfaction *and* conflict so that eventually the child inhibits touching and operates on a symbolic level. This is said to lead to ego development. Frank further states: "Since living in a symbolic world of ideas and concepts is a most difficult and subtle achievement, denial or deprivation of primary tactile experiences may be revealed as crucial in the development of personalities and character structure, and also in the configuration of a culture." (9, p 230)

Initial tactual experiences assist in the development of internal homeostasis. Without internal homeostasis, there will not be an adequate awareness of the external world; thus there arises an inability to shift from tactual dependency to linguistic-symbolic communication. Therefore, with early deprivation we see not only the physical manifestations of speech retardation, learning disabilities, and other gross disturbances, but also emotional and affective problems such as schizophrenia (8,9).

Tactual contacts begin to diminish at about ages five to six in our culture, with the evasion or denial of touch directed more strongly toward the male. The desire to touch and be touched suddenly increases at puberty, first between members of the same sex and then heterosexually. However, in our adult culture, it is reserved primarily for that most intense of human experiences, the sexual process (8-12). Frank indicates that, in this sexual form of interpersonal communication, the primary mode of tactile communication is reinstated "provided the individuals have not lost the capacity for communication with the self through tactile experiences." (9, p 233)

We learn the boundaries for tactual communication culturally. These boundaries vary from culture to culture. Those of Anglo-Saxon origin, especially the English and German, are relatively nontactual. Those of Latin, Russian, Black, Jewish, and primitive cultures are highly tactile peoples. People in the United States are generally considered nontactile (7-16). There are even laws that legislate against touching. Within these cultural groups there will be individual variations that appear to be somewhat dependent on one's experiences within child rearing practices. The need for tactual input is there, however, and may be one explanation for the plethora of pets found in the American culture. Touching and being touched by a pet is acceptable when human touch interaction is denied.

The American culture tends to substitute verbal interaction for body contact with specific distances delineated for various types of communication. Hall has found these verbal interaction distances to be up to 1.5 feet for intimacy; 1.5 to 4 feet for personal subject matter; 4 to 12 feet for nonpersonal, social information; and 12 feet or more for public disclosures (8,11,12,17). It is much easier to talk with an individual or a small group than with a larger one because of the greater distance involved and the smaller amount and kind of feedback received as distance increases.

Goffman (18), however, indicates that middle class Americans are handling one another all the time, if we keep our eyes open to see it. Handling punctuates communication at times when there can only be one meaning received. Thus, the context is all important. It is also involved with status (10,13). For example, it is all right for an adult to touch a young child and for a doctor to touch a patient (high status to touch low status). However, it is generally not acceptable for the patient to reach for the doctor. A group of therapists recently said to me that it was all right to touch the patient, but it was not all right to touch others. In the psychoanalytical tradition it is even taboo for the doctor to touch the patient.

The fact that touching goes on all around us and is ignored indicates our attitude toward it. We equate tactual contact with sex unless it is perfectly clear there is no connection. Thus we use it sparingly to express warmth, affection, understanding, and acceptance. Contact tends to be perfunctory between individuals of the same sex, between parents and their grown children, and in medicine, including the occupational, physical, and speech therapies. The touch is often mechanical and without feeling for fear of revealing too much of oneself or being misinterpreted, especially if that contact occurs on any part of the body other than the upper extremities. Unless involved in lovemaking, most of us tend to be disembodied, with our bodies disappearing from our experience. We suffer from "skin hunger" (10, p 139) as children, as adolescents, and throughout the adult years. Fortunately, child-rearing practices are changing with breast feeding, child backpacks, and the use of cradles on the increase. Rocking chair use by adults is also on the increase, but that form of tactual input, important as it is, is still an impersonal one because it involves only one person. Encounter groups are positive attempts to help us get in touch with our bodies and those of others through various experiential activities.

Perhaps the elderly in our society are deprived the most because of impersonal care in nursing homes and the loss of loved ones. Their distance receptors of vision and hearing decrease in functional capacity; thus limiting experiential capability. These disabilities, compounded by the lack of meaningful touch with others, make their isolation even more acute. The elderly cling to those possessions that can be handled or that evoke memories of lost contact.

A recent, informal survey of 12 individuals in a comprehensive retirement home included the following questions. What is your most valuable possession? Why? The group consisted of eight women and four men; three are still married (two men, one woman), five are widows, two are widowers, and two are single women. Their status include six in fair to very good health, two who are ambulatory with cardiac problems, three with cataracts, one with emphysema, and three in wheelchairs either because of rheumatoid arthritis, multiple sclerosis, or brain stem, cerebellar involvement.

I found their responses quite revealing. The single women responded with "my health," because it permitted them to do the things they wanted to, which included enjoying their friends. One of the married men also indicated his health. His wife was quite ill and I felt it significant that he did not respond to the question until about two hours later, after he had been to visit his wife. He was not asked "why."

One of the men, a minister, replies "my Faith because I have built my life on it and it keeps me going." The lady with multiple sclerosis gave a dual answer. "My husband because I love him the most, and my Bible because it is my hope and inspiration." This woman is quite dependent on her husband for care as the only movement she has is in her right hand.

Of the nine people whose spouses or children or both are still living, six responded that their most valuable possession was their spouse or their children. Their words were different but the basic reason for this was that they are "a part of me, make me feel needed and wanted, and are there if I need help."

One lady's response to the question was her diamond ring because her husband gave it to her. A widower replied "The picture of my wife. I loved her very dearly." Finally one widow with two married daughters said, "If we had a fire I'd grab the picture of my husband and two girls because it can't be replaced."

All of the responses are expressions of a loving, reciprocal relationship that, in one form or another, includes touch, although the word "touch" was never used. (Money and other material possessions as such were not mentioned.)

As Americans we have tended to make a distinction between mind and body. The products of the mind, which rely heavily on the distance receptors, are considered clean, trustworthy, and good. Conversely, those products of the body, which depend on touch, taste, and smell, are considered unworthy—even bad. Some have said that the current sexual revolution will change our tactual habits. But touching is even more basic than sex as a primary drive. Until there is a change in early contact experiences between parent and child, it will be difficult, but not impossible, to change adult behavior (10).

Other cultures and eras placed a great emphasis on touch for healing, destruction, power, or the transference of a life force. Primitive cultures construe the use of touch as magical in curing both mental and physical illness. Many of history's great healers cured their patients by a "laying on of the hands." Galen, Mesmer, Greatrakes the Stroaker, and others in the early history of European medicine wrote of the healing powers of touch. Why then did the strong taboo regarding touch found in the psychoanalytical tradition emerge? Mintz (19) provided us with some historical insight. She thought one of the reasons for the taboo might be that Freud developed his theories during the Victorian era, which, in contrast to the Elizabethan era, was one of sexual prudery with a strong emphasis on the products of the mind. Freud and his associates probably had a strong desire to dissociate themselves from magic and religion in order to be established as scientists. Freud originally used stroking, hypnosis, and therapeutic massage in this practice. However, since he and his associates were viewed as sexual perverts because of their practices, it became important to avoid any contact with the patient no matter how neutral its intent. Although external circumstances at least played a role in the establishment of the taboo, two basic principles of the traditional psychoanalytic approach do seem to contraindicate touching: the rule of abstinence; transference should occur with minimal influence by the real personality of the therapist.

Many contemporary therapists have moved away from the traditional principles of psychotherapy. A review of their tenets finds a variety of attitudes toward touching ranging from nontouch to somewhat mechanical use of tactual input; to the use of contact as a natural part of the relationship; and to its use as a means of knowing through feeling. The literature is replete with the controversy—space not permitting, the reader is referred directly to the literature (8,16,19-38).

The nursing literature has been the most productive in providing controlled studies on the effects of touch (20, 39-41); theoretical concepts (42-44); guidelines for the use of touch in a variety of settings (17,45-48); and student reactions (20,46,49).

Generally, it has been found that the areas most often touched are the patient's forehead, shoulder, and hand. McCorkle's (40) study on seriously ill patients indicated a significant difference between those patients who are touched and those who are not touched during verbal interaction. Ninety-three percent of the experimental group (those who were touched) versus 70% of the control group (those who were not touched) responded positively to the interaction. The analysis indicated that, although the patient may be unaware of the touch, he seems to be more aware of the nurse's concern, interest, and caring when touch is used.

Aguilera's controlled study in a psychiatric setting showed that the use of touch "resulted in increased verbal interaction, rapport, and approach behavior" (20, p 13), especially with the schizophrenic patients. Since the patient population was relatively small and some variables were not controlled, she suggests further study. She does not suggest that touch be used indiscriminately, but that the judicious use of touch may be one means of nonverbal communication with psychiatric patients.

Krieger's (39) research indicates that there is a significant change ($p > .001$) in hemoglobin values as a result of therapeutic touch. Research with plants and animals, where understanding by the recipient is not a factor, has shown significant changes in enzymes when therapeutic touch is used (50). So there *is* more to touch than just the emotional aspect of being accepted and cared for by someone who understands.

Burnside (45) and Preston (47) directed their interests toward the geriatric population with chronic brain syndrome. The basic premises of these studies are, that:

1. In a regressed patient the inability to communicate has led to isolation;
2. Unless repeated contact is made with him he will continue to withdraw;
3. With a nonintact nervous system there is difficulty with the registration, retention, and recall of information;
4. Since tactual input has the characteristic of a conditioned response learned very early in life, the ability to use this system appears to remain viable (47).

Burnside's (45) goals were to:

1. Decrease inappropriate behaviors such as babbling, withdrawal, hallucinations, exhibitionism, and refusing to make eye contact;
2. Encourage appropriate behaviors such as laughing, smiling, spontaneous behavior, expression of negative feelings, display of affection, and tenderness;
3. Develop an awareness of clothes, food, and other people through eye contact and touching.

Touch was the primary method used to reach a small group of six patients. She used an Indian handshake at the beginning and end of each session; a hand on the shoulder when speaking to them; simple hand games; dancing; and other contact activities. And what were the results? The patients began touching each other and the group leader; there was an increase in appropriate verbal communication and eye contact; and they began to respond to music. She noted that they like polkas the best! I believe Ruesch's statement is most apropos. "Nonverbal language takes on prime importance in situations where words fail completely."(51, pp 189,190)

For some time we have heard that under stress there is a tendency for the individual to regress. This has been said in regard to reflex activity when the primitive reflexes reappear, to emotional reactions, and to behavior patterns of the mentally ill and geriatric populations. Can you, from your own professional experience, think of other instances in which this supposition has been used? The scientific literature supports this premise (8,14,17,18,20,30,42,43,46,52-54). Under stress the individual reverts to an earlier, more primitive method of coping, which at some point has been successful. This occurs whether we are healthy or ill physically, mentally, or emotionally. Since the nervous system acts holistically, and ultimately controls our physical, mental, and emotional states, stress can affect any or all three areas of function. Just as we need food, water, and sleep for physical survival, we have a constant emotional need for comfort, reassurance, and security. These needs are particularly active when there is increased stress. The need for body contact, which signifies being loved, comforted, accepted, and protected, can be affected by illness, anger, anxiety, and depression. Due to cultural influences, body contact may be seen by the individual as unavailable, inappropriate, or childish, and therefore, he tries to conceal his need or seeks satisfaction through sex. However, if the person's sexual activity is looked at carefully, it may be seen that being held is really what is being sought (53,54). Could this be one explanation for the increased popularity of massage parlors? It has been suggested that one reason people depend on drugs may be because they do not receive enough body contact, which is the first tranquilizer we experience (14).

Implications

If touch is as therapeutic and necessary for homeostasis as the literature appears to indicate, then what are the implications for us as therapists? How can we learn to use a caring touch? How do we learn to give and receive it comfortably?

At this point in the history of occupational therapy there is a great deal of emphasis on the sensorimotor treatment approaches of Ayres, Rood, Bobath, Knott, and Brunnstrom in both physical and psychosocial dysfunction. All of these include, to some degree, handling of the patient. As I taught these approaches to students and clinicians, I have become aware of those who learned the mechanics of application but were unable to use the approaches effectively. It is not uncommon to have therapists to students able to discuss the basic principles and, on paper, plan good programs. Yet, when provided with the opportunity to "lay on the hands," they sit back and wait for someone else to do it. I have also observed those who perform the treatment in a perfunctory way. They do not use their tactual sense to perceive the changes or lack of change in the patient and thus modify their approach accordingly. For a long time I wondered why this was so.

In other areas of occupational therapy, such as general medicine and surgery, orthopedics, geriatrics, psychiatry, and education, how is touch used, and is there a place for the caring touch? Based on my own professional and personal experience, I reply to that question with an unequivocal "yes," there is a place for the caring touch.

During my own hospitalizations, I became very sensitive to the difference between perfunctory touch and a caring touch, and their effect on my homeostasis. During a one-month stay two years ago, I was the recipient of physical and occupational therapy as well as the care of many nurses, aides, and physicians. I became aware of the fact that most communication was carried on in the 4- to 12-foot social distance range. When it was necessary to be close, the nonverbal message was still, for the most part, that of the greater distance. When touch was necessary, it was mechanical and gave no message of caring. Instead, it was a job to be performed. Being on complete bed rest and knowing that they really did not know what the problem was or how to treat it, I became acutely aware of the effects of sensory-tactual-deprivation. My salvation was one aide and the occupational therapist who were comfortable within the intimate and personal zones and whose hands conveyed a caring touch. They were the only two I perceived as caring for me as a total person and not just another problem occupying a bed. I was experiencing what Dominian (43) calls the "anxiety of disintegration," since my body refused to perform its daily tasks. At such times, physical contact is of great importance.

During my last hospitalization for surgery, I was able to compare the effect on my psyche by an intern who had not yet learned the caring touch, with the effect created by my primary physician who had learned it. I was distressed by the intern who invaded my intimate space with indifference. He appeared to be very uncomfortable. When the surgeon came to see me the day after surgery, he approached the bed, placed his hand on my knee, and asked me how I was doing. I knew immediately that he cared about me as a human being. "The behavior of caring can elicit the feeling of caring."(30, p 173)

It has been observed that most patients coming out of anesthesia or some other unconscious state first begin their reorientation through tactual exploration. They reach for the bed rails or the nearest person and hold on tenaciously (42). My own experience was no exception. I shall be forever grateful for the presence of three people whose touch conveyed "I care." It is interesting to note that these three were not a part of the hospital staff but were two occupational therapy students and a retired nurse. The entire staff, with the exception of my surgeon, were quite distant throughout my hospital stay. I find this rather frightening.

Professionally, I have been aware of the number of individuals of all ages who have demonstrated the anxiety of disintegration and in one way or another reached out for understanding and acceptance. Does anyone hear their cries, or has the medical machine grown so large and impersonal that it zeroes in on the specific problem, ignoring the broader aspects of the total human being? Occupational therapists have said that they treat the total person, that mind and body cannot be separated. And yet we, too, get caught up in the specialization process and concentrate on the problem presented by the patient. The educational process encourages this with compartmental learning. We may talk about the necessity of total care, the acceptance of the individual and the use of therapeutic touch, but our actions reinforce the cultural taboo regarding the touch. Goffman (18) has said that touching can occur in an acceptable way when there is a medical perspective, but we still find that practitioners are uncomfortable using it. Following discussions about the effects of touch, students and colleagues have said to me, "Intellectually I can understand the importance of touch, but how can I learn to use it when my culture says no?" That question haunts me.

It is obvious from the literature and my own experiences that talking about it may be necessary, but talk alone is not sufficient. There must be experiential learning to reinforce it. I am also convinced that we must first experience it with our peers and understanding instructors who can help us sort out our feelings. Second, we must experience it with those in distress and be able to discuss it with a clinician who understands.

Touching involves risk. It is a form of nonverbal communication and, therefore, may be misunderstood by one or both parties involved. It invades intimate space and may be a threat. If we are not in tune with ourselves and the one we touch, it may be inappropriate. However, nontouch may be just as devastating at a time when words are insufficient or cannot be processed appropriately because of disintegration of the individual.

Some of us have had to learn to use therapeutic touch the hard way. Some use it and are not aware of the fact until someone points it out to them. Some perhaps assume that it "goes along with the job" and give it no thought, while others unconsciously fight it and wonder why they are so tense. There have been individuals who have told me that the kind of treatment I do is physical therapy, not occupational therapy, because I handle the patients. Could this possibly be an unconscious reaction to their own discomfort in touching and being touched by others? At the other end of the continuum, there are some therapists who experience an energy flow between themselves and the clients as they work with them.

How, then, can we learn to use touch appropriately? It is not feasible for all of us to participate in encounter groups. For those who do, it can be a very rewarding experience. What can we, as educators and clinicians, do to help our students, colleagues, and ourselves tune in to this vital form of communication?

I believe it is important first to be aware of our own use of and feelings toward nonverbal communication before we can use touch effectively with others. There are many techniques from Gestalt therapy and the Encounter movement that can be used either individually or in small groups. Books, such as *Joy* by Schutz (16), *Awareness* by Stevens (37) and *Sense Relaxation* by Gunther (55), can be very helpful in providing direction in experiential activities.

I would like to share with you some of the activities that I have found helpful. One very simple way to begin to look at your own feelings is to take time to write your name as slowly as you can. When you are finished, reflect on what you felt while doing this. Can you correlate your feelings with some of the reactions you have seen in your clients? One student said to me, "Now I can really understand the frustrations of the patient when he has to concentrate consciously on every movement he makes! No wonder he feels frustrated!"

A period of time spent relating with others without verbal communication can be very revealing. We tend to conceal ourselves behind the use of words, but when forced to communicate without them, we have to share our feelings and thoughts through body language. This can be very difficult for some, enjoyable and easy for others. But again, whatever your reactions, consider them thoughtfully and relate them to your experiences with clients.

There are many people who find it difficult to make contact with others. "Small talk" is threatening ("How do I make a meaningful contact?" "What do I do or say?"). For some it is easier to withdraw, saying "I don't care," and then to live with the agony of loneliness. Others may overreact, becoming boastful or boorish, to cover up their insecurity. All of this may occur quite subconsciously.

One technique that helps to alert us to the conflict of being alone and together is called *Feeling Space* (16). The group sits close together. For five minutes, with eyes closed and hands outstretched, they feel the space all around themselves. They are instructed to feel their reactions to this space and to the contact made with others. Do they prefer to stay in the empty space and resent any intrusion of it by others? Do they feel uncomfortable when invading space of others? Do they enjoy the touch contact? Do they seek it out or withdraw from it? What are the reactions of those around them? This is followed by a discussion of those feelings.

Similar but more generalized feelings about a total group awareness of others as human beings and one's role in a group can be experienced by milling around the room with eyes closed. There should be no verbal communication. When people meet they explore each other for however long and in whatever way they wish. Discussion follows the experience.

The blind walk is extremely helpful in awakening one's senses, and becoming aware of one's dependence on others, and one's reactions to touching and being touched. The participants pair up with someone they trust. One is blindfolded. They are not allowed to communicate verbally. It is the responsibility of the sighted partner to provide an opportunity for as many varied experiences as possible, including the senses of taste, touch, smell, and movement, as well as to provide for the safety of his partner. The blindfolded person is instructed to experience his environment and to identify those individuals with whom he comes into contact. At the end of the allotted time, 30 minutes or longer, they trade places. The immediate reaction upon reconvening is a flood of verbiage. Some have found it extremely difficult not to talk during the experience. They find that their senses of touch and smell are extremely important in orienting themselves and that touch is very meaningful in relating to others, developing trust, and a sense of caring, as well as being necessary for communication with their partner. This can lead to a discussion of the use of touch with their clients.

These are only a few of the many experiential activities that might be helpful. You are urged to explore further.

In our educational process, sensitivity to the effects of touch could be incorporated into many different courses, and the earlier it is begun the better. The faculty, as a group, should first explore their own feelings through experiential activities. It would not only make us better instructors but also better coworkers, since we would be able to sense the feelings and reactions of ourselves and others. The experiential activities could then be incorporated into courses such as kinesiology, neuroanatomy, evaluation procedures, growth and development, physical and psychosocial dysfunction treatment theories, group process, community relations, and administration-supervision. As clinicians explore and become comfortable with a caring touch, it could be then incorporated into the students' fieldwork assignments as well.

To assist the clinicians in their development, this course material could be included in many of the existing continuing education workshops. State associations could sponsor workshops for this purpose. Finally, we can also learn from our clients once we are tuned in to observe our behavior and theirs.

Conclusion

I believe that a concerted effort on our part could make a difference in our own lives and in the lives of those with whom we live and work. If we, as occupational therapists, would begin to use touch in a caring manner, in time we could make a difference in our culture.

Occupational therapists have the necessary academic background in the biological and behavioral sciences to be cognizant of the implications of a caring touch. What we need is an awareness of our feelings as human beings. We need to experience the touch that releases the energy that can refresh, regenerate, and revitalize us whether we are well or ill. "In the hands of a person who understands, touch can sometimes be as effective as drugs or surgery." (55, p 112)

We must learn that touch can be an effective means of nonverbal communication as long as it is acceptable to the touchee and the toucher, together with the understanding that it has a unique meaning to those involved (20).

I urge you to not only review some of the literature, but, more importantly, to experience the caring touch.

> Reach out and touch
> Somebody's hand
> Make this world
> A better place if you can.(56)

REFERENCES

1. Barr ML: *The Human Nervous System*, 2nd Edition. New York: Harper and Row, 1974
2. Noback CR, Demarest RJ: *The Human Nervous System—Basic Principles of Neurobiology*, New York: McGraw-Hill Book Co., 1975

3. Williams PL, Warwick R: *Functional Neuroanatomy of Man*, Philadelphia: W.B. Saunders Co., 1975
4. Ayres AJ: *Sensory Integration and Learning Disorders*, Los Angeles: Western Psychological Services Corp., 1972
5. Moore JC: Behavior, bias, and the limbic system. *Am J Occup Ther* 30:11-19, 1976
6. Leboyer F: *Birth Without Violence*, New York: Alfred A. Knopf, 1975
7. Gibson JJ: *The Senses Considered as Perceptual Systems*, Boston: Houghton Mifflin Co., 1966
8. Montagu A: *Touching—the Human Significance of the Skin*, New York: Columbia University Press, 1971
9. Frank LK: Tactile communication. *Genet Psychol Monogr* 56:209-255, 1957
10. Davis F: *Inside Intuition*, New York: The New American Library, Inc., 1973
11. Hall ET: *The Silent Language*, Garden City, New York: Anchor Press/Doubleday, 1959
12. Hall ET: *The Hidden Dimension*, Garden City, New York: Doubleday & Co., Inc., 1966
13. Gorney R: *The Human Agenda*, New York: Simon & Schuster, 1972
14. Jourard SM: An exploratory study of body accessibility. *Br J Soc-Clin Psychol* 5:221-231, 1966
15. Lomranz J et al: Communicative patterns of self-disclosure and touching behavior. *J Psyhol* 88 (2d half): 223-227, 1974
16. Schutz WC: *Joy—Expanding Human Awareness*, New York: Grove Press Inc., 1967
17. Durr CA: Hands that help—but how? *Nurs Forum* 10:392-400, 1971
18. Goffman E. *Relations in Public*, New York: Basic Books, Inc., 1971
19. Mintz EE: Touch and the psychoanalytic tradition. *Psychoanal Rev* 56:365-376, 1969
20. Aguilera D: Relationship between physical contact and verbal interaction between nurses and patients. *J Psychiatr Nurs* 5:5-21, 1967
21. Burton A, Heller L: The touching of the body. *Psychoanal Rev* 51:122-134, 1964
22. Carvell P: The loving touch. In *Man and Woman. The Encyclopedia of Adult Relationship*, Vol. 1. London: Greystone Press, 1970
23. DeThomaso MT: "Touch power" and the screen of loneliness. *Perspect Psychiatr Care* 9:112-118, 1971
24. Fromm-Reichman F: *Principles of Intensive Psychotherapy*, Chicago: University of Chicago Press, 1950
25. Horner A: To touch—or not to touch. *Voices* 4:26-28, 1968
26. Linden JI: On expressing physical affection to a patient. *Voices* 4:34-38, 1968
27. Lowen A.. *The Betrayal of the Body*, New York: MacMillan, 1966
28. Mercer LS: Touch: Comfort or threat? *Perspect Psychiatr Care* 4:20-25, 1966
29. O'Hearne JJ: How can we reach patients most effectively? *Int J Group Psychother* 22:446-454, 1972
30. Pattison J: Effects of touch on self-exploration and therapeutic relationship. *J Consult Clin Psychol* 40:170-175, 1973
31. Perls FS, Hefferline RF, Goodman P: *Gestalt Therapy*, New York: Dell Publishing Co., 1965
32. Rogers CR, Stevens B et al: *Person to Person—The Problem of Being Human*, New York: Real People Press, 1967
33. Rogers CR: *On Encounter Groups*, New York: Harper & Row, 1970
34. Seagull AA: Doctor don't touch me, I'd love it! *Vocies* 4:86-90, 1968
35. Searles H: Transference psychosis in the psychotherapy of schizophrenia. In *Collected Papers on Schizophrenia*, New York: International Universities Press, 1965
36. Spotnitz H: Touch countertransference in group psychotherapy. *Int J Group Psychother* 22:455-463, 1972

37. Stevens JO: *Awareness: Exploring, Experimenting, Experiencing*, New York: Bantam Books, 1971
38. Warkentin J, Taylor JE: Physical contact in multiple therapy with a schizophrenic patient. *Voices* 4:58-61, 1968
39. Krieger D: Therapeutic touch: The imprimatur of nursing. *Am J Nurs* 75:784-787, 1975
40. McCorkle R: Effects of touch on seriously ill patients. *Nurs Res* 23:125-132, 1974
41. Rubin R: The maternal touch. *Nurs Outlook* 11:828-831, 1963
42. Barnett K: A theoretical construct of the concepts of touch as they relate to nursing. *Nurs Res* 21:102-110, 1972
43. Dominian J: The psychological significance of touch. *Nurs Times* 67:896-898, 1971
44. Luckman J: What patients' actions tell you about their feelings, fears and needs. *Nursing* 5:54-61, 1975
45. Burnside IM: Caring for the aged: Touching is talking. *Am J Nurs* 73:2060-2063, 1973
46. Johnson BS: The meaning of touch in nursing. *Nurs Outlook* 13:59-60, 1965
47. Preston T: Caring for the aged: When words fail. *Am J Nurs* 73:2064-2066, 1973
48. Riehl J, Chambers J: Better salvage for the stroke victim. *Nursing* 6:24-31, 1976
49. Amacher NJ: Touch is a way of caring—and a way of communicating with an aphasic patient. *Am J Nursing* 73:852-854, 1973
50. Grad B: Some biological effects of the laying on of hands; A review of experiments with animals and plants. *Human Dimensions*, 52:27-38, 1975
51. Ruesch J, Kees W: *Nonverbal Communication*, Berkeley: University of California Press, 1956
52. Barthol RP, Ku ND: Regression under stress to first learned behavior. *J Abnorm Soc Psychol* 59:135-136, 1959
53. Hollender MH: The need or wish to be held. *Arch Gen Psychiatry* 22:445-453, 1970
54. Hollender MH et al: Correlates of the desire to be held in women. *J Psychosom Res* 14:387-390, 1970
55. Gunther B: *Sense Relaxation—Below Your Mind*, New York: MacMillan, 1968
56. Ashford N, Simpson V: *Reach Out and Touch (Somebody's Hand)*, Hollywood, CA: Jobete Music Co., 1970

The 1978 Eleanor Clarke Slagle Lecture

Toward a Science of Adaptive Responses

Lorna Jean King

An "asset almost peculiar to occupational therapists is their high tolerance for puzzlement, confusion and frustration." (1) Ten years ago this was the opinion of Dr. J. S. Bockoven, one of our profession's most vocal admirers. Today one might argue about the tolerance, but who could dispute the puzzlement, confusion, and frustration as we look back on a good many years of effort to define practice, to structure theory, and to build philosophies of occupational therapy.

Need for a Comprehensive Theory

And, as we look toward an era of increasing specialization, we are soberly aware that, without a unifying theory to ensure cohesiveness, specialization could easily become fragmentation. In fact, back at the time when the profession's definition began "Occupational therapy is any activity, mental or physical, . . . ," (2) recreation, art, music, and dance all fell under the rubric of occupational therapy. The responsibility for the fact that these modality-based specialties have become separate professions can be assigned in large measure to the lack of unifying theory.

It seems readily apparent that splintering into small professions results in watering-down of job development effectiveness, the scattering of progressively scarcer financial resources for education, and the loss of political "clout." The economics of the health care delivery system will not indefinitely support professional proliferation and duplication of effort. To allow future specialization to result in further fragmen-

Reprinted from *The American Journal of Occupational Therapy*, Vol. 32, No. 7, 1978

tation might well be suicidal. Therefore, we need a framework that will give specialists the bond of a common structure.

We must also cope with the fact that today's consumers, far more sophisticated than in the past, expect to understand what they are paying for. They will no longer accept "on faith" what they are told. This underscores the need for a coherent theoretical model understandable, not just to the professional initiate, but also to the consumer. We may develop complex theories, but, in order to be really useful, they will need to be based on a straightforward structure that can be widely understood, and is clearly related to the client's life functions.

Difficulties in Constructing a Science of Occupation

As a prelude to an attempt to identify a usable theoretical framework, let us look at the roots of some of our difficulties in achieving a science of occupation. One of the difficulties is related to the fact that occupational therapy was born of common sense; and common sense is, by definition, "what everyone knows." Everyone knows that it is a good thing to keep busy. There is the old proverb, "The devil finds mischief for idle hands." Carlyle said it with great feeling, "An endless significance lies in work; in idleness alone is there perpetual despair."(3) One must reach far down on the evolutionary ladder to find organisms that are not active, that simply exist. Occupation, or employment, or activity, is quite literally bred in our bones. Occupational therapy, then, deals with purposeful behavior—with people *doing*. But isn't this what people are engaged in during most of their waking hours? It is hard to see what is significant about such a commonplace fact of life, and that is precisely the problem, or one of them—something so ever present is hard to grasp conceptually. Whitehead is credited with saying that the more familiar something is to us, the more difficult it is to subject it to scientific inquiry (4). As a commonplace example, consider how many eons must have gone by before Man even thought to wonder about the nothingness that surrounded him. A great many more eons probably passed before Man realized that it was *not* nothingness, and named it atmosphere. I am suggesting, then, that the very universality of the filling or occupying of time with purposeful behavior has made it difficult to form concepts that would help us to construct a theory or science of occupation.

Who has not had the experience of trying to explain occupational therapy to someone, only to realize that people think they know all about it because, of course, they have *experienced* occupation and activity. They are thinking about it in everyday terms, and the therapist is, we hope, thinking about it scientifically and analytically. So, although words are exchanged, frequently no communication takes place.

Another problem in constructing models is the difficulty that therapists sometimes have in communicating with each other because of the many levels on which purposeful behavior can be organized. One can talk about the effects of activity on the biochemistry of cells, or about its place as an essential component of neurodevelopment. Purposeful behavior is also basic to cognitive processes; and on the still broader scale of cultural anthropology, an individual's role in the cultural milieu can be thought of as determining purposeful behavior. Conversely, behavior may determine cultural roles. So, whether one looks at biochemical Man, psychological Man, social, economic or ecological Man, purposeful behavior is inextricably woven into the total fabric of human function. However, if one therapist looks at occupation solely in terms of its psychological implications, while another looks only at the cognitive issues, and a third describes chiefly the neurophysiological consequences, a situation results much like that of the blind men examining the elephant. One described the leg, another the ear, and another the trunk. Finally, they were convinced that they could not possibly be talking about the same creature. Certainly an outsider would be hard-pressed to find a principle unifying work simplification, sensory integration, hand splints, and acceptable outlets for aggression, to name just a few of the topics with which therapists may be concerned.

Naturally, attempts have been made to deal with this disparity of viewpoints. Development frameworks are appropriate for many clients, but are not particularly helpful with the normally developed adult who is suddenly faced with trauma or disabling disease. Other models deal with occupation in terms of chronic conditions or the sequelae of disease—a rehabilitative context. These are not readily applicable to developmental problems or acute, as contrasted with chronic, conditions. Few models that I am aware of have spelled out what it is that is peculiar to occupational therapy as contrasted with physical therapy or vocational counseling, for example. What *is* that factor which makes occupational therapy so uniquely valuable that, as Dr. Reilly says, if the profession were to disappear tomorrow, it would have to be quickly reinvented? (5)

General systems theory teaches that systems share common features, that large inclusive systems tend to recapitulate the features found in more specific units. As Laszlo says, "A system in one perspective is a subsystem in another."(6) It seems, then, that our task in finding a theoretical frame for occupational therapy is to identify a level of system that is not so specific as to shut out some of our areas of specialization, nor yet so general as to include a great many more areas than are applicable.

In short, in order to satisfy the profession's current needs, a theory or science of occupational therapy should provide a unifying concept that will apply to all areas of specialization; a framework that will clearly distinguish occupational therapy theory and techniques from those of other disciplines; a model that is readily explainable to other professionals and to consumers; and a theory that is adequate for scientific elaboration and refinement.

Adaptation as a Unifying Concept

While mulling over some of these considerations, I read Konrad Lorenz's recent book, *Behind the Mirror, A Search for a Natural History of Human Knowledge* (7). Lorenz deals essentially with the evolutionary and individual processes of adaptation that are involved in Man's active acquisition of knowledge and techniques. I was struck with the implications of his work for occupational therapy. Then Kielhofner and Burke's recent review of the ideological history of occupational therapy (8) drew my attention to Dr. Ayres' phrase, "eliciting an adaptive response," (9) which seemed a succinct and accurate description of what an occupational therapist does. I was at this time going over the occupational therapy literature, and suddenly the words *adaptation* and *adaptive* seemed to leap out from almost every page. In fact, few of our professional articles fail to mention adaptation, regardless of the author's specialty or point of view. I was struck, like Cortez, with "a wild surmise" (10); could the *adaptive process* be an adequate synthesizing principle for our profession? Is it too nebulous a concept to be useful? Surely it is too simple an idea—or is it? Has its very familiarity, like that of the word *occupation* blinded us to its true significance?

Certainly the words *adaptation* and *adaptive* are well-known to us. We advertise on bumper stickers that occupational therapists are adaptive; we have large investments in adaptive equipment; and assumptions about adaptation are implicit in our literature. Adolph Meyer began his treatise on "The Philosophy of Occupation Therapy," in 1922, by defining disease and health in terms of adaptation (11). But I have not found evidence that we have rigorously analyzed the concept or used it consciously to explain our functions in any broad sense. Perhaps it is time that some of our implicit assumptions about adaptation be made explicit. Only when these assumptions are articulated can their validity be examined through research.

At the outset we must distinguish between adaptation as an evolutionary concept and the process of individual adaptation. Evolutionary adaptation refers to changes in the structure or function of an organism or any of its parts that result from the process of natural selection (12). Natural selection, in turn, is the process by which a differential survival advantage is transmitted to successive generations. The process of evolutionary adaptation is very slow, requiring at the minimum hundreds of thousands of years for significant changes in form or function to occur.

Individual adaptation refers to adjustments made by the individual that primarily enhance personal rather than species survival, and secondarily contribute to actualization of personal potential. Tinbergen says, "Adaptedness is a certain relationship between the environment and what the organism must do to meet it."(13)

The idea of using adaptation as a model in a health-related profession is reinforced by Dr. Rene Dubos in his book, *Man Adapting* (14). He says "states of health or disease are the expressions of the success or failure experienced by the organism in its efforts to respond adaptively to environmental challenges."

Rappaport, the general systems theorist, says "Science is clearly a systematized search for simplicity." He adds, "Seek simplicity, and distrust it."(15) I would invite you, then, to keep a healthy skepticism as we explore the concept, a relatively simple one, that the adaptive process constitutes the core of occupational therapy theory, and that specific attributes of adaptation are also the significant and characteristic attributes of occupational therapy. This will make explicit and specific and testable some of our heretofore unexamined assumptions.

Characteristics of the Adaptive Process

Initially, let us discuss four specific features of individual, as opposed to evolutionary, adaptation. The first characteristic of adaptation is that it demands of the individual a positive role. The adapting person is defined as "adjusting himself to different conditions or environments."(12) In doing this he is acting, not being acted upon. An adaptive response cannot be imposed, it must be actively created. To quote Nobel prize-winning ethologist Tinbergen again, "Living things do not move passively through the physical processes of the environment; they do something against it."(13) Active participation of the client in the treatment process has long been recognized as characteristic of occupational therapy.

Alexei Leontiev, Chairman of the Psychology Faculty of the University of Moscow, reminds us that "Even seemingly simple human functions develop as an interaction between sensory stimulation from the environment and the *person's own activity.*"(16) (Italics by this author)

Even unprofitable or maladaptive adjustments to change are actively entered into. Withdrawal, for example, which is often considered a negative condition, is actually an active response, sometimes appropriate, sometimes maladaptive.

Secondly, adaptation is called forth by the demands of the environment. The challenge of something the individual needs or wants to do—obstructed by change or deficit in the self or the environment—calls forth a specific adaptive response. We could say that occupational therapy consists of structuring the surroundings, materials, and especially the demands, of the environment in such a way as to call forth a specific adaptive response. Another way of saying this is that occupational therapy uses the demands of tasks or other goal-oriented activities in a specially structured environment to trigger the unfolding of a need adaptation.

Among the healing sciences, occupational therapy is unique in its utilization of the demands of the real-life environment. An adaptive response cannot truly be said to have occurred until the individual consistently carries it out in the course of ordinary activities. Thus an amputee may practice opening the hook of the prosthesis over and over, but has not truly adapted to it until the prosthesis is used habitually in a daily routine. The occupational therapist uses this knowledge by providing the amputee with many real-life activities in which to use the prosthesis. The therapist knows that pure exercise, no matter how repetitive, often does not generalize into daily activities, and therefore fails to be adaptive.

This brings us to the *third* characteristic of the adaptive response, namely that it is usually most efficiently organized subcortically, and, in fact, often can *only* be organized below the conscious level. Conscious attention to a task or an object permits the subconscious centers to integrate and organize a response. Dr. Yerxa, in her 1966 Slagle Lecture (17), gave an example that can hardly be improved upon. She said,

"A year ago I helped evaluate a brain damaged client's function. She was asked to open her hand. No response occurred, except that she was obviously trying. Next she was moved passively into finger extension while the therapist demonstrated the desired movement. This time the client responded with increased finger flexion. In frustration she cried, 'I know, I know.' Finally she was offered a cup of water. As the cup was perceived, her fingers opened almost miraculously to grasp it." It would be hard to overemphasize the importance of the therapist's using his or her cognitive powers to structure situations that will elicit a subcortical adaptive response from the client. We tend to rely too much on the client's cognitive processes.

Another example of the importance of subcortical adaptive learning is less familiar to the therapist, but popular with the sports enthusiast. It is to be found in such concepts as "inner tennis." Gallweg, author of *The Inner Game of Tennis* (18), says, "There is a far more natural and effective process for learning and doing almost anything than most of us realize. It is similar to the process we all used but soon forgot as we learned to walk and talk. It uses the so-called unconscious mind more than the deliberate "self-conscious" mind, the spinal and mid-brain areas of the nervous system more than the cerebral cortex. This process doesn't have to be learned, we already know it. All that is needed is to unlearn those habits which interfere with it, and then to just *let it happen*." This approach recognizes the frequently *dis*organizing effects of analyzing consciously what should be automatic sequences of movement.

I stress this point because it is another essential reason why occupational therapists use purposeful activity instead of exercise: namely, that tasks, including crafts, or other goal-directed activities, such as play (where the goal is fun), focus attention on the object or outcome, and leave the organizing of the sensory input and motor output to the subcortical centers where it is handled most efficiently and adaptively. I am suggesting, then, that the distinguishing characteristic of occupational therapy, derived from a similar truth about adaptation, is that *there is always a double motivation:* first, the motivation of the activity itself—catching the ball, creating the vase, making the bed; and the second motivation, recovering from illness, maintaining health, preventing disability—in short, adapting. Now no *animal* recognizes the need to "adapt." It sets out to do something specific—escape a pursuer, or find food. The immediate objective provides the motivation. Adaptation is a secondary and unrecognized goal. But in dealing with humans we need to recognize that the double motivation of therapeutic activity may or may not need to be brought to the client's awareness, depending on age, cognitive function, and so forth. The therapist should see to it, however, that other professionals and the client's family are made aware of *both* motivations, and of how the direct motivation of the activity subserves the indirect, but *primary* motive of therapy.

The implications of the foregoing definitions of the nature of occupational therapy practice are important in light of certain current problems. As mentioned earlier, the profession has been concerned with role definition—how to delimit the boundaries that separate our practice from that of physical therapy or other professions. In a recent report of an American Occupational Therapy Foundation board meeting, to which Washington area therapists were invited, concern was expressed about occupational therapists "infringing on" exercise, the territory of physical therapy (19). And well may we be concerned, for it is *our* professional identity that will be diluted by this infringement, not theirs. Obviously all disciplines that are working with a client should work together cooperatively, but it seems equally obvious that it is uneconomic if there is duplication of function. Exercise has its important place, so also does purposeful activity as a producer of adaptive responses, and this latter is the realm of the occupational therapist. We need to be able to explain in terms of the principles outlined above why purposeful behavior can elicit adaptive responses that exercise alone cannot. Defining our role in this way will be much more satisfactory than the old way of dividing the patient in the middle and giving the top half to the occupational therapist and the bottom half to the physical therapist.

The *fourth* characteristic of the adaptive response is that it is self-reinforcing. In animal behavior the reward for successful mastery of environmental demand is survival, and the penalty for failure is death. In humans the results are seldom so immediate and stark. Nevertheless, mastery of environmental demand is a powerful reinforcer and Maslow lists the drive to master the surroundings as one of Man's innate needs (20). Mastery of one demand is rewarding and serves as a stimulus for attention to the next necessary response at a higher level of challenge. This is the genius of occupational therapy—that, as the old adage has it, "nothing succeeds like success." As the occupational therapist plans and structures successful efforts, each success serves as a spur to a greater effort. Exercise, psychotherapy, behavior modification are all means to an end. But with purposeful activity, the activity itself is an end, as well as being a means to a larger end, therapy or adaptation, hence the double motivation mentioned before.

To summarize the thesis thus far, I am implying that the essential purpose of occupational therapy is to stimulate and guide the adaptive processes through which an individual may best survive and develop. I have suggested that the basic characteristics of occupational therapy derive from the corresponding elements of adaptation: *first*, that it is an active response; *second*, that it is evoked by the specific environmental demands of needs, tasks, and goals; *third*, that it is most efficiently organized below the level of consciousness, with conscious attention directed to objects or tasks; and *fourth*, that it is self-reinforcing, with each successful adaptation serving as a stimulus for tackling the next more complex environmental challenge.

Having tried to identify the basic characteristics of the adaptive process from which the significant features of occupational therapy derive, let us look at some familiar aspects or categories of practice in the light of adaptation, and also at the adaptive process as an organizing principle in two newer or less familiar areas of practice.

In broad general terms we can divide individual adaptation, on the one hand, into the phase that is synonymous with developmental learning, and, on the other hand, the process of adjusting to change or stress.

Developmental Learning as an Adaptive Process

The organizing of sensory input into information, and the subsequent integration of an appropriate motor response, is a continuous adaptive process. As mentioned earlier, Leontiev suggests that human functions consist of the interaction of sensory input and individual activity. For example, we learn to see by seeing. The visual figure-ground skills of a child raised in the green leafy lights and shadows of the jungle will be different from those of the child raised in the clear light and great vistas of the Navajo reservation. Each child begins with similar, basic visual equipment, but the process of learning to see in each environment is a process of adaptation in which available stimuli, combined with active sorting and filing, produce patterned vision.

There are a number of theoretical frames for considering the adaptive processes of early childhood, and the occupational therapy profession can be proud of the several outstanding developmental theorists among its ranks. It is not the intention here to recapitulate developmental theories, but to emphasize the fact that "eliciting an adaptive response," in Dr. Ayres' apt phrase, is, in essence, eliciting goal-directed or pur-poseful behavior. This may be as basic as enticing an infant to lift its head to look at a toy, or more complex, such as suggesting to a child that he shovel sand into a wheelbarrow to trundle across the playground to a sandbox. The child's goal is playing with the sand; the therapist's goal is stimulating cocontraction, heavy work patterns, and so forth, in the service of integrating and organizing sensory input and motor be-havior.

The role of the occupational therapist in stimulating this sequence of integration and response appears deceptively simple to the consumer who cannot be expected to understand, without explanation, that it takes considerable knowledge and professional finesse to know which adaptive response is needed and to provide the proper setting and stimuli for a given action at the opportune moment when the individual's develop-ment makes it possible for him to make a successful response.

We have been considering the well-known field of developmental learning in children. However, it is not only in childhood that one must organize sensory data and respond appropriately. This process goes on throughout life. Afferent, or incoming impulses, particularly those char-acterized as proprioceptive feedback, play a crucial role in sensory in-tegrative processes in adults as well as in children. The key concept is that sensory input is the raw material for adaptation at *any* age. If de-velopmental adaptation does not take place normally in childhood, the adult will show various disabilities ranging, as an example, from mild motor planning problems to severe disabilities such as process schizo-phrenia. Recent studies, suggesting that the adult brain is relatively plas-tic, give some hope that even in adulthood developmental adaptations can be facilitated.

The role of sensory data in the adult has been strikingly illuminated in the last 25 years by a large number of sensory deprivation studies, which have, as a matter of fact, strengthened the theoretical base for sensory integration theory. However, the critical relationship between these studies and the health of the average citizen is just beginning to be appreciated. As an example, consider the scenario for an all too familiar tragedy that goes something like this. An elderly man, in some-what precarious health, must undergo major surgery. As a precaution, he is kept somewhat longer than usual in the intensive care unit. When he is moved to a room, he is kept very quiet, sedated, curtains drawn, and visitors restricted. Somewhere between the third and fifth day, postsurgery, the nurse's notes show that the patient appears to be confused and disoriented. The following day he is hallucinating and has to be restrained because he is trying to get out of bed. There are no family members who are willing to care for him in his apparently deranged state, so he is transferred to a nursing home where he continues in a state of relative sensory deprivation, and his mental and physical condition deteriorates rapidly.

The tragedy is that this kind of occurrence is often preventable. And in the instances where confusion or disorientation occur in spite of precautions, it is important to note that it is often reversible if suitable sensory input is provided. Lipowski, whose studies (21) suggest the reversibility of deprivation-caused psychiatric symptoms, also warns that around age 55 vulnerability to the effects of sensory deprivation increases quite sharply. Thus it is apparent that it is not just the very old who are at risk.

It is also important to note that the effects of deprivation are cumulative, and that the more sensory modes that are understimulated, the faster confusion and disorientation result. One of Lipowski's most significant findings appears to be that immobilization is the most disabling form of deprivation, and that, if added to other sensory losses, is very likely to produce psychiatric symptoms in the vulnerable.

In terms of the emphasis of this discussion on adaptation, we may think of confusion and disorientation as *dis*-adaptation—failure of organization and response. Hallucinatory and delusional phenomena, on the other hand, represent *mal*-adaptation; the sensory data is organized, but incorrectly, and therefore, of course, the response seems inappropriate. So-called unpatterned stimuli are as bad or worse than complete absence of stimuli. "White noise," such as the constant hum of a motor, is an auditory example, while the test pattern on a television set is an instance from the visual domain. Kornfeld, Zimberg, and Malm, in a paper on psychiatric complications of open heart surgery (22), report that "The patient might first experience an illusion involving, for example, sounds arising from the air conditioning vent or the reflection of light from the plastic oxygen tent. Many experience a rocking or floating sensation. These phenomena were often not reported to the staff and could then develop into hallucinatory phenomena and associated paranoid ideation." Kornfeld and his group confirm the harmful effects of immobilization, noting that many patients interviewed after recovery remembered as one of their chief discomforts not being able to move. Let us emphasize again that *sensory input is the raw material for adaptation*. Without adequate sensory data, the individual's adaptive capacity is greatly curtailed.

Motivational loss is another aspect of hospital-induced sensory deprivation that is of critical importance in rehabilitation or therapy. Zubek, in a report on electroencephalographic correlates of sensory deprivation (23), reports that not only were alpha frequencies progressively decreased during 14-day deprivation experiments, but this was also accompanied by severe motivational losses. The abnormal encephalograms persisted for a week after the subjects returned to normal living conditions, *but the motivational losses lasted even longer*. These findings have profound implications for all medical personnel who are trying to motivate patients toward independence. Perhaps the cart has been ahead of the horse! Perhaps the first thing to do is to provide sensory stimulation, particularly of the proprioceptors, through whatever degree of mobility is possible. Then motivation for independent behavior might follow more quickly and spontaneously.

I am indebted to Lillian Hoyle Parent for discussing with me some of the material on sensory deprivation, and, as she points out in her recent helpful summary of the deprivation studies (24), occupational therapists are better prepared than any other health care professionals to make use of this information. A dozen exciting research projects come readily to mind in reference to hospital-induced deprivation. For example, a control group receiving the usual postoperative care could be compared with an experimental group receiving systematic meaningful sensory stimulation under an occupational therapist's supervision. Comparisons could be made of number of hospital days postsurgery, incidence of complications, and amounts of pain and sleep medications.

We have suggested that sensory input and motor output are the essentials of individual adaptation as seen in the familiar field of developmental learning, and we have looked at the less familiar concept of sensory deprivation as a prime factor in *dis*-adaptation or *mal*-adaptation.

Therapeutic Adaptation to Change or Stress

The second general category of adaptive response is adaptation to change or stress. One aspect of response to change is represented by a very active current field of specialization in occupational therapy, namely the field of physical disabilities. This field concerns itself with the individual's adaptation to physical change.

Changes within the person can be of many kinds; what they have in common is they demand that the individual alter habitual responses. Arthritis, heart disease, amputations, spinal cord injuries, stroke, and blindness are a few examples. The use of adaptive equipment, work simplification, splinting, development of strength and skill in residual body segments are among the adaptive considerations in this area of practice. Sometimes the acquiring of appropriate adaptive responses may actually be a matter of survival, as with the cardiac client. More often adaptation means the possibility of actualizing potential that would otherwise be wasted.

While the concepts of adapting to physical change are very familiar to us as therapists, we have had less direct experience with the relatively new field of adaptation as it relates to stress medicine. The role of activity in adapting to or coping with stress is an old idea whose scientific time has come. Dr. Hans Selye, who is considered the "father" of stress medicine, comments, "The existence of physical and mental strain, the manifold interactions between somatic and psychic reactions, as well as the importance of defensive-adaptive responses, had all been more or less clearly recognized since time immemorial. But stress did not become meaningful to me until I found that it could be dissected by modern research methods and that individual tangible components of the stress response could be identified in chemical and physical terms."(25) Dr. Selye called this stress response the "general adaptation syndrome." Today few literate people are unaware of the fact he demonstrated: that any stimulus which appears to pose a threat to survival elicits a response that includes the secretion of the cortico-steroids which prepare the body for a fight or flight reaction. The heightened blood pressure, pulse, and respiration that follow a danger signal had a distinct survival value when the appropriate reaction was running, or climbing, or hand-to-hand combat. In our present culture, running, climbing, or fighting are seldom considered appropriate responses, and threats are often perceived as long continued, like the danger of losing one's job, or the daily stress of driving through rush-hour traffic. There are well-known stress diseases such as ulcers, high blood pressure, and heart disease, to mention the most common, that follow chronic stimulation of cortico-steroid secretion. The current vogue for jogging, marathon running, and other strenuous sports owes part of its very real usefulness as a health maintenance measure to the fact that exercise metabolizes and renders harmless the stress hormones that otherwise might accumulate and cause permanent damage to the body.

What is not so often considered is the effect of either subtle or overt stress on an already over-taxed system. A person who is already feeling ill is told he must enter the hospital. Whether it is for surgery or for tests, or for nursing care, everything about the experience spells danger: the strangeness, the uncertainty, the painful or uncomfortable procedures, but most of all the feeling of helplessness. Stress hormones are poured into a system that not only is already reacting to the stress of illness, but also has few opportunities for activity that might help to metabolize and dissipate the cortico-steroids. Stress hormones can make the sick person sicker and can retard recovery.

It is often assumed that *rest* is what is needed in the hospital, but, as Dr. Selye points out, unless the organism is completely exhausted, activity of some sort is much more appropriate to stress dissipation than too much rest. Many years ago an occupational therapist frequently stopped into a hospital room and made available purposeful, goal-directed activities that allowed the patient an adaptive response to stress. If we had known then what we know now, we might have called it *stress management* or *stress reduction therapy*. Instead, someone used the word *diversional*, with the result that the whole area of human needs has been virtually abandoned, and the word *diversional* has become the equivalent of profanity. In fairness we must point out that few third-party reimbursement agents are willing to pay for something labeled *diversional*.

To turn to another aspect of this subject, before the stress hormones and their physiological effects had been identified by Dr. Selye, we often spoke of *tension*, and in the mental health field were able to recognize the usefulness of activity, even though the reasons were vague. Dr. Roy Grinker writes of the treatment of *battle fatigue* or *war neuroses* (26) and says, "In their free time physical activities are encouraged in order to dissipate accumulated tensions. Enforced idleness and rest are bad therapy for these states." Later he comments, "The patients are busy the whole day with physical and mental activities and various aspects of occupational therapy."

The high hopes held for the usefulness of the psychotropic drugs led to the serious curtailment of other forms of treatment such as those described by Grinker. Now that there is widespread disillusionment with the major tranquilizers, which seem to cause almost as many problems as they solve, perhaps the efficacy of what might be called *adaptational therapy* will be rediscovered.

The psychiatric disorders provide excellent examples of the interrelatedness of the various aspects of the adaptive process. In some instances, as in autism or in process schizophrenia, we are probably dealing with inadequate developmental adaptive learning and the attendant severe problems in perception and communication. These problems inevitably produce stress and the concomitant physical changes produced by the stress hormones. These, in turn, probably further derange the sensory-integrative processes. Many of the symptoms seen in the psychoses represent either disadaptations or maladaptive behavior. As the therapist is able to facilitate adaptive development, that is, sensory integration, coping behaviors improve. Activity also helps to metabolize stress hormones and thus increases the client's feeling of well-being. Though basic biochemical causes may ultimately be found for some of the major psychoses, there will probably always be a need for facilitating adaptive or coping skills in a society that seems increasingly stressful.

Psychologists Gal and Lazarus, it seems to me, have made the strongest case of activity as an adaptive response to stress. Their article, "The Role of Activity in Anticipating and Confronting Stressful Situations" (27), spells out the physiological correlation of activity with the reduction, or metabolism, of the stress hormones. They point out that while activity which is related to the cause of the stress is best, yet activity of any kind is better than none. Their useful analysis of the literature concludes with these words: "Regardless of the interpretation, it seems quite evident that activity during stressful periods plays a significant role in regulating emotional states. We are inclined to interpret activity as being a principal factor in coping with stress. As has been repeatedly argued by Lazarus a person may alter his/her psychological and physiological stress reactions in a given situation simply by taking action. In turn this will affect his/her appraisal of the situation, thereby ultimately altering the stress reaction."

To summarize, we may divide adaptation in response to change or stress into three major components of concern to the occupational therapist:

1. Adaptation to physical change (which includes a component of adaptation to stress because the physical changes are in themselves stressors);

2. Adaptation to the stress of hospitalization or acute illness;

3. Adaptation to reduce stress reactions in psychiatric conditions.

We have engaged in a lengthy exploration of stress and adaptation because it seems that in the foreseeable future coping with or adapting to stress is going to be one of the major health challenges facing humanity. Toffler, in his book *Future Shock* (28), makes a good case for the thesis that the extremely rapid rate of change in almost all of our cultural institutions is a significant cause of stress for large segments of humanity, certainly including our own. Ethologist Tinbergen warns, "The amounts of strain now imposed on the individual may well overstretch man's capabilities to adjust."(13) If it is true that stress is a major health problem for modern man, and if, as Gal and Lazarus propose, activity is of major importance in stress adaptation, then occupational therapy has a major role to play in health maintenance and disease prevention as well as in health restoration.

One of my colleagues (Roene Shortsleeve) once drew a cartoon that expressed this rather well. She drew a bearded figure in the white robes of a prophet. In his hand was a placard which read, "The world is NOT coming to an end; therefore, you had better come to occupational therapy and learn to cope."

Conclusion

I have attempted to demonstrate in this paper that the adaptive process can provide a theoretical framework for occupational therapy that meets the criteria suggested at the outset: that it can be applied to all the specialty areas as a unifying concept; that it will differentiate occupational therapy from other professions; that it is readily explainable to other professionals and to consumers; and that it is adequate in depth to allow for scientific elaboration and refinement.

The adaptive process is probably not the only tenable model for occupational therapy. If this paper spurs others to articulate a more suitable theory, it will have served its purpose.

Toffler, in concluding *Future Shock*, comments that, as yet, there is no science of adaptation. Is it too ambitious to suggest that occupational therapists are uniquely prepared to begin constructing *a science of adaptive responses?* It is a challenge worthy of our best.

REFERENCES

1. Bockoven JS: Challenge of the new clinical approaches. *Am J Occup Ther* 22:24, 1968
2. Dunton WR: *Prescribing Occupational Therapy*, Springfield, IL: Charles C Thomas, 1947

3. Carlyle T: *Past and Present*, Boston: Houghton Mifflin, 1965, p 196
4. Thayer L: Communications systems. In *The Relevance of General Systems Theory*, E Laszlo, Editor. New York: Braziller, 1972, p 96
5. Reilly M: The educational process. *Am J Occup Ther* 23: 300, 1969
6. Laszlo E: *The Systems View of the World*, New York: Braziller, 1972, p 14
7. Lorenz K: *Behind the Mirror: A Search for a Natural History of Human Knowledge*, New York: Harcourt Brace Jovanovich, 1977
8. Kielhofner G, Burke JP: Occupational therapy after 60 years; An account of changing identity and knowledge. *Am J Occup Ther* 31: 657-689, 1977
9. Ayres AJ: *Southern California Sensory Integration Tests Manual*, Los Angeles: Western Psychological Services, 1972
10. Keats J: On first looking into Chapman's Homer. In *Century Readings in English Literature*, JW Cunliffe, Editor. New York: The Century Company, 1920, p 639
11. Meyer A: The philosophy of occupation therapy. *Arch Occup Ther* 1: 1-10, 1922
12. Stein J (Editor): *Random House Dictionary of the English Language*, Unabridged. New York: Random House, 1966
13. Tinbergen N, Hall E: A conversation with Nobel prize winner Niko Tinbergen. *Psychol Today*, March: 66, 74, 1974
14. Dubos R: *Man Adapting*, New Haven: Yale University Press, 1965, p xvii
15. Rappaport A: The search for simplicity. In *The Relevance of General Systems Theory*, E Laszlo, Editor. New York: Braziller, 1972, pp 18, 30
16. Leontiev AN, cited by Cole M, Cole S: Three giants of Soviet psychology, conversations and sketches. *Psychol Today* 10: 94, 1971
17. Yerxa E: Authentic occupational therapy. *Am J Occup Ther* 21: 2, 1967
18. Gallweg WT: *The Inner Game of Tennis*, New York: Random House, 1974, p 13
19. The Foundation. *Am J Occup Ther* 31: 114, 1978
20. Maslow AH, Murphy G (Editors): *Maturation and Personality*, New York: Harpers, 1954
21. Lipowski ZJ: Delirium, clouding of consciousness and confusion. *J Nerv Ment Dis* 145: 227-255, 1967
22. Kornfeld DS, Zimberg S, Malm JR: Psychiatric complications of open-heart surgery. *New Engl J Med* 273: 287-292, 1965
23. Zubek JP: Electroencephalographic changes during and after 14 days of perceptual deprivation. *Science* 139: 490-492, 1963
24. Parent LH: Effects of a low-stimulus environment on behavior. *Am J Occup Ther* 32: 19-25, 1978
25. Selye H: *The Stress of Life*, New York: McGraw-Hill, 1956, p 263
26. Grinker R: *Men Under Stress*, 2nd Edition. New York: McGraw-Hill, 1962, pp 30, 218
27. Gal R, Lazarus RS: The role of activity in anticipating and confronting stressful situations. *J Human Stress* 4: 4-20, 1975
28. Toffler A: *Future Shock*, New York: Random House, 1970

Remember?

L. Irene Hollis

Being named an Eleanor Clarke Slagle lecturer brings many problems, especially for someone who is about to retire. The delight in being named for this high honor is tempered by the reality of the responsibility involved. Choosing a topic for the lecture is especially difficult. From the moment the letter from the President of the Association arrives with the news that you have been selected—asking whether you will accept—your mind races along trying to choose a topic that will be of general interest.

As most of you know, my last 15 professional years have been involved in hand rehabilitation. The 20 before that had been much more diversified. I went into occupational therapy in 1944 after nine years of teaching home economics. One might say that Lorna Jean King, last year's Slagle Lecturer, and I are "late bloomers" since she, also, has had about 35 years of experience. Checking back over the list of recipients of the Slagle award I found that June Sokolov, who gave the second Slagle Lecture in 1956, had only nine years of experience in occupational therapy when named to the honor. Josephine Moore, the 1975 Lecturer, had 11. The average number of years of experience of the 21 lecturers, so far, was 19.

During the period of time that I was struggling to decide on a topic for my lecture, I was on one of my numerous flights to or from a city where I had been teaching. I was reading the magazine supplied at each seat and enjoyed an article entitled "Memory" reprinted from the August 1978 issue of *Fortune Magazine*. This helped me decide on the topic. I had been considering the idea of how important one's professional roots are and how much one is indebted to the people who have been influ-

Reprinted from *The American Journal of Occupational Therapy*, Vol. 33, No. 8, 1979

ential through the years. In 1675 Sir Isaac Newton said: "If I have seen further . . . it is by standing on the shoulders of giants." It has been my good fortune to have many giants in our profession to boost me along the way. If you will indulge me, I would like to relate some of the meaningful memories I have accumulated these 35 years. It is said that one remembers things better and longer if they are pleasant, so the memories I relate will be the ones that brought pleasure. In general, my years in occupational therapy have been exciting and fulfilling, and I only hope that those of you who are young in the field will get as much satisfaction from your work as I did. My enthusiasm still runs high.

In 1944 I was happily teaching high school home economics only 30 miles from a large Army hospital in central Texas. World War II was raging. There was an announcement in the local paper asking for volunteers to help thread looms in the Occupational Therapy Department of this Army hospital. Since I had studied weaving in my home economics textiles courses, I drove over each Saturday to help out. Clinics were open six days a week then, and, in some instances, seven days a week in the psychiatric sections. While threading looms, I observed the other activities going on in the clinic and was quite intrigued. When the therapists informed me that the Army was setting up some war emergency courses to help relieve the shortage of occupational therapists, I applied and was accepted.

There were 30 Army hospitals at that time and all of them were in need of staff. Mrs. Winifred Kahmann, a lively lady who had been an occupational therapist since 1917, was recruited to set up the War Emergency Courses. Six hundred carefully selected students with degrees in related subjects were enrolled in seven schools of occupational therapy over the next several years. I was sent to the University of Southern California where I had my initial encounter with Los Angeles smog. Margaret Rood was head of the occupational therapy program at U.S.C., and that was an encounter of quite a different kind—a very exciting one. She and Mrs. Kahmann saw to it that we were well indoctrinated as to what occupational therapy was all about. A good foundation was laid and a good dose of enthusiasm for occupational therapy was given. I was in the first class, starting July 1944, and as far as I know I am the only person with a certificate in occupational therapy from one of those abbreviated, but intensive, courses who has been selected as an Eleanor Clarke Slagle Lecturer.

I returned to Texas from California and had two enjoyable years working at the amputee center where I had been a volunteer. Several thousand soldiers were being treated there, so that I worked with many patients who had lost one or more extremity. Nothing can make one appreciate the marvelous instruments—the human hands—more than working with patients who have lost one or both. Could this have had an influence on the direction of my interests in later years so that I was led to work in the special area of hand rehabilitation?

In 1946 the amputee center was closed and I was sent to San Antonio to work at Brooke Army Hospital in the physical disabilities section. At that time, the occupational therapists in Army hospitals were civilians, classified as subprofessionals. The War Department, at Mrs. Kahmann's insistence, requested that Civil Service reclassify occupational therapists to professional status. This was done!

In 1947, through Mrs. Kahmann's influence and a resultant Act of Congress, commissions were granted occupational therapists in the Army. Since it was optional, I chose to remain a civilian, and had five memorable years there at Brooke.

Soon after I arrived, Virginia (Ginny) Bond Scardina came. She had been at the University of Southern California working on her master's degree and was all fired up. In her inimitable fashion she organized an in-service training program for the staff. She assigned topics and we studied hard to be prepared to present our material to our coworkers. There was a large staff with unequal knowledge bases so that this program was beneficial to all of us. Ginny's leadership ability assured its success.

During my years at Brooke the burn unit was set up in the section where I had a clinic. Before that we had treated the few burn patients on the wards. If they had survived severe injuries, they were among the most difficult patients with whom to work. There had been no way to control infections until the introduction of antibiotics in the late 1940s. The odor around a badly burned patient before the advent of antibiotics is a memory I cannot erase. It was always a difficult decision for me to make regarding whether I would go to see such a patient before lunch and ruin my appetite, or go after I had eaten and lose my lunch. The management of the burn patient has undergone numerous changes through the years, but nothing else has had the impact of antibiotics. It was a welcome change.

Another challenge that came about while I was at Brooke Army Hospital was to pioneer in setting up a cerebral palsy treatment unit for dependents of Armed Forces personnel. San Antonio in the late 1940s had no facility for treatment of these children. One of the medical residents who wanted a pediatric residency in the Army approached me to work with him on such a project. None of us knew how far-reaching this project would be. Dr. George Deaver, a consultant from New York, came to speak to the staff, and he arranged for me to visit various facilities in the New York area. As a civilian attached to the Army, I could get time off, but it was at my own expense that I flew up to the big city to start learning the necessary details of how to set up a cerebral palsy treatment program.

With the help of a talented aide and several volunteers, we soon had the essential equipment constructed, space was made available, and patients were waiting to be treated. The Army extended the use of the facility to Air Force personnel in the vicinity as well as to the children of civilian employees on the bases. We had an active half-day program underway quite soon. A physical therapist who had been working at the Kabat Kaiser Institute in the Washington area came to Brooke to do her two-week reserve duty. Sharing her experiences with the early neuromuscular facilitation concepts, which were associated with the Institute where she had worked, helped us in handling some of our more difficult patients. We managed to have her two-week stay extended to more than a month. This was a marvelous learning experience. I studied hard, returned to New York to take a course offered by United Cerebral Palsy, and was active in the State Crippled Children's Society. Although the cerebral palsy treatment program was only on a half-time basis, it was very engrossing, and for more than two years I made a special effort to be an effective therapist with this group, in addition to carrying on the regular treatment program.

Before I conclude the discussion of my years with the Army program, I would like to pay tribute to Col. Ruth A. Robinson, whom I was fortunate to get to know since she came to Brooke soon after I arrived. The Army hospitals had very liberal budgets and plentiful supplies for occupational therapy. We even had sterling silver for our patients to use. But Col. Robinson taught us all to use the supplies judiciously. Her favorite statement: "Remember, this is the taxpayers' money," has influenced me through the years. True, we should have a budget for equipment and supplies in our work, but we should never overestimate the need for expensive equipment and supplies since they are not necessarily indicative of a good treatment program.

After I left the Army program, working with polio patients was my next challenge. As you may recall, it was through Franklin D. Roosevelt, himself a victim of polio, and his influential friends that the Warm Springs, Georgia, treatment center for poliomyelitis was organized. The annual March of Dimes brought in funds to use for research, for payment for treatment, and for stipends that were made available to doctors, nurses, occupational and physical therapists, and social workers so that they could attend courses where special training prepared them for work with polio patients. I applied for the Georgia Warm Springs course, was accepted, and began in October 1952. There was an epidemic of poliomyelitis in the world then, and the hospital was full. Patients came from all over the United States and from many foreign countries. Therapists and doctors from other countries came to take the course also.

The first three months of the course were devoted to acute care, and the second three months to functional training. Again, my good fortune held and I was exposed to some excellent instructors. The polio virus usually affects only the anterior horn cells in the spinal column, so patients with poliomyelitis had intact sensation and very discrete muscle involvement. In order to work effectively with these patients, one needed detailed knowledge of anatomy and kinesiology, refined muscle testing techniques, and, in addition, ability to relate to these people in a way that helped them adjust to their period of restricted activity. Protection of the affected parts was considered most important during the acute phase. The temptations the patients had to carry on with functional activities, even though such activities called for abuse of the involved muscles and substitution patterns that were detrimental, required stern discipline by the therapist. In so many areas of treatment we urge patients to become more functionally independent, but in treating the acute polio patient, much of our emphasis was on the curtailment of physical activity. Supportive and protective devices were applied to restrict undesirable motion. The psychological impact was devastating, so that every therapeutic skill was recruited.

I was asked to serve as instructor in the postgraduate courses at Warm Springs and stayed on after completing my six months of training. The upper extremity was mainly the responsibility of the occupational therapists, so that teaching these units was fun. After two years, I moved back to Texas to work with respiratory polio patients in Houston. Warm

Springs did not accept patients who required breathing aids, so that this was an added dimension to the problem. I became accustomed to working with patients who slept in an iron lung or on a rocking bed and were made mobile by donning chest respirators so that they could come to occupational therapy in wheelchairs. This group was wonderful to work with, and taxed every bit of ingenuity one could muster. John Gardner's book, *No Easy Victories*, describes so well the way I felt when working with these severely involved patients and the way I feel about occupational therapy today. "What could be more satisfying than to be engaged in work in which every capacity or talent one may have is needed, every lesson one may have learned is used, every value one cares about is furthered?" (1, p 32)

Fortunately, the Salk vaccine was perfected during the years I worked at Warm Springs. The intensive public effort to vaccinate everyone paid off and polio is now a rarity. However, the recent outbreak in an Amish community in Pennsylvania is cause for renewed concern and effort toward prevention.

By late 1956, the vaccine had polio under control so that the acute need for therapists in that specialty area waned. I then moved to the Houston Veterans Hospital and had a small clinic where hand cases were treated: fractures, and other types of trauma, peripheral nerve problems, and numerous quadriplegic patients. All my experience to date was made use of in this particular setting.

I had been there a year when AOTA announced that a grant-financed position was being established for a Field Consultant in Physical Disabilities. That was just the job I wanted and that was just the job I got! AOTA offices were in New York during that period and Marjorie Fish was the executive director. Establishing that new service would have been impossible without her able guidance. Helen Willard and Wilma West, as presidents of AOTA during those years, gave their support and assistance. Many other therapists helped me also. My sincere thanks go to all of them for their willingness to advise and consult along with me. Frequently, I merely served as a means of getting the ones who wanted help in touch with therapists who could supply the needed guidance.

The entire United States was my territory, and I was presented with an enormous range of problems within the field of physical disabilities in occupational therapy. Many of the problems we have today are the same ones that we had when I was a consultant. I doubt that the profession will ever be problem-free. Again Gardner's *No Easy Victories* offers the premise that problems serve to stimulate and spark us toward our best performances. A life with no problems would be so dull that an intelligent person would go out and set up a situation that would provide him or her with a problem—a challenge. That, according to Gardner, is why people play golf or other sports. Artificial problems sought out by the bored person do not call upon one's full resources, though. The problems in occupational therapy certainly do. They "interest the whole mind, the aggregate nature of man more continuously and more deeply." (1, p 32) Isn't it consoling to think that all our problems might be quite therapeutic for us!

I had taken this job as consultant for three years and stayed on for five. At the end of those five years I felt somewhat drained, and I took a year off to go to Europe. What a rejuvenating year that was! I had promised myself that I was on a vacation, but was tempted from time to time to look in on some interesting occupational therapy programs. My first three months were spent in the deep snows of southern Switzerland, in the French-speaking section. Friends of mine had a cerebral palsy treatment center in a small Swiss village where I was. They used Bobath methods in their treatment program, and it was all I could do to keep from becoming involved. How I wished I could have known about some of their interesting concepts during the years I had worked with children with cerebral palsy. Instead of working in the therapy sessions, I volunteered to mend and sew for them. That gave me more freedom to take off on a beautiful sunny day to ride the lift to the top of a ski area nearby. Needless to say, I rode the lift back down the mountain, too. I tried skiing, but since I was 50 that year, my better judgment made me give up the idea because I was afraid I would break a leg.

When I returned to the United States I went to the AOTA offices to check on positions available in North Carolina. During my five years of consulting I had gone to nearly all of the states and had selected the Chapel Hill-Durham area as a favored location. I could hardly believe it, but there was an opening in Chapel Hill for a therapist to work with a hand surgeon. That sounded pretty good to me. So my start in hand rehabilitation was not a premeditated move on my part, but an act of fate. It does illustrate that, with our broad basic preparation in occupational therapy, if, in the drama of our professional lives, the casting director should put us in one particular role or another, we can perform adequately. At times we may be fortunate and have preparation meet opportunity. This role in hand rehabilitation suited me as an individual and suited my talents. I grew in it, and it continued to provide challenges for 15 years. The flexibility made possible by our broad humanistic base in occupational therapy enables us to build up into peaks of professional excellence or into specializing at times. The base should not be ignored, even though attention might be temporarily focused on the elegant points of the peaks.

In 1958, Carlotta Welles had an article in *The American Journal of Occupational Therapy* with the intriguing title "DaVinci is Dead! The Case for Specialization." She stated that Leonardo daVinci had been dead for more than 400 years and that he was possibly the "last single individual to possess a significant portion of existing knowledge."(2, p 289) Today there is so much to be known about such a wide variety of subjects. The quantity of published information rapidly increases: libraries keep expanding; information is put on microfilm in order to consolidate it for storage. Ideas used to outlive people. Now people often outlive ideas. There is a proliferation of new ideas—some good and some bad. Keep in mind the questions that T. S. Eliot asked, in his poem *The Rock*, "Where is the wisdom we lost in knowledge? Where is the knowledge we have lost in information?"(3, p 81) What we need is a good system to filter this mass of information so as to capture the knowledge that will be beneficial and to screen again to help select those things that will make us wise, at least in one area of concern.

Acquisition of new knowledge might well rank below the formulation of a new attitude toward, or a better understanding of, old knowledge. Many so-called specialties in occupational therapy are nothing more than a special arrangement of things that are already familiar to us, or a reorganization of our services to meet the needs of a specific group. How often I have found this to be true in my own career. In the first issue of the Physical Disabilities Specialty Section *Newsletter* last summer, there was an open letter from Louise Elfant expressing her concern about the danger of overspecialization. She feared that one might sometimes trade off treating the whole person for treating the parts more effectively. This, in my opinion, will not happen if one remembers to consider what the illness or trauma means to the patient. The therapist's special competence must be combined with compassion at all times. An extremity with a slight residual deformity might well serve, but a warped and crippled mind or personality can never be useful. Helping the patient put an injury or illness into proper perspective is fundamental to occupational therapy. We would be remiss in our responsibilities if we neglected this important aspect of treatment, even though we might be concentrating on a particular segment. We know full well that patients must become involved and rehabilitate themselves. This is impossible unless we help them understand and adjust to their conditions.

Being a clinician has been my way of functioning as an occupational therapist. We clinicians are on the front line and are more often than not the ones from whom the public formulates an image of our profession. This is quite a responsibility and one that I have never taken lightly. Flexner, when addressing a national conference on social work in 1915, stated the criteria by which a profession could be identified (4). He also developed the thesis that what matters most is professional spirit. He thought that trades carried on with such spirit might rise toward the professional level. Conversely, accepted professions might sink toward the trade level if people within the group lose such a spirit. That really emphasizes the importance of the role of the clinician and the spirit in which the duties of the clinician are carried out.

Rather than thinking of myself as a specialist, I prefer to rank myself as a master clinician. There have been numerous suggestions through the years favoring the use of such a designated title, and I find it rather pleasing to the ear and to the ego. One does not become a master of anything without putting forth some concentrated effort in the right direction. One needs to become more deeply committed and to make an effort toward acquiring definitive knowledge in the particular sphere selected. As Martha Moersch quoted (from Richard L. Kenyon) in her summary of the Curriculum Revision Study in 1966, ". . . academic training is the base for founding a professional career and it is the quality of growth thereafter that builds the professional."(5, p 57) Continuing education as a means of growth, whether it be by reading extensively, by attending workshops and courses, or by communicating with others personally must be an active ongoing process. One statement that sticks in my mind is that continuing education is active exercise, not massage. An accumulation of intellectual facts is of little value. One must absorb the material and have a change in attitudes and behavior in order to grow. Every single day one should give oneself a chance to be a good occupational therapist—the very best! In anticipation of an unusual problem a patient might present, therapists should be confident of their ability to deal with that problem. If they feel inadequate, they should make a concerted effort to read a ready reference or call in a consultant to help them solve the problem—to grow professionally. A patient or client will more likely be impressed by the honesty of the therapist who admits to an inadequacy and demonstrates a desire to get help than to have the therapist attempt treatment in an area in which the therapist lacks competence. All of us have had times when we needed to turn to someone for advice. The less experienced the therapist is, the more important it is to be working in a clinic under supervision. Help is readily available then. Getting out on one's own too soon or going into a specialty area of practice prematurely may put one in a compromising situation and arrest professional development. One should give serious consideration to these matters as one embarks upon a career.

As I said in my introductory remarks, being named the Eleanor Clarke Slagle Lecturer is quite an honor. I have never aspired to national acclaim. My main goal has been to work with patients to help them improve and to help them assume responsibility for caring for themselves. I have never felt guilty about working in a medical setting. Much of what I do is preventive in nature, even though it might be categorized as secondary rather than primary prevention. The medical setting enabled me to save energy and time since case-finding was simplified. The people who needed my services were gathered in one spot. I always did enough community work to let it be known what my program entailed, and at the Hand Rehabilitation Center I could take direct self-referrals. In this way, people could come to a convenient location to have services rendered. I was comfortable in this environment and I am sure that helped me to be productive.

All I did was "to do the common things uncommonly well," as some advertisement has said. That is what brought success. May I give an example of how only one aspect of treatment was developed with some measure of success?

When there is edema in the hand, we know that reducing it is of primary concern. The small joints of the fingers cannot tolerate the presence of this scar-producing fluid in and around the soft tissues that surround these compact joints. Limited motion results and the stiffness that follows can turn an otherwise delicate instrument like the hand into a clumsy tool.

Through the years we have had an opportunity to study the effectiveness of a variety of ways in which edema reduction routines have been carried out in both occupational and physical therapy. Methods of monitoring the size of the hand such as water displacement, as suggested by Dr. Paul Brand (personal communication), as well as circumferential measurements by tape or ring size, have enabled us to determine the effects of various treatment approaches. Massage, heat, cold, whirlpool, application of the Jobst intermittent pressure unit, active exercise, exercise in elevation, elevation alone, and a variation on string wrapping have been among the approaches evaluated. Some patients reacted adversely to massage and the same was true of the Jobst unit or other approaches.

If we found that any one of these modalities led to an increase in volume, it was discontinued in favor of one or more of the other more effective techniques. As a general rule, we found that warm whirlpool was most often detrimental, but active exercise in an elevated position was most effective in edema reduction. Sanding projects positioned at or above shoulder level, cord knotting similarly placed, and leather lacing with a long strip of lacing are ideal occupational therapy projects. Close supervision is essential to get the correct routine established. The combination of fine motion of the fingers that involves use of the intrinsic muscles of the hand as well as movement of the entire arm so as to get active involvement of forearm and upper arm muscles will bring the best results. The contraction of the muscles is what gets the pumping action started to mobilize the fluid, and the elevated position facilitates flow from distal to proximal areas of the arm.

During waking hours, rather than have the patient place the arm in a sling, which would encourage inactivity of the arm muscles, we found that it was far better to teach the patient to elevate the hand above the head frequently, using his or her own muscle power; to rest the hand on top of the head, up on an elevated surface or door frame; as well as to use a cane or crutch to position the hand at the desired level. Most patients watch television for several hours daily throughout their convalescent period. One speaker I recall suggested that the patient should be instructed to raise the arm toward the ceiling each time a commercial came on. Actively making a fist and relaxing it while the hand is in elevation during these numerous times works wonders to control edema. What a simple approach to a complicated problem!

All of us are aware of fluid accumulation during sleeping hours. Eyes get puffy, fingers feel stiff upon awakening, and some time is required to mobilize the so-called normal hand. Think how much more difficult it is to mobilize the hand when one has any pathology. We tried various things to help keep edema out of the hand while the patient is in bed. One was a special sling into which the arm could be strapped. It held the hand elevated with the elbow flexed and the forearm in a vertical position. Bunk beds in our center facilitated hanging the sling since it could be attached to the upper bunk, but I.V. stands, hat racks, or constructed L-shaped frames with one section to slip in under the mattress could be provided for home use.

Another item suggested for night use was some type of external pressure. The company that makes the intermittent pressure unit also makes custom-fitted gloves from two-way stretch fabric. These gloves are fine but they are expensive and it takes some time to order and have them delivered. Since I am so cost conscious I found that used surgical gloves, which were available to us free of charge from the nearby hospital, sufficed. Too, the Thrift Shop had stretch nylon gloves at a minimal cost. The colors of the gloves did not matter since they were to be worn at night, and if only one of a pair was available, that was fine, also. A patient usually needs only one. If my supply of gloves consisted only of those for the left hand and my patient had an injured right hand, I would turn the glove wrong-side out. This proved fortuitous since the seam on the outside made it more comfortable for the patient. Necessity is truly the mother of invention. A word of caution here: do not put a glove that fits too snugly on the edematous hand since circulation might be impaired. Always try the glove for at least 30 minutes, then remove it to check on the circulation in the fingertips.

Another way to provide external pressure is to make a Temper-foam sandwich splint. Two pieces of Temper-foam, a NASA by-product, can be used next to the hand and heavy cardboard can be put outside, top, and bottom. The splint can be strapped together around the hand. This type of external pressure is excellent for use with any hand with the combined problem of edema and a tendency toward flexion contracture. The hemiplegic's hand responds well since this splint reduces edema as well as holding the fingers in extension. It also provides neutral warmth which, according to Miss Rood, encourages relaxation.

I have gone into some detail in discussing this aspect of treatment to point out how unsophisticated these methods are, but how very effective. Occupational therapy is commonplace and unsophisticated often, and therapists are frequently apologetic about this aspect. Instead, we should take pride in our use of the ordinary and commonplace to bring about desired results when more sophisticated modalities have failed. I take frank delight in being innovative.

None of us has any idea what the world, and specifically occupational therapy, will be like in 2020 AD. About that time a beginning therapist of today will have reached my age. Remarkable changes have taken place during my time—television, jet airplanes, credit cards, computers, synthetic fabrics, frozen foods, drug abuse problems of great proportions, Medicare, too many people, Blue Cross-Blue Shield, Velcro, transplantations, space travel, holography, bio-plastics, antibiotics—the list could go on and on. Some of these things affected me and my profession directly—others indirectly—but the shocks came in small, adaptive doses. We were hardly aware of how important each one was.

The young will more than likely face as many or more changes in their lifetimes. Their opportunities will be cleverly disguised with seemingly insoluble problems. I only hope that we can all help them to grow and handle their futures. In my senescence—notice that I am avoiding the use of the term senility—I want to volunteer my efforts along the way.

In conclusion, I would like to quote an excerpt from a poem written by another occupational therapist, Edward Dunning. This appeared in the December 1973 *AJOT*:

> . . . We've better things to do than reruns of old projects,
> Better scripts to write than catalog the past
> Or lose the present by condemning it.
> You've got a future to invent! How about it? (6, p 472)

REFERENCES

1. Gardner JW: *No Easy Victories*, New York: Harper & Row, 1968
2. Welles C: DaVinci is dead: The case for specialization. *Am J Occup Ther* 12: 289, 1958
3. Eliot TS: *The Wasteland and Other Poems*, New York: Harvest Books, 1934
4. Flexner A: Is social work a profession? In *Proceedings of the National Conference of Charities and Correction*, Chicago: Hildmann Printing Co., 1915
5. Moersch M: Implications of the occupational therapy curriculum study. In *Proceedings of Final Conference*, New York: AOTA, 1966; Quote from Kenyon RL: Designing professional education. *Chem Eng News*, 1966
6. Dunning RE: Vibrations on two instruments. *Am J Occup Ther* 27: 472, 1973

Occupational Therapists Put Care in the Health System

Carolyn Manville Baum

I address you today with a sense of pride and great thanks for your recognition for this most singular honor. I am also thankful for the opportunity to have experienced the year of growth the responsibility of this honor imposed.

I hope to share with you my perspective of occupational therapy and its position in the health system. Occupational therapists' tremendous commitment to Man and to his ability to shape his destiny through activity and accomplishment puts us in a very favorable position because we provide a service that the health care system is reorganizing to assure it is delivered. Our responsibility as a profession is to implement a broader perspective of health care delivery—one that places its values on individuals as they accept the responsibility for their own health status.

To accomplish this task, I want to lead you through a process of assessment, recognition, and strategy development. For my framework, I will use the process each of us uses daily in our service delivery.

Assessment: The Referral Has Been Received

"The health care system must be directed at improving the health of the American people by encouraging health, providing constructive behavior and improving the effectiveness of our medical care system." (1, p iii) This mandate (our referral) came from President Jimmy Carter in his introductory remarks in the Department of Health, Education, and Welfare's publication, *Health and United States*, 1978 (1).

Reprinted from *The American Journal of Occupational Therapy*, Vol. 34, No. 8, 1980

The Problems Requiring Management

1. High quality health care at a reasonable cost is often inaccessible.
2. Health care is beyond the means of many.
3. The system is focusing on hospital acute care rather than ambulatory and preventive care.
4. Technology has been exploited.
5. There is poor distribution of medical personnel.
6. Human beings are not allowed to control their own health status (2).

The Goal. Organize and humanize the system.

Requested Service. Develop a plan for implementation to effect change as quickly and as simply as possible.

To meet this challenge our profession must develop a plan—thus we need a "treatment plan."

We always perform an assessment before establishing a plan. Only when we have a sense of the total picture can we have vision. The health care system is very complex and involves many characters. Our first process, that of assessment, involves seeking to understand each of the characters and their contributions to the current health care dilemma.

The Characters

The Consumer. As a framework for the consumer, I have chosen the work of Hadley Cantril (3). He describes humanistic characteristics that must be considered by Man in relating to Man. Man requires that his survival needs be satisfied and wants security in physical and psychological meaning to provide orientation and integration through time. Security protects gains made and allows Man to look to the future. It is also important to have enough order or certainty in life to enable Man to judge with some accuracy what will or will not occur. Human beings have the capacity to make choices. People perceive only what is relative to their choices and make choices accordingly. Humans require the freedom to exercise the choices they are capable of making. Humans must know they are valued by others. The individual must have values and beliefs to which he or she can commit himself with some certainty (3).

These are the humans who get sick, have accidents, and appear at the door of the health care system. They are in jeopardy of losing control of themselves and they are afraid. As professionals we must recognize their tremendous vulnerability and offer them services in which they have choices and control.

To describe the consumer, I would say: . . . some are saved, . . . some are used, . . . some are passive, . . . some want control, . . . some are sick, . . . some are well, . . . some are disabled, . . . some are crocks. Yet *all* are *human* and *all* are *individuals*.

Consumers feel that health care has become a right. The current situation is governed by a "more is better" attitude—that is, more resources, more facilities, more manpower, more of what it will take to provide what "I" need with no thought to how the services will be paid for. Human life is considered priceless and no amount of money is too much to devote to "my" life (4).

The Federal Government. The federal government is a multibillion-dollar operation organized to protect the consumer at the expense of the consumer. Federal involvement in health care began in 1907 when the Hygienic Laboratory was formed to work toward the eradication of public health problems in food and water. From this laboratory, the National Institutes of Health (NIH) were developed. The NIH is the biomedical research center of the country. It houses 11 institutes that study specific diseases and organ systems. The NIH is the main support of the majority of medical teaching institutions. Medical schools' dependence on federal subsidies encourages specialization and emphasizes technology as the answer to health problems (4). The public health service no longer focuses on health promotion and disease prevention.

The following represents the major dates that led to the current federal regulation of health care:

> **1935**—The Social Security Act of 1935 put the federal government in the health business. It gave grant-in-aid to states to provide Maternal and Child Health Assistance and Assistance to Crippled Children. It has led now to more than 1,000 specialized programs.
>
> **1940**—The start of third-party reimbursement—basically so that hospitals and doctors would be assured of being paid.
>
> **1943**—The start of Health Manpower training, with grants to educational institutions to prepare manpower.
>
> **1946**—Hill Burton construction grants were initiated and to date have totalled more than 4 billion dollars.
>
> **1959**—Government employees were given health insurance.
>
> **1960**—Medical schools were having difficulty surviving so that the government provided support through manpower funds, thus increasing revenue to the schools.
>
> **1965**—Medicare and Medicaid provided help to the poor and elderly to obtain health service.

As expenditures for health care increased so did the government's concern, and eventually its involvement shifted from purely contributory to regulatory. The major controls placed on the health industry today are:

The Occupational Safety and Health Act (OSHA) enacted in 1970 was designed to protect the worker in the work environment. It has provided some protection, but it has also increased costs.

The Professional Standards Review Organization (PSRO) initiated in 1972 also had a humanistic goal—to assure that appropriate care was given to individuals by qualified professionals. This program has had a major impact on delivery of services by imposing control, restricting access to care, and increasing costs.

In 1974, the National Health Planning Resource Act (HSA) presented in law the concept that health care is a "right." Its impact has been on the control of capital expenditures, and the creation of a political football game with providers and consumers on opposing teams. The government serves as referee, and occasionally can be accused of making poor calls on the plays.

The transition from public health promotion and disease prevention to a high technological mode has been influenced by the federal government in the following ways: the sponsorship of high technology biomedical research; the sponsorship of programs to produce specialization; money for training nearly 200 health professionals; and the construction of facilities.

The Physician. Early health care was concerned with the individual. Public health and prevention were emphasized and dominated most thinking until the early 1900s. Until that time, the state of medicine was primitive and lacked a scientific base. Also, health problems were primarily a result of poor sanitation, poor living conditions, and contaminated water.

Health care has changed because medicine has become a scientific discipline as well as a political force. Specialist societies were formed for scientific and educational purposes. Most physicians initially were general practitioners, but focused on a specialty part time. A particularly strong influence for change in medicine was the publication of the Flexner report in 1904, where the disparities in the quality of education and the standards of performance in teaching institutions were exposed. This led to the development of medicine as a science.

Physicians generally are trained to think science and to think "sick." Most are dedicated to saving life at all costs. Few are oriented to the humanities and social sciences. The profession requires a tremendous time commitment to ensure competence.

The physician is the person each of us turns to for guidance and direction when we have a health problem. Physicians are in powerful positions and play a critical role in the delivery of care and in any changes in health care delivery.

Medical School. Medical schools for the most part continue to separate the art and the science of medicine. They remain elite and do not use community resources for health delivery. The schools continue to prepare specialists and do not emphasize the social and behavioral sciences.

The Health Care Administrator. This individual is taught to be decisive and in control, and the measurement of his or her performance is best described by the following "want ad" for a health facility administrator:

Wanted: Health Facility Administrator
The position requires a person with the ability to maintain an average occupancy rate of at least 96% on medical/surgical nursing units, 63% on ICU/CCU units, and 63% on obstetrics units, while scheduling all emergency surgical patients and, on the average, 21 out of the 100 medical patients each week. No more than 5 scheduled patients out of every 1,000 can be cancelled and no more than 15 out of 1,000 ICU/CCU patients, 5 out of 1,000 OB patients, or 10 out of 1,000 emergency patients can be turned away.

In addition, the person in this position is responsible for allocating nurses to each of these nursing units (1) so that an average of 5.0 hours of nursing care is maintained for each patient each day, (2) so that registered nurses, licensed practical nurses, and aides are assigned to each unit to utilize their skills fully, (3) so that the nurses' individual work stretches with or without 3-day weekends, and (4) so that quality nursing care is provided.

Applicants must have knowledge or skill in setting up systems for physicians to control patient placement in appropriate levels of care, and to control medical necessity of patient services (5).

These are the people who run our systems and our resources for implementing our concepts. They manage a complex system and are rarely trained or oriented in the concepts of human service delivery.

Allied Health Professionals. This group in general is striving for professional status and is very competitive in the health services marketplace. The knowledge base of most allied health professionals has grown to the point that they seek recognition as independent health practitioners. The skills of the allied health professional are rarely used fully to support the delivery system. In our assessment process I will look in depth at one of the allied health professional characters; namely, occupational therapists.

Our profession started with the basic premise that Man has control over his health status by having control over his use of time, body, and mind. In the early 1900s, when our profession was conceived, society did not have specific knowledge in biochemistry, neurology, or behavior. Modern medical science was in its infancy when the original paradigm of occupational therapy was developed. By today's standards, the body of knowledge was minute and, although research had begun to be a part of medicine, it was greatly limited. In the second half of the 19th century, the bacterial origin of many infectious diseases had been demonstrated. This led to the concept of asepsis, which made surgical management a possibility. From World War I to World War II, progress in medical science quickened. The sulfonamides were introduced in 1934, and penicillin was discovered in the 1930s. After World War II, the antibiotic era came into its own. A by-product of this era was the realization by the American people of the impact of research on the creation of knowledge. As a result, the public's expectations about medicine changed dramatically (6).

Occupational therapy was initially associated with and today continues to be a profession closely allied with medicine. We are not a medical model profession but we do have a medical base. The scientific inquiry in medicine as a science has had a major impact on our profession. Rather than take an active role in the scientific inquiry, we have relied on the work of others to provide direction to our principles. Thus by not directly addressing the concepts of activity and its impact on the nervous systems, behavior, or the cardiovascular system, we have not based our principles on the scientific movement.

We must do more than speak about our theories. We must develop a rage for knowledge and document our principles as a scientific discipline.

In 1969, the President of AOTA (Ruth Brunyate Wiemer) challenged the profession to address questions that would document the relationship between deprivation or affluence of play and teenage aggression; deprivation of work or enforced retirement and the onset of illness after age 65; the lack of work and recreation and the apathy of the slow learner; and the inescapable uselessness of the terminally ill and longevity (7). Do we wish to continue to talk about the effect of activity or do we wish to do something about it? Now 11 years later, if we want to make a mark in both the humanistic and scientific movements, we must address questions like these and support the people who ask them.

As a profession we are not to date unlike the Bakhtiari Tribe of Persia. This is a nomadic tribe of goat herders who daily move their entire tribe to new grazing land. They have taught us that a group cannot refine a culture on the move. The Bakhtiari life has changed very little since 10,000 B.C. They have only the simple technology that can be carried on daily journeys. The simplicity is not romantic, it is a matter of survival (8). In applying this analogy to occupational therapy, I have to ask the question, When are we going to stop following the grazing trail and develop the technology to plant our own fields?

As a profession we have seen our nearly singular roles in vocational rehabilitation, basic living skills, and use of activity come and go. Other professions have implemented what initially were our roles, but we have survived! This means that the health care system is looking to us for a special emphasis on health care delivery. We must internalize this positive concept of us. I think we can develop a fertile strain that will allow our fields to be very fruitful. We have something very unique to harvest. We must master our own product, understand it, and use that understanding to mold the living environment.

Within our profession there are many capable people in education and clinical practice yet we have difficulty developing a master plan for and getting started on a program to define our practice in scientific terms. I want to share with you my perspective of a conflict that I think has our profession at a standstill and is preventing us from developing our "fertile strain."

Our professional organization, the American Occupational Therapy Association (AOTA), has supported the development and continuance of a structured pluralism with education and practice being separate in structure and function. Two prevailing thoughts have developed out of this relationship.

The first thought is: *Because occupational therapy educators do not practice clinical occupational therapy, they do not have the knowledge, attitude, or skill to produce students trained in current practice.*

Since the middle 1960s, therapists in clinical practice have been working their way into the changing health system. To do this required the following eight activities:

1. Acquire third party reimbursement.
2. Establish collaborative working relationships with other professionals involved in direct service.
3. Define practice standards for professional review.
4. Establish cost-effective services.
5. Identify patient populations and develop services to support program implementation.
6. Develop treatment methodologies that can be included in short-term care facilities.
7. Establish networks for referral of the patient to long-term or community services to obtain maximum benefit for occupational therapy.
8. Design activities and intervention that support the theory of occupational therapy.

Treatment interventions have been established by practitioners to provide remediation to impaired areas of function as well as to promote healthful behaviors. For us to gain identity as a scientific discipline each area of function must be supported by research supplied from the basic sciences.

Some of the fields that relate to *motor and sensory-integrative function* are neuropathophysiology, neurology, anatomy, physiology, neurophysiology, neuroanatomy, chemistry, and physics. Some of the fields that relate to *cognitive, psychological and social function* are psychology, sociology, psychopathology, and chemistry.

I think therapists in practice have stimulated their own growth by graduate study in areas to support understanding of function—not exclusively relying on advanced occupational therapy education to provide it, possibly because occupational therapy educators are not publishing information to answer the basic questions needed to be answered about the body systems' ability to respond to the demands required to function in these areas. The professional dialogue for practitioners is primarily with others in clinical practice through publication and continuing education experiences. Because of this I believe practitioners have adopted the following notion: Because occupational therapy educators do not practice clinical occupational therapy, they do not have the knowledge, attitude, or skill to produce students trained in current practice.

Now I will describe the second thought that has developed. The practitioner is ignoring his or her responsibilities and compromising the field of occupational therapy by collaborating with other professionals and not demonstrating occupational therapy as an independent health profession.

In 1977, a report of the Ad Hoc Committee on Education was submitted to the Executive Board of the AOTA and eventually published in *The American Journal of Occupational Therapy* (9). The stated purpose was to raise issues that influenced our attempt to become a fully recognized profession. I will present the education description from the Ad Hoc Committee Report.

Faculty Characteristics and Responsibilities. Faculty are operating autonomously with minimal involvement with university missions, which undermines efforts to continue association with these institutions.

Faculty generally give up patient treatment and remove themselves from the practice of occupational therapy.

Faculty engage in repetitive and time-consuming requirements for accreditation that deprive faculty of valuable time, some of which might be spent in research, scholarly activities, and other endeavors expected of all university faculty members.

Faculty Shortage. There is a serious shortage of qualified faculty members at every academic level. The Association efforts and resources are focused on baccalaureate and associate degree entry-level preparation and exclude resources to clinical specialization and graduate education.

Multiple Entry Routes Leading to Certification as an OTR. Our multiple entry points serve to support the thesis that occupational therapy is a semi-profession or a technical profession. The value of our educational preparation is negated by multiple entry routes that do not rely upon a liberal arts base. "The processes of acquiring and assuming knowledge ... unique to occupational therapy, are seldom the priorities of our educational programs, ..."

Lack of Research. "The lack of research related to hypotheses supporting our theoretical foundations, treatment modalities, and modes of intervention seriously impedes all aspects of education and practice."

External Influences and Forces. "Actions and decisions made by external agencies continue to have a negative influence and impact on our development." Examples cited are the limitation of funding of health programs, especially at the postbaccalaureate level, and the control that the American Medical Association has over our education programs.

AOTA Member Readiness to Decide on Semiprofessional or Professional Status. The committee reported that members do not focus in either education or practice upon those functions and behaviors that are traditionally identified with the status of a profession. The authors state the following behaviors are necessary by the membership to reach professional status:

1. Willingness and responsibility for diagnosing problems;
2. Providing service without referral from physician;
3. Working without physician supervision or members of other disciplines;
4. Conducting one's own professional assessment;
5. Accepting the necessity for research to substantiate or refute the principles upon which treatment is based (9).

This completes my description of the Ad Hoc Committee on Education Report.

Thus we have documentation of the pervasiveness of the second idea: *The practitioner is ignoring his or her responsibilities and compromising the field of occupational therapy by collaborating with other professionals and not demonstrating occupational therapy as an independent health profession.*

I have now described those six I think are the main characters in the health system and described in depth my perception of the character of occupational therapy. From these descriptions, I perceive that the entire system is in conflict. Each character has its own values, knowledge, structure, and personality. This causes the system, which should be a team of specialists organizing to develop a network of interactions, to be at a stalemate resulting in power struggles and strained communications.

The patient is frequently the victim of the isolation caused by this poor communication. The definition of a closed system is that the system is isolated from its environment and the final state is determined by the initial conditions. Certainly the health system is made up of many closed systems (10). The patients unfortunately become a closed system also because they have no mechanism for being in a dynamic state with their environment and in control of their own status.

The prejudices harbored by each of the characters in the health system seek to maintain the independent status of each character rather than focusing on the individual human being who is paying for the service to change his or her health status.

I have now completed the assessment process of our plan. I see three separate problems that the profession has to address to meet its responsibilities in organizing and humanizing the health care system:

The three problems are a perceived conflict between occupational therapy practice and occupational therapy education, to actually destroy what I perceive as myths; a focus on health services delivered within the acute care model; and the health system's lack of orientation toward the human being.

Now that we have completed the assessment by looking at the characters and identifying the problems, let us take each problem one at a time and develop our treatment plan.

Treatment Plan

Problem I. A Perceived Conflict between Practice: Education.

GOAL: Resolve the Conflict between Practice and Education. It is important that our profession reduce the social distance between education and practice and move from pluralistic positions into one of integration. We need a link between education and practice with the purpose of further developing occupational therapy as a scientific discipline. This focus will remove the need for maintaining the conflict and move us toward integration and further away from fragmentation—thus, we will destroy the myths.

In investigating methods to resolve the conflict, I went to C.P. Snow's lecture on "Two Cultures." Snow perceives that there is conflict between the scientist—who believes that literary intellectuals are totally lacking in foresight, peculiarly unconcerned with humanity—and the nonscientist—who has a rooted impression that the scientist is shallowly optimistic and unaware of Man's condition (10). I wondered whether occupational therapy housed any scientists, so I found myself engulfed in *The Search*, also by C.P. Snow, a novel that describes the scientist through a number of behaviors ranging from unending curiosity to the need to understand things even if they can't be controlled (12). It became clear to me that the educational preparation of the occupational therapist does not encourage the scientist.

For the profession to ascend, we will need to produce true professionals who are skilled in inventing, inferring, and analyzing, and who can communicate with basic researchers in a collaborative relationship to investigate areas of our clinical practice as well. We must prepare professionals who possess the humanistic qualities to relate to an individual who requires our service. Since these qualities are not mutually exclusive, the educational preparation of the occupational therapist must develop both qualities.

As I became more aware of the lack of basic scientists in our profession, I explored ways to approach the production and distribution of knowledge.

According to Machlup, a profession must be responsible for producing two types of knowledge:

1. Internal knowledge, which answers questions to measure the effectiveness of our service—this knowledge is developed by daily dialogue with each other and through our newspapers and journal.
2. New knowledge that assists society in expanding its understanding (13).

I believe the profession must contribute societal knowledge in the following areas:

1. The activity process and activity's effect on the human body;
2. The process of adaptation and its effect on the human body;
3. The process of integration of human function through activity and adaptation.

To produce discoveries through inventing, inferring, analyzing, or evaluating is not enough (13, p 30). For discoveries to be valuable, they must be conveyed. Knowledge is produced in three basic ways, all under the general category of research.

Research is defined as a systematic intensive study directed toward fuller knowledge of the subject studied.

Basic Research is directed toward the increase of knowledge. It is research where the primary aim of the investigation is a fuller understanding of the subject under study rather than the practical application thereof.

Applied Research creates directly applicable knowledge. The researcher looks for results which promise to be of ultimate use in practice.

Development is the systematic use of scientific knowledge directed toward the production of useful materials, systems methods, or process (13, pp 146-147).

Within the profession two of these three types of research can and are being accomplished—applied research and development. Our greatest lack is in basic research. To do basic research requires a scientist with not only the scientific approach, but also the scientific background. I do not know of a profession that performs basic research entirely for themselves—certainly medicine does not—and I do not know why we should continue to struggle with the idea of performing our own basic research to the detriment of our educational process.

I propose that educators and clinicians formulate collaborative relationships with social scientists to address the social, cognitive, and psychological aspects of function and with biological scientists to address the motor and sensory integrative aspects of function.

A research team should inspire a collaborative relationship between the occupational therapy educator, the basic scientist, and the clinician or clinicians. The occupational therapy educators must assume the role of coordinator and facilitator of research projects. The clinician should function as a clinical scientist who logs observation and inferences, and communicates with the educator who can organize teams to design and implement research to answer pertinent questions.

One reason these research teams have not yet developed is that educators and practitioners have not been interested in addressing common questions. The stability and then the ascent of our profession depends on the establishment of common goals for research and a commitment on the part of the educator and the clinician to collaborate on research questions of interest to both. By including the appropriate basic science researchers, the gap in the basic sciences on the part of both the educator and the clinician can be narrowed so that questions can be addressed as they relate to the human body and mind and its response to activity.

We can no longer afford to destroy each other with words and lack of action. The profession must make a commitment to action using a team collaborating for the outcome of producing internal knowledge for the benefit of our patients and societal knowledge for the benefit of mankind. We must develop the skill and accept the responsibility to critically analyze our work and not react defensively to criticism but realize that criticism will help the profession grow.

We must recognize that too few of us have the skills or resources to do basic scientific research. However, it has to be done if we are to attain a credible status with the public in the subject areas we do know— that of adaptation and integration. I predict that, through the experience of collaborative relationship with the basic scientist, many of us will develop the skills necessary not only to do the basic research ourselves, but also to teach these skills to others within our profession. I think we would then attract more students interested in a scientific discipline. We also would have greater strength as a profession in relating to other groups who are infringing on our territory because we would have a strong theory base for our service delivery. Our confidence would be strong knowing that we are the profession to deliver our services—this would be built into our images of ourselves as professionals. The issues from the practice arena and the issues from the education arena would all be given a tremendous boost and be closer to resolution if the credibility of our profession was housed in research methodologies that are strong. It is important for clinicians and educators to recognize the extreme pressures facing each group as each works to gain a stable position within the health system. Perhaps we can all feel that we are approaching the problems together. It is critical that we channel our energy away from conflict and into research. I believe funding for research would be forthcoming from the government for coordinated projects that demonstrate a link with the basic sciences.

Time is a problem for all of us. However, well-designed and funded research projects should provide resources to support the clinician and educator in research activities. We have to organize and order our priorities to accomplish basic research for the sake of professional stability. Looking outside the profession, I find that similar conflicts between education and practice are not uncommon. Survival of the profession is an issue whether one is from the university structure or a clinical facility. The missing link in destroying this conflict is collaborative research with a commitment to the growth of our profession. Some persons might not agree that the social or biological scientist must enter the picture, but I am now convinced that the skills and attitude of those individuals are critical for the process to proceed.

Now we must develop a treatment plan for the second problem.

Problem II. The Health Services Delivery Primarily within the Acute Care Model.

GOAL: Expand the Delivery of Occupational Therapy Service from the Acute Care Model of Service. Hospitals initially were a shelter for the socially unfit whether due to severe disability, mental illness, or indigence. The hospital was set apart from the medical community. This was the population served when occupational therapy was initiated as a profession. Private patients were not treated in hospitals until the turn of the century. Insurance did not pay for hospital care until the 1930s and then for only a few. Not until the late 1950s was there a major breakthrough in third-party reimbursement. Social forces and the scientific revolution have produced many changes in hospital care. These forces have grown so strong, coupled with government regulations and escalating costs, that a new organizational structure for hospital systems has been mandated. Hospitals are being forced to become more and more responsive to community health needs, and more accountable to the community for their performance (14).

The economic forces of high cost, capital equipment obsolescence, cost containment directives, reimbursement, and government control are generating pressure on hospitals to share services within a geographic area.

The social forces of population shifts to the cities while health resources move to the suburbs, the push for consumer rights, the increase in the elderly and chronic disease population coupled with a declining birthrate, have forced consideration of role modifications in hospitals.

Political forces of government involvement, more pressures to achieve regionalization, cost containment, and the requirement for quality control ensure more comprehensive services. We can expect to see an alteration in the thinking of institutions that will yield a more effective and accessible delivery of care for consumers (15). This means for occupational therapy that we can assist our institutions in their survival while expanding our services into a community model that supports the basic concepts of our profession.

We have many hospital-based occupational therapy programs currently functioning within the community model of occupational therapy service delivery. Two that we can use as models are Memorial Hospital in Sarasota, Florida, directed by Louise Sampson, OTR, and Research Medical Center, Kansas City, Missouri, directed by Sharon East, OTR, and Gloria Scammahorn, OTR. Both programs are in community hospitals of 600 to 700 beds.

At Memorial Hospital, the occupational therapy department contracts with the county school system, Head Start, the Public Health Department, the Home Care Team, the Guidance Center, two extended care facilities, and an outpatient rehabilitation center. Groundwork has been laid for the community's outpatient dialysis unit. Future programs include a private facility for the mentally retarded, day care centers, service programs for the elderly, and a hospice.

At Research Medical Center, the occupational therapy department contracts with schools, nursing homes, and small rural community hospitals. Future programs include industry and home health services.

I asked each of these program directors to respond to the following questions: How do you view outreach in terms of your philosophy of Occupational Therapy practice?

> **Louise Sampson:** I believe that a hospital-based program is the most effective way to provide "outreach" occupational therapy services. If services are planned and accomplished properly, we do not have to remain a "medical model" and can serve the expressed needs of the community. I feel that the solid base has many advantages including decreasing the fragmentation and isolation of therapists, being cost effective with full utilization of staff and equipment providing more flexible opportunities for professional growth and a general consistency otherwise unavailable (16).

> **Sharon East, Gloria Scammahorn:** The outreach concept has certainly facilitated the growth and expansion of occupational therapy into new markets. Our association with a medical center has been an important aspect to the success of occupational therapy's involvement in outreach. Had there been no association with the medical center, I feel certain occupational therapy's efforts would have been stifled early on.
>
> The whole outreach approach has provided so much stimulation and remotivation for the staff involved that regardless of the outcome the experience for the staff has been well worth all the effort. That is not to say that we're not concerned with the outcome—we still maintain the same standards and quality of care for the outreach contracts as we do for the patients at our facility (17).

The outreach concept provides a stability for services that promotes creativity. It also will assure the continuance of our profession in modern economic times. It expands occupational therapy concepts into a community model with the hospital functioning as the base unit. It reduces the fragmentation and isolation of therapists, it is cost effective, it fully uses staff and equipment, and it promotes professional growth. It allows therapists with specialized skills to use their skill to fill contract hours using their expertise. It also allows facilities that otherwise would not have occupational therapy to obtain the services to fulfill needs.

Public Law 93-641 of 1974, The Health Planning and Resource Development Act, establishes the following priorities for national attention:

1. The provision of primary care services for medically underserved populations, especially those in rural or economically depressed areas.

2. The development of multi-institutional systems for consideration of institutional health services.
3. The development of medical group practices, especially those services that are appropriately coordinated or integrated with institutional health services and health maintenance (18).

Occupational therapists, we have a mandate: break down those walls. We have been accustomed to patients coming to us—we have to go to them. Let us establish occupational therapy as a viable community service implementing the basic philosophy of our profession and help our hospitals survive in the process. The challenge is here now—let us respond and further develop our profession in the process.

Now we will develop our treatment plan for problem three.

Problem III. The Health System Is Not Oriented Toward the Human Being.

GOAL: Develop Human Oriented Programs Encouraging Man to Explore his Potential in Producing a Change in his Own Health Status. The human that enters the health system has little knowledge of this situation and the health professional little of the individual's situation. We are nothing more than a bystander in the life of that individual until a relationship is formed.

Our service delivery is initiated by assessment with a resulting relationship that has the potential of making impact on that individual.

It would be difficult to expect an individual to be at home in a sterile and unfamiliar environment that has produced chaos. The individual must establish some control over the forces of chaos. In establishing control the client demonstrates a variety of behaviors, either by an internal mental operation or by external activity (19). Occupational therapists have the skills, attitude, and knowledge to provide the relationship and the structure through activity to introduce meaning to that individual and thus giving him control.

In *Anatomy of an Illness,* Norman Cousins tells of a personal experience with Pablo Casals that had a profound impact on him. I want to share it with you because it so poignantly expresses activity and its ability to produce meaning in the human.

> I learned that a highly developed purpose and a will to live are among the prime raw materials of human existence. I became convinced that these materials may well represent the most potent force within human reach. . . .

I met him for the first time at his home in Puerto Rico just a few weeks before his ninetieth birthday. I was fascinated by his daily routine. About 8 A.M. his lovely young wife Marta would help him to start the day. His various infirmities made it difficult for him to dress himself. Judging from his difficulty in walking and from the way he held his arms, I guessed he was suffering from rheumatoid arthritis. His emphysema was evident in his labored breathing. He came into the living room on Marta's arm. He was badly stooped. His head was pitched forward and he walked with a shuffle. His hands were swollen and his fingers were clenched.

Even before going to the breakfast table, Don Pablo went to the piano—which, I learned, was a daily ritual. He arranged himself with some difficulty on the piano bench, then with discernible effort raised his swollen and clenched fingers above the keyboard.

I was not prepared for the miracle that was about to happen. The fingers slowly unlocked and reached toward the keys like the buds of a plant toward the sunlight. His back straightened. He seemed to breathe more freely. Now his fingers settled on the keys. Then came the opening bars of Bach's *Wohltemperierte Klavier,* played with great sensitivity and control. I had forgotten that Don Pablo had achieved proficiency on several musical instruments before he took up the cello. He hummed as he played then said that Bach spoke to him here—and he placed his hand over his heart.

Then he plunged into a Brahms concerto and his fingers, now agile and powerful, raced across the keyboard with dazzling speed. His entire body seemed fused with the music: it was no longer still and shrunken but supple and graceful and completely freed of its arthritic coils.

Having finished his piece, he stood up by himself, far straighter and taller than when he had come into the room. He walked to the breakfast table with no trace of a shuffle, ate heartily, talked animatedly, finished the meal, then went for a walk on the beach.

After an hour or so, he came back to the house and worked on his correspondence until lunch. Then he napped. When he arose, the stoop and the shuffle and the clenched hands were back again . . . . As before, he stretched his arms in front of him and extended his fingers. Then the spine straightened and his fingers, hands, and arms were in sublime coordination as they responded to the demands of his brain for the controlled beauty of movement and tone. Any cellist thirty years his junior would have been proud to have such extraordinary physical command.

Twice in one day, I had seen the miracle. A man almost ninety, beset with the infirmities of old age, was able to cast off his afflictions, at least temporarily, because he knew he had something of overriding importance to do. There was no mystery about the way it worked, for it happened every day. Creativity for Pablo Casals was the source of his own cortisone. It is doubtful whether any anti-inflammatory medication he would have taken would have been as powerful or as safe as the substances produced by the interaction of his mind and body . . . He was caught up in his own creativity, in his own desire to accomplish a specific purpose, and the effect was both genuine and observable (20). (Excerpt reprinted from *Anatomy of an Illness,* by Norman Cousins, with the permission of the publisher, W.W. Norton & Company, Inc., New York, New York. Copyright© 1979 by W.W. Norton & Company, Inc.)

We all can recount of patients with strong wills. With the introduction of activity, we too have seen miracles.

As a profession, occupational therapy harnesses will and gives the individual control through activity. That is human, that is care. We are respected by physicians and the health care system for that caring, perhaps because we have a strong background in the physical and biological dimensions of life, as well as the psychological and social. Most importantly we have respect for the human and the unknown. This is empathy.

Brian Hall describes empathy as:

> The capacity for one person to enter imaginatively into the sphere of consciousness of another, to feel the specific contour of another experience, to allow one's imagination to risk entering the inner experiencing process of another (19, p 162).

Through our professional relationships we reach out and with empathy show that we care, hoping that from this caring the person will find his or her own strength.

The humanistic approach to patient care is the initial reason most health professionals entered their respective careers. Each of us is supposed to remember why we entered the human services system rather than have coursework that would intensify our commitment to the human being by the introduction of theories of humaneness, motivation, and values. I would like to see our curricula increase their program content in the area of values and motivation.

There are other groups of professionals, especially medical sociologists, who are trying to work their way *into* the health system to effect change from within. They desire the position that fields such as occupational therapy hold—that of a primary service, professionally recognized by physicians and reimbursed by third-party payment—because we are in the position to implement a total concept of health, a concept of caring. Also we are a recognized part of the health delivery system.

Those who do understand and support the humanism of health delivery must exert their control and influence in shaping the system in that direction. Health programs must be designed that support the patient's need to have control of his life, especially while he is receiving health care. Clinical studies can be designed by occupational therapists' relating to the outcome of care when the individual has control over his environment and is valued for his contribution to his care as opposed to giving up control.

A growing body of evidence indicates there are limits to what medicine can be expected to accomplish. There are still many unknowns.

There is still healing, there is still coping, and there is still the individual who must survive with dignity.

The major chronic conditions must be dealt with and outside the strict medical model. Improvements in these conditions require significant changes in personal life-style, habits, and environmental conditions.

Roger M. Battistella, in his essay "The Future of Primary Health Services," states:

> A strong foundation of simple and inexpensive services, for the treatment of routine illness and the care of illness apart from the relief of suffering, is essential.
> The importance of personalized relationships for the treatment of illness in which psychological and physical factors are heavily interconnected, the necessity to influence life-styles in the management of chronic illness, and the compelling obligations for the humane care of the incurable long-term ill and dying indicates that the relationship between the patient and the health professional displaced by progress in scientific medicine has to be restored . . . . (21, pp 315-316).

We must move prevention *into* the curative model as we contribute our skills and performance to the population served by the medical care system.

A humanistic health care system is possible—the possibility, however, requires much out of each professional, which decreases the probability. Occupational therapists have unique skills and a tremendous commitment to Man and his abilities. We must show great confidence in implementing our concepts of caring.

I have now presented strategies for three problems the profession must address.

By directing professional energies toward solving these problems we will:

1. Develop our services as scientific discipline, thus gain a stronger position with a strong professional identity;
2. Increase the dialogue of educators and clinicians toward common goals;
3. Expand the acute-care model of service to include an ambulatory and health prevention model;
4. Extend occupational therapy manpower by expanding services into intercity and rural delivery through multihospital systems;
5. Assist the individual in gaining control over his health status by having control of his environment and engaging in activity.

I want to share with you a very important thought of Bronowski's, from the *Ascent of Man:*

> Man is a singular creature. He has a set of gifts which make him unique among the animals so that, unlike them, he is not a figure in the landscape. He is a shaper of the landscape . . . His imagination, his reason, his emotional subtlety and toughness, make it possible for him not to accept the environment, but to change it (8, p 19).

This thought is true for us. It is true for each patient or client we serve. Are we a profession that supports change? I believe so.

Another quote from Bronowski:

> We are all afraid—for our confidence, for the future, for the world. That is the nature of the human imagination. Yet every man, every civilization, has gone forward because of its engagement with what it has set itself to do. The personal commitment of a man to his skills, the intellectual commitment and the emotional commitment working together as one, has made the Ascent of Man (8, p 438).

As a profession and as professionals, let us put our resources, intelligence, and emotional commitment together and work diligently toward the ascent of our profession. The health care system, the clients we serve, and each of us individually will benefit from our commitment.

REFERENCES

1. *Health and United States*, U.S. Department of Health, Education, and Welfare, Public Health Service, Health Resource Administration, 1978, p iii
2. Brown JHU: *The Health Care Dilemma*, New York: Human Sciences Press, 1978, pp 10-12
3. Cantril H: *Challenges of Humanistic Psychology*, New York: McGraw-Hill, 1967, pp 14-16
4. Battistella RM, Rundell TG: *Health Care Policy in a Changing Environment*, Berkeley: McCutcheon, 1978, pp XV-VXIII
5. Warner DM, Holloway DC: *Decision Making and Control for Health Administration*, Ann Arbor: Health Administration Press, 1978, pp 337-378
6. Glaser RJ: Some Thoughts of Medical Education and Medical Care, Health Manpower Education and Distribution, The Carnegie Commission Report, The Dedication Proceedings, Oct. 12, 13, 14, 1977, pp 65-66
7. Weimer R: *Educational Aspects of The Changing Role of Occupational Therapy*, Committee on Basic Professional Education Educational Forum, Oct. 31, 1969, "O.T." Community Health Alienation vs. Non-alienation, p 9
8. Bronowski J: *The Ascent of Man*, Boston: Little, Brown and Co., 1973, pp 62-64
9. Ad Hoc Committee on Education (Nationally Speaking) Issues in Education. *Am J Occup Ther* 32: 355-358, 1978
10. Von Bertalanffy L: *General Systems Theory*, New York: George Brazier, 1963, p 39
11. Snow CP: *The Two Cultures and a Second Look*, Cambridge: University Press, 1964, p 5
12. Snow CP: *The Search*, New York: Charles Scribner and Sons, 1968, p 49
13. Machlup F: *The Production and Distribution of Knowledge in the United States*, Princeton: Princeton University Press, 1962, p 122
14. Sheps CG: Trends in hospital care. In *Multi Hospital Systems: Strategies for Organization and Management*, Germantown, MD: Aspen Systems Press, 1980, pp 3-4

15. Brown M: Current trends in cooperative ventures. In *Multi Hospital Systems: Strategies for Organization and Management,* Germantown, MD: Aspen Systems Press, 1980, pp 14-19
16. Sampson L: Written Interview with Carolyn Baum, January 1980
17. East S: Scammahorn G, Conery W: Written Interview with Carolyn Baum, January 1980
18. Brown M: Sharing: An overview. In *Multi Hospital Systems: Strategies for Organization and Management,* Germantown, MD: Aspen Systems Press, 1978, pp 96-97
19. Hall BP: *The Development of Consciousness A Confluent Theory of Values,* New York: Paulistic Press, 1976, p 83
20. Cousins N: *Illness as Perceived by the Patient,* Toronto: W.W. Norton and Co., 1979, pp 72-75
21. Battistella RM, Rundell TG: *Health Care Policy in a Changing Environment,* Berkeley: McCutcheon, 1978, pp 315-316

Occupational Therapy Revisited: A Paraphrastic Journey

Robert K. Bing

I wish to dedicate the 1981 Eleanor Clarke Slagle Lectureship:

To my parents, who provided me with those cumulative experiences and values that inevitably led me to the decision to become an occupational therapist;

To a very great woman, Beatrice D. Wade, OTR, FAOTA, who has been my valued teacher and beloved mentor for more than 30 years;

To my cherished colleagues, Lillian Hoyle Parent and Jay Cantwell, both occupational therapists, who constantly stimulate me and insist on a high level of constructive activity;

To Charles H. Christiansen, OTR, whose personal and professional qualities and insistence on excellence from himself and others assure me of the future of occupational therapy.

Without the examples, teachings, guidance, counseling, and friendship of these individuals, I could never have achieved this exalted opportunity.

Try as one might, it is impossible to recount the evolution of occupational therapy so that it resembles the cliff-hanging biographies of Butch Cassidy and the Sundance Kid. Masters and Johnson, as well as Kinsey, who took years to amass their stories, had something going for them that does not exist for us. Somewhat puckishly I was tempted to entitle this paper, *Everything You've Ever Wanted to Know About Occupational Therapy, but Were Afraid to Ask*. That would not have been altogether misleading. Because of my part German heritage, and true to that cultural bias and tendency, I thought I should take us back to the Thirty

Reprinted from *The American Journal of Occupational Therapy*, Vol. 35, No. 8, 1981

Years' War and bring everyone up to date. After all, it is important territory occupational therapy has won and lost.

The title, *Occupational Therapy Revisited: A Paraphrastic Journey*, prevailed because this paper is a tour to what should be familiar historical landmarks and progenitors. For some of us, it will renew old friendships and acquaintances. For others, it will be a second-hand account of certain ancestors, not unlike those stories that emanate from grandmothers. For some, it will only be like an endurance of those pictures that inevitably get projected on the screen by vacationers returning home.

Because of the relative youthfulness of those of us in practice (most have entered within the past decade), now seems the time to critically examine our ancestral roots and subsequent grafts to determine the nature of the present and to offer some speculations about why we (and the profession) developed as we did through several generations. This is not the history of occupational therapy nor of the Association that supports our endeavors. Nor is it a history like someone else might well find it. It is not a detailed, definitive account of how we multiplied, divided, and invaded several areas of medicine and health care. It is one person's way of telling the story of who we are and citing some lessons to be learned. That is important! After several months of submergence just off the coast of Texas (as my colleagues in Galveston will attest), I have at long last come up for air and am ready to declare my findings.

This is a statement of how an idea, born in a philosophical movement, became activated through *the good works of men and women* who inalterably believed in the ideal that those who are sick and handicapped can regain, retain, and attain some semblance of function within the fundamental limitations of the human organism and the expectations of the society in which all must exist: that this may occur through the most obvious means of all—*one's reorganization through occupation, through activity, through leisure, and through rest.*

This journey about occupational therapy, its evolution and development, presents vexation: one must accept a fair number of ambiguities, something some today consider a fundamental problem in occupational therapy; a more than reasonable amount of astonishment; and a certain degree of messiness, closely akin to what is created by the beginner in finger painting. What can it all mean? What was taking place at the time? Will the patient recover? Most significantly, does it make any difference? To answer these and related questions I wanted to conduct some scholarly research that could be equally interesting, helpful, and valuable to students, occupational therapy assistants, occupational therapists, and others who are interested in our profession. This is how I interpret the intent of the originators of the Eleanor Clarke Slagle Lectureship.

Such a historical presentation should be long enough to say something, yet short enough to be tolerated.

To give you some idea of the continuing dilemma I encountered these past several months in preparing the lecture and in limiting its scope and length, I wrote:

> There once was a historian named Dan,
> Whose prose no one could scan,
> When, once, asked about it,
> He said, "I don't doubt it,
> Because I try to cram as many facts and dates into each sentence as I possibly can."

Significant Landmarks

Let us start this paraphrastic journey and take note of some significant landmarks along the way—those recurring patterns and themes of the past 200 years that give us today's relevance:

1. There is an inextricable union of the mind and the body; the employment of activity or occupation must be based on this precept, which is unique to occupational therapy.
2. Activity, inherently, contains modes the patient may employ to gain understanding of and ascendancy over one's feelings, actions, and thoughts. These modes include the habits of attention and interest; the perceived usefulness of occupation; creative expression; the processes of learning; the acquisition of skill; and evidence of accomplishment.
3. Activity provides a balance between the practical and intellectual components of experience; therefore, a wide variety of activities must be accessible to meet human objectives for work, leisure, and rest.
4. One's approach to the patient is as significant to treatment and rehabilitation as is the selection and utilization of an activity.
5. Essential elements of occupational therapy practice are continuous observation, experimentation, empiricism, and analysis.
6. An appreciation of the pain that accompanies an illness or disability; a strong desire to reduce or remove it; a gentle firmness;

and a knowledge of the patient's needs are fundamental characteristics of the provider of therapeutic occupations.
7. Therapeutic processes and modes of treatment are synonymous with the processes of learning and methods of education.
8. The patient is the product of his or her own efforts, not the article made nor the activity accomplished.

A Theory of Experience

We could go back to the Garden of Eden to begin this story, if time permitted, since occupational therapy could well have started in that idyllic spot. Dr. Dunton, one of the founders of the 20th century movement, insisted that those fig leaves had to have been crocheted by Eve, who was trying to get over her troubles. They had something to do with her being beholden to Adam and his rib. We will unfortunately pass over all of that and begin the modern epoch with a brief description of what was taking place in Europe approximately 200 years ago.

It was the *Age of Enlightenment*, or, as some prefer, the *Age of Reason*. The roots of 20th century occupational therapy are visible in the empiricism of John Locke, an English philosopher and physician, who fostered confidence in human reason and human freedom; in Etienne de Condillac, a French philosopher, who advanced the dualism of body and mind; and in Pierre Cabanis, a French physician and theorist, who offered an explanation of the importance of the moral and social sciences in perfecting the art of medicine. These three, together with others, popularized the new ideas. Indeed, it was the *best of times*, a clear demarcation in the emergence of the modern world.

If one were to combine the thoughts of these three, one would arrive at a *theory of experience*. John Locke, in his famous *Essay Concerning Human Understanding*, published in 1690 (1), examines the nature of the human mind and the processes by which it learns about and comes to know the world. When born, the human is a blank tablet (tabula rasa). Because of an innate ability to receive sensations from the outside world, the human can assimilate and organize impressions. As contact with the environment stimulates the senses and causes impressions, the mind receives and organizes these into ideas and concepts. Since the human mind does not already contain innate ideas, all must come from without (2, p 287).

There is a second source for the accumulation of experience, according to Locke. It is the mind itself: ". . . the perception of the operations of our own mind, . . . [such as] thinking, doubting, believing, reasoning, knowing. . . . this source of ideas every man has wholly within himself."(3, p 74) Locke strongly held that the body and mind exist as real entities and they interact. He spent a great deal of time developing his perspective. He spoke of the aim of education as the process of knowing and learning through experience and in striving toward happiness. Ideally, he contended, one should work toward a sound mind in a healthy body. To achieve this ideal, Locke advocated physical exercise as a hardening process, and an exposure to a wide variety of sensations from the physical and social worlds.

Condillac was Locke's apologist. He tried to simplify Locke's fundamental theory by arguing that all conscious experiences are the result of passive sensations; these sensations are the raw materials from which one forms complex and interrelated ideas. Learning is the noting of incomplete ideas, considering each separately, combining them into relationships, and ordering them. This process results in retaining the strongest degrees of association. Condillac asserted: "Then we shall grasp (ideas) easily and clearly and shall understand their origins entirely." (see 3, p 7)

Elsewhere in his writings Condillac presented his thoughts on analysis. One cannot have the proper conception of a thing until one is in a position to analyze it. "To analyze," claimed Condillac, "is nothing more than to observe in successive order the qualities of an object, . . . the simultaneous order in which they exist."(4, p 17)

The third philosopher, Pierre Cabanis, tended to apply medicine to philosophy and philosophy to medicine. Cabanis considered illness and its impact upon the formulation of values and ideas. Through the social sciences, which emerged in the *Age of Enlightenment*, he explained *moral* as a psychological phenomenon on a physiological base. He concluded that moral impressions can have both physiological and pathological results. At last, there was a rational explanation for the psychological production of disease in which the so-called moral (emotional) passions play a significant part (5, pp 37-38). Cabanis contributed a socially based theoretical explanation of human experience that became the cornerstone for the moral management of the insane.

Age of Enlightenment and Moral Treatment

Moral treatment of the insane was one result of the *Age of Enlightenment*. It sprang from the fundamental attitudes of the day, a set of principles that govern humanity and society; faith in the ability of the human to reason; and the supreme belief in the individual. The rapid changes caused by this new philosophy advanced the disappearance of the notion that the insane were possessed of the devil. Mental diseases became legitimate concerns of humanitarians and physicians. The discontinuance of the idea that crime, sin, and vice were at the core of insanity brought forth humane treatment. Up to this time the insane had been housed and handled no differently than were criminals or paupers—often in chains.

Two men of the 18th century working in different countries, and unknown to each other, initiated the moral treatment movement. "No two men could possibly have been chosen out of all Europe at that time of whom it could be said more truly that they were cradled, and nursed, and educated among widely differing social, political, religious influences . . . ."(6, pp 24-25) Philippe Pinel was a child of the French Revolution, a physician, a scholar, and a philosopher. He is described as ". . . far exceeding the bounds of pure humanitarianism . . . to encompass the goals of a naturalist, . . . a reformer, a clinician, . . . and, above all, a philosopher."(7, *Intro*) William Tuke was a devout member of the Society of Friends (Quakers).

Philippe Pinel: Physician-Reformer

Whenever Philippe Pinel's name comes up in a conversation among health professionals, he is immediately mentioned as the *striker of the chains* at two French hospitals. His efforts and contributions go way beyond that reformational act. As a physician, he began his most serious work in 1792 as superintendent of Bicêtre, the asylum for incurable males in Paris.

As a natural scientist, Pinel achieved exceptional skill in the observation of human behavior and the bringing of ". . . some order into the chaos of . . . treatment methods by means of critical and objective investigations."(5, p 12) Pinel says this about himself:

> Desirous of better information, I resolved for myself the facts that were presented to my attention; and forgetting the empty honours of my titular distinction as a physician, I viewed the scene that was opened to me with the eye of common sense and unprejudiced observation (8, p 109).

From his own experience, he urged that observations ". . . be the basis upon which (one) should decide what opinions to believe."(9, pp 74-75) Throughout his work, he held constantly before him his own motto of independent thought: "Chercher à èviter toute illusion, toute prè-vention, toute opinion adoptèe sur parole" (to seek to avoid all illusion, all prejudice, all opinion taken on authority) (10, pp 8-9).

Pinel's descriptions of the mentally deranged provide insight into his own compassionate nature. For him, the loss of reason was the most calamitous of human afflictions. The ability to reason principally separates the human from other living forms. Because of mental illness, the human's ". . . character is always perverted, sometimes annihilated. His thoughts and actions are diverted. . . . His personal liberty is at length taken from him. . . . To this melancholy train of symptoms, if not early and judiciously treated . . . a state of the most abject degradation sooner or later succeeds." (8, pp *xv-xvii*)

What Pinel entitled *revolution morale*, or moral revolution, is the ultimate insight of the insane into the delusional and absurd nature of their experiences (7, p 256). This, to him, was the basis for treatment. Some historians believe that he was stating that moral treatment is synonymous with the humane approach. His own writings do not bear this out. Pinel believed that each patient must be critically observed and analyzed; then treatment should commence. "To apply the principles of moral treatment, with undiscriminating uniformity, would be . . . ridiculous and unadvisable."(8, p 66) The moral method is well reasoned and carefully planned for the individual patient.

According to Pinel, moral management is a maintained continuity of approach; a predictable routine, infused with vigor by personnel who inspire confidence. Moreover, moral treatment calls for a constant, observed study of patient behavior and performance. It included a gentle, but firm approach. Each patient is given as much liberty within the institution as he or she can tolerate. The approach is designed to give the patient a feeling of security as well as a respect for authority. Pinel asserted: "The atmosphere should be the same as in a family where the parents are quite strict. To establish this relationship, the doctor must convince the patient that he wishes to help him and that recovery is a real possibility." (9, p 76)

Occupations figured prominently in Pinel's conception of moral treatment. He used activities to take the patients' thoughts away from their emotional problems and to develop their abilities. He considered literature and music as effective in altering patients' emotions. Physical exercise and work should be part of every institution's fundamental program and be employed in accord with individual tastes. He concluded: "The (occupations) method is primarily designed and intended to reach man at his best which . . . means human understanding, intelligence, and insight."(3, pp 63-64)

The concept of *moral treatment* belongs solely to Philippe Pinel. His fundamental belief was that its purpose is to restore the patient to himself, ". . . to use the patient's own emotions to balance his emotional excesses."(9, p 76) Truly, Pinel and his efforts, rooted in the *Age of Enlightenment*, mark the beginning of the modern epoch in the care of the mentally ill.

William Tuke: Philanthropist-Humanitarian

Across the channel, in England, things were astir at the same time. King George III, who was giving the American colonies fits, was himself in similar trouble. In 1788 it became public knowledge that the King was seized with mania. Questions arose about his fitness to continue ruling. Nevertheless, public sentiment was on his side. For the first time, insanity and its treatment formed a topic of public discussion: "The subject had been brought out of concealment in a way which defeated the conspiracy of silence."(11, p 42) This being the *Age of Enlightenment*, the public openly sympathized with the sufferer; there was no condemnation. No one suggested that the King was being visited by the Devil, or that he was being punished for his sins.

The Society of Friends, derisively called Quakers, originated in 17th century England and became one of the most distinctive movements of Puritanism: "They arose out of the religious unrest of England . . . and stood for a radical kind of reform within Christendom which contrasted sharply with Protestant, Anglican and Roman patterns alike." (12, p 118) George Fox, founder of the Society, discovered ". . . the spirit of the living Christ and knew that it was an experience open to all men. 'This was the true light that lighteth every man that cometh into the world!' " (13, p 1)

William Tuke, a devout Quaker, wealthy merchant, and renowned philanthropist, was made aware of the deplorable conditions in the insane asylum in York, England. There were tales of extreme neglect and possible cruelty. He was an unusual man, not given to listening to sensational reports and acting rashly (14, p 12). In true Quaker fashion Tuke presented a concern at a Friend's Quarterly Meeting in the spring of 1792—that an institution for the insane be established in York under the direction of the Society. At first, he was met with considerable resistance by those who believed that there were too few mentally ill Quakers, and that no one would want them concentrated in such a lovely, quiet locale (15, p 58).

The York Retreat

Initially, Tuke was disheartened; yet, he pressed on, and within six months *The Retreat for Persons* afflicted with *Disorders of the Mind*, or simply, *The Retreat* came into being. Up until then the term *Retreat* had never been applied to an asylum. Tuke's daughter-in-law suggested the term to convey the Quaker belief that such an institution may be ". . . a place in which the unhappy might obtain refuge; a quiet haven in which (one) . . . might find a means of reparation or of safety."(16, p 20) The cornerstone simply stated the purpose of the institution: "The charity or love of friends executed this work in the cause of humanity."(15, p 19)

William Tuke became the superintendent. Thomas Fowler, an unusually open-minded man, was appointed visiting physician. After a trial-and-error period, they came to believe that moral treatment methods were preferable to those involving restraint and use of harsh drugs. The new approach was a product of Tuke's humanitarianism and Fowler's empiricism.

Several fundamental principles became evident within a short time. The approach was primarily one of kindness and consideration. The patients were not thought to be devoid of reason, feeling, and honor. The social environment was to be as nearly like that of a family as possible, with an atmosphere of religious sentiment and moral feeling (16, p 35).

Tuke and Fowler strongly believed that most insane people retain a considerable amount of self-command. Upon admission, the patient was informed that treatment depended largely upon one's own conduct. Employment in various occupations was expected as a way for the patient to maintain control over his or her disorder. As Tuke reported: ". . . regular employment is perhaps the most efficacious; and those kinds of employment . . . to be preferred . . . are accompanied by considerable bodily action."(16, p 156) The staff endeavored to gain the patient's confidence and esteem, to arrest the attention and fix it upon objects opposite to any illusion the patient might have. The fundamental purpose of employment and recreation was to facilitate the regaining of the *habit of attention*, as Tuke called it. Various learning exercises were used, such as mathematical problems, to help the patient gain ascendancy over faulty habits of attention.

Tuke and Fowler determined that "indolence has a natural tendency to weaken the mind, and to induce ennui and discontent. . . ."(16, pp 180-181) A wide range of occupations and amusements was available. Patients not engaged in useful occupations were allowed to read, draw, or play various games. Tea parties, walks, and visitations away from the institution were planned regularly in preparation for the patients' returning home. All activities were closely analyzed through observation in order to individualize patients' needs.

The pioneer work of William Tuke and his son, Samuel, who wrote the definitive treatise on *The Retreat,* opened a new chapter in the history of the care of the insane in England. Mild management methods, infused with kindness, and building self-esteem through the judicious use of occupations, resulted in the excitation and elicitation of superior, human motives. Patients recovered, left *The Retreat,* and rarely needed to return for further care. The entire regimen was carefully patterned ". . . to accord (patients) the dignity and status of sick human beings."(17, p 687)

Moral Treatment Expansion

As soon as Pinel's major work on moral treatment (1801) and Samuel Tuke's description of *The Retreat* were published (1813), there was a rush toward implementing many reforms in other hospitals, particularly in England and the United States. In both countries occupations were introduced as an integral part of moral treatment (18, pp 83-84). Some unusual experiments were undertaken by Sir William Charles Ellis, a physician, who became the superintendent of a pauper lunatic asylum. The mainstay of his asylum management was useful occupations. He moved well ahead of mere amusements and "introduced a gainful employment of patients on a large scale and even had them taught a trade." (19, p 62) Ellis and his wife undertook other reforms. She organized the women patients into groups under the supervision of a *workwoman* to make useful and fancy articles.

Another Ellis innovation was the development of what would eventually be called *halfway houses.* Keenly aware of environmental and social influences on insanity, Ellis suggested ". . . aftercare houses and night hospitals as a stepping stone from the asylum to the world by which . . . the length of patients' stay would be reduced and in many cases the cure completed. . . ."(17, p 871) He insisted that convalescing patients should go out and mix with the world before discharge. His proposals were made in the 1830s!

In the United States, few public and private asylums existed in the post-Revolutionary era: however, institutional reforms were needed. Any recounting of this period must include two very important individuals and their work: Benjamin Rush and Dorothea Lynde Dix. Their efforts did not overlap: they did not know one another, nor was one influenced by the other. Just as in the cases of Pinel and Tuke, no two individuals this side of the Atlantic could have been more unlike one another in background, education, or experience. Nevertheless, each recognized the hapless plights of the institutionalized insane and set out to alleviate dire conditions and the inauguration of moral treatment, including occupations and exercise.

Benjamin Rush: Father of American Psychiatry

Benjamin Rush, often referred to as the *father of American psychiatry*, was a Philadelphia physician in the latter half of the 1700s. Through his training in Europe and several visits there, he adopted many of Pinel's practices; however, Rush did not adopt moral principles until later. As a member of the staff of Pennsylvania Hospital, he was placed in charge of a separate section set aside for the insane, the first hospital in America to reserve such a section. He was appalled by the conditions and he appealed to the staff and the public for change. Change did come and humane treatment was instituted. Rush saw to it that "certain employments be devised for such of the deranged people as are capable of working. . . ."(20, p 257) This approach was based upon his philosophical stance that man, by his very nature, is meant to be active; "Even in paradise (Garden of Eden) he was employed in the health and pleasant exercises of cultivating a garden. Happiness, consisting in folded arms, and in pensive contemplation . . . by the side of brooks, never had any existence, except in the brains of mad poets, and love-sick girls and boys."(21, pp 115-116)

In his major writing, *Medical Inquiries and Observations Upon the Diseases of the Mind,* Rush clearly differentiates between goal-directed activity and aimless exercise: "Labour has several advantages over exercise, in being not only more stimulating, but more endurable in its effect; . . . it is calculated to arrest wrong habits of action, and to restore such as regular and natural. . . ."(21, pp 224-225)

Dorothea Lynde Dix: Humanitarian-Reformer

Dorothea Lynde Dix, a reform-minded humanitarian during the middle 1800s, vehemently pressed for improved conditions of the insane who were incarcerated in jails and almshouses. She presented a number of *Memorials* to state legislatures, believing that the public had an obligation to care for such individuals. By 1848 numerous states had responded to her efforts, and she decided to tackle a more formidable object—the Federal government. Dix envisioned the sale of public lands to finance the building of a federal system of hospitals for the indigent blind, deaf and mute, as well as the insane. For six years she wheedled and cajoled members of the Congress. Finally, in 1854, the bill was ready for President Franklin Pierce's signature. He was a close friend of Miss Dix and she felt highly confident of the outcome. The President vetoed the bill claiming unconstitutionality: ". . . every human weakness or sorrow would take advantage of this bill if it became law. . . . It endangers states' rights."(22, p 20) Through her contacts with physicians in several states, Miss Dix embraced moral treatment as the most humane method. She strongly advocated ". . . decent care, quiet, affection and normal activity (as) the only medicine for the insane."(22, p 11)

United States: Individual Treatment, Occupations, Education

The Quakers brought moral treatment to the United States as part of their intellectual and religious luggage. Through published accounts about *The Retreat* in York, some private asylums were established in which moral principles were practiced. A number of public institutions altered their programs to include individualized treatment, occupations, and education. Those patients who had remained for years unimproved and listless, even on the verge of apathy ". . . are seen in encouraging instances, when transferred to attendants who have more disposition to attend to them, . . . to waken (them) from their torpor, to become animated, active and even industrious. . . ."(23, pp 487-488)

Moral management also was taking on a new facet: The influence of a sane mind upon the insane mind. Those who daily attended the sick were to impress upon the insane the influences of their own character, designed to specifically improve the patients' behavior. Personnel must possess a number of traits: observational skills to see the ". . . actual condition of the patient's mind . . . and a faculty of clear insight. . . ." (23, p 489) Other traits: ". . . seeing that which is passing in the minds of (patients). . . . Add to this a firm will, the faculty of self-control, a sympathizing distress at moral pain, a strong desire to remove it. . . ." (23, p 489)

Arguments appeared in the literature relative to the moral use of firmness and gentleness. Strong cases were made for both extremes; however, it took two alienists (the precursor to psychiatrist), John Bucknill and D. Hack Tuke, grandson of Samuel Tuke, in 1858 to settle the dispute: "The truth, as usual, lies between; and the (individual) who aims at success in the moral treatment of the insane must be ready to be all things to all men, if by any means he might save some." (23, p 500) They elaborate on their thesis by stating: "With self-reliance, . . . it requires widely different manifestations, to repress excitement, to stimulate inertia, to check the vicious, to comfort the depressed, to direct the erring, to support the weak, to supplant every variety of erroneous opinion, to resist every kind of perverted feeling, and to check every form of pernicious conduct." (23, p 500)

Bucknill and Tuke also wrote that moral treatment included the gaining of the patient's confidence, fixing his or her attention on interesting and wholesome objects of thought, diverting the mind from introspection, and loosening the hold on concentrated emotion. They explain: "For (these) purposes useful occupation is far superior to any form of amusement. The higher the purpose, and the more appellant the nature of the occupation . . . the more likely it is to draw him from the contemplation of self-wretchedness, and effect the triumph of moral influences." (23, p 493)

The next step in institutional occupations emphasized education. Those occupations that require a process of learning and thought were determined far preferable, from a curative point of view, than those that require none. "Moral treatment is as wide as that of education; . . . it is education applied to the field of mental phenomena. . . ." (23, p 501) Therefore, it was not unusual to find specific mental activities included with occupations. The purpose was to educate the individual in order to provide him or her with "the power of controlling his feelings, and his thoughts, and his actions." (24, pp 166-167)

With continued experience, a number of alienists decided that occupations and amusements also could serve as a prophylactic against insanity. One interesting prescription for the return and maintenance of sanity was: ". . . rest in bed, occupation, exercise, and amusements." (25, p 14) D. Hack Tuke declared: "If idleness is a curse to the sane, it is the parent of mischief and ennui to the insane, especially to the pubescent and adolescent."(26, p 1315) He urges that the same approach be taken with the sane and the insane: "Employment, Nature's universal law of health, alike for body and mind, is specially beneficial, . . . seeing that it displaces ideas by new and healthy thoughts, revives familiar habits of daily activity, restores (and maintains) self-respect while it promotes the general bodily health." (26, p 1315)

Decline of Moral Treatment

Moral management and treatment by occupations reached its zenith in the United States just before the outbreak of the War Between the States (Civil War). Corporate, private asylums continued to expand their efforts. State- and public-supported institutions withdrew their programs, so that by the last quarter of the 19th century, virtually no moral treatment was taking place.

Several reasons for this decline and eventual disappearance can be identified, including a nation at war with itself. Bockhoven cites others:

1. The founders of the U.S. movement retired and died, leaving no disciples or successors;
2. The rapidly increasing influx of foreign-born and poor patients greatly overtaxed existing facilities and required more institutions to be built with diminished tax support;
3. Racial and religious prejudices on the part of the alienists, beginning to be called psychiatrists, reduced interest in treatment and cure; and
4. State legislatures became increasingly more interested in less costly custodial care (27, pp 20-25).

Essentially, there was no place in the public institutions for moral treatment. "The inferior physical plants and facilities, poorly trained and insufficient staff, . . . and, worst of all, overcrowding, prohibited any attempts to practice moral management."(28, p 128) A belief emerged that many insane were incurable. One eminent psychiatrist stated: "I have come to the conclusion that when a man becomes insane he is about used up for this world."(29, p 155) Such pessimism was predominant for a century in this country. Custodial care had come to stay for a very long time.

As we shall see next, moral principles and practices emerged in the early years of the 20th century through the efforts of individuals, then by a group who founded an organization dedicated to those principles. This group, in collaboration with others, established a definition and fundamental principles that have carried over through several generations of specifically educated practitioners of occupational therapy.

Once again, as with Pinel and Tuke, Rush and Dix, the individuals who founded and pioneered the 20th century occupational therapy movement could not have been more diverse in their backgrounds, experience, and education. They included a nurse, two architects, a physician, a social worker, and a teacher.

Susan Tracy: Occupational Nurse

Susan Tracy was this century's first proponent of occupations for invalids. A trained nurse, she initiated instruction in activities to student nurses as early as 1905 as part of their expanding responsibilities. She also developed the term *occupational nurses* to signify specialization (30, p 401). By 1912 she decided to devote all her energies to patient activities and she distinguished herself by applying moral treatment principles to acute conditions. As Tracy stated, "The application of this most rational remedy to ordinary, everyday sick people, as found in the general hospital, is almost unknown." (31, p 386) She strongly claimed that remedial treatments "are classified according to their physiological effects as stimulants, sedatives, anesthetics . . ., etc. Certain occupations possess like properties." (31, p 386) The physician may select stimulating occupations, such as watercoloring and paper folding; or sedative occupations such as knitting, weaving, and basketry.

Throughout Tracy's many years of work she employed experimentation and observation to enhance her practice. Her carefully worded writings provide ample evidence of her intense desire to bring scientific principles to the application of invalid occupations. In 1918 she published a remarkable research paper on 25 mental tests derived from occupations; for example, by instructing the patient in using a piece of leather and a pencil, "require him to make a line of dots at equal distances around the margin and at uniform distances from the edge. This constitutes a test of *Judgment* in estimating distances." (32, p 15) Continuing with the same piece of leather, the patient is instructed to punch a hole at each dot. "In order to do this he must consider the two sides of leather, the two parts of his tool and bring these together thus making a *Simple Coordination* test." (32, p 16) Other tests in the fabrication of the leather purse include *Aesthetic Coordination and Rhythm, Differentiation of Form and*

Size, Purposeful Relation. In all 25 tests, she stressed a completed, useful and "not unbeautiful" object.

Tracy's other writings state the value and usefulness of discarded materials to successful ward work (33, p 62). She also emphasized high quality workmanship: "It is now believed that what is worth doing at all is worth doing well, and that practical, well-made articles have a greater therapeutic value than a useless, poorly made article."(34, p 198) A premium is placed upon originality and the "... adoption of the occupation to the condition and natural tastes of the patient." (35, p 63) Further, she believes that "... the patient is the product, not the article that he makes."(33, p 59)

Tracy's major work, *Studies in Invalid Occupation*, published in 1918 (36), is a revealing compendium of her observations and experiences with different kinds of patients, for instance: "the child of poverty and the child of wealth, the impatient boy, grandmother, the business man."

By 1921, Susan Tracy had adopted the term *occupation therapy* originally coined by William Rush Dunton, Jr., and defined it and differentiated it from vocational training. She felt this was necessary because of the arising confusion between the two concepts following World War I. She wrote: "What is occupation? The treatment of disease by occupation.... The aim of occupation is to get the man well; that of vocational training is to provide him with a job. Any well man will look for a job, but the sick man is looking for health."(37, p 120)

Throughout all of her writings she stated that nothing is "... too small to be pressed into the service of resourceful mind and trained hands toward... the establishment of a healthy mind in a healthy body." (33, p 57)

George Barton: Re-education of Convalescents

George Edward Barton, by profession an architect, contracted tuberculosis in his adult life. This plagued him for the remainder of his years. His constant struggle led him into a life of service to the physically handicapped. Out of his own personal concerns came the establishment of Consolation House, an early prototype of a rehabilitation center. He was an effective speaker and writer, often given to hyperbole; he gained his point with the listening or reading public.

Barton's central themes were hospitals and their responsibility to the discharged patient; the conditions the discharged patient faces; the need to return to employment; occupations and re-education of convalescents. These were intense concerns to him because of his own health problems.

His first published article, derived from a speech given to a group of nurses, points out a weakness he perceived in hospitals: "We discharge from them not efficients, but inefficients. An individual leaves almost any of our institutions only to become a burden upon his family, his friends, the associated charities, or upon another institution." (38, p 328) In the same article, he warms to his subject: "I say to discharge a patient from the hospital, with his fracture healed, to be sure, but to a devastated home, to an empty desk and to no obvious sustaining employment, is to send him out to a world cold and bleak. . . ."(38, p 329) His solution: ". . . occupation would shorten convalescence and improve the condition of many patients."(38, p 329) He ended his oration with a rallying cry: ". . . it is time for humanity to cease regarding the hospital as a door closing upon a life which is past and to regard it henceforth as a door opening upon a life which is to come."(38, p 330)

Barton established Consolation House in Clifton Springs, New York. Those referred to his institution underwent a thorough review, including a social and medical history, and a consideration of one's education, training, experience, successes, and failures. Barton believed that "By considering these in relation to the condition (the patient) must presumably or inevitably be in for the remainder of his life, we can find some form of occupation for which he will be fitted. . . ."(39, p 336) He claimed that Consolation House was "getting down to our social difficulties."(39, p 337)

By 1915, Barton had adopted Dunton's term, *occupation* therapy, but preferred the adjectival form: occupational therapy. He declared: "If there is an occupational disease, why not an occupational therapy?" (40, p 139) He expansively stated: "The first thing to be done . . . is for occupational therapy to provide an occupation which will produce *a similar therapeutic effect to that of every drug in materia medica.* An exercise for each separate organ, joint, and muscle of the human body. An exercise? An occupation! An occupation? A useful occupation! Then [occupational therapy] can fill the doctor's prescriptions . . . written in the terms of materia medica."(40, p 139) He even advocated curing constipation by *occupation.*

Re-education entered Barton's terminology with the aftermath of World War I. He viewed hospitals as taking on a mission different from that previously adopted. A hospital should become ". . . a re-educational institution through which to put the waste products of society *back and into the right place.*" (40, p 139) Using alliteration, he declared: ". . . by a catalytic concatenation of contiguous circumstances we were forced to realize that when all is said and done, what the sick man really needed and wanted most was the restoration of his ability to work, to live independently and to make money." (41, p 320)

Barton's major contribution to the re-emergence of moral treatment was the awakening of physical reconstruction and re-education through the employment of occupations. Convalescence, to him, was a critical time for the inclusion of something to do. Activity ". . . clarifies and strengthens the mind by increasing and maintaining interest in wholesome thought to the exclusion of morbid thought . . . and a proper occupation . . . during convalescence may be made the basis of the corollary of a new life upon recovery . . . I mean *a job, a better job, or a job done better* than it was before. (42, p 309) With Susan Tracy, Barton held that the major consideration of occupations ". . . should be devoted to the therapeutic and education effects, not to the value of the possible product." (43, p 36)

William Rush Dunton, Jr: Judicious Regimen of Activity

Of the founders of the 20th century movement, William Rush Dunton, Jr., was the most prolific writer and the most influential. He published in excess of 120 books and articles related to occupational therapy and rehabilitation: served as president of the National Society for the Promotion of Occupational Therapy; and, for 21 years, was editor of the official journal. As a physician, he spent his professional career treating psychiatric patients in an institutional setting. Key to his treatment methods is occupational therapy, a term he coined to differentiate aimless amusements from those occupations definitely prescribed for their therapeutic benefits. Before embarking on what he called a *judicious regimen of activity*, he read the works of Tuke and Pinel, as well as the efforts of significant alienists of the 19th century.

From his readings and from observations of patients in Sheppard Asylum, a Quaker institution in Towson, Maryland, Dunton concluded that the acutely ill are generally not amenable to occupations or recreation. The acutely ill exhibit a weakened power of attention. Occupations at this time would be fatiguing and harmful. The prevailing prescription is ". . . to let the patient alone, meanwhile improve (his) condition, restore and revivify exhausted mental and physical forces. . . ." (44, p 19) Later, activities should be selected that use energies not needed for physical restoration. Stimulating attention and directing the thoughts of the patient in regular and healthful paths would ensure an early release from the hospital. Dunton developed a wide variety of activities from knitting and crocheting to printing and the repair of dynamos, in order to gain the attention and interest, as well as to meet the needs, of all patients.

Dunton's proclivities for history and research led him to extensive readings and experimentations—all related to the human, his need for work, leisure, rest, and sleep; the causal factors of mental aberrations; various cures of mental illness. Each excursion brought him back to a *judicious regimen of activity* as the treatment of choice, regardless of whether the patient was mentally or physically ill. He became more and more convinced that attention and interest in one's work and play are as efficacious, if not more so, than the many and varied other medications available. He stated it this way: "It has been found that a patient makes more rapid progress if his attention is concentrated upon what he is making and he derives stimulating pleasure in its performance." (45, p 19)

At the second annual meeting of the National Society for the Promotion of Occupational Therapy (AOTA) in 1918, Dunton unveiled his nine cardinal rules to guide the emerging practice of occupational therapy, and to ensure that the new discipline would gain acceptance as a medical entity: 1. any activity in which the patient engages should have as its objective a cure; 2. it should be interesting; 3. it should have a useful purpose other than merely to gain the patient's attention and interest; 4. it should preferably lead to an increase in knowledge on the patient's part; 5. curative activity should preferably be carried out with others, such as in a group; 6. the occupational therapist should make a careful study of the patient in order to know his or her needs and attempt to meet as many as possible through activity; 7. the therapist should stop the patient in his or her work before reaching a point of fatigue; 8. encouragement should be genuinely given whenever indicated; and 9. work is much preferred over idleness, even when the end product of the patient's labor is of a poor quality or is useless (46, pp 26-27).

The major purposes of occupation in the case of the mentally ill were outlined in Dunton's first book (47, pp 24-26). The primary objective is to divert the attention either from unpleasant subjects, as is true with the depressed patient; or from daydreaming or mental ruminations, as in the case of the patient suffering from dementia praecox (schizophrenia)—that is, to divert the attention to one main subject.

Another purpose of occupation is to re-educate—to train the patient in developing mental processes through ". . . educating the hands, eyes, muscles, just as is done in the developing child." (47, p 25) Fostering an interest in hobbies is a third purpose. Hobbies serve as present, as well as future, safety valves and render recurrence of mental illness less likely. A final purpose may be to instruct the patient in a craft until he or she has enough proficiency to take pride in his or her work. However, Dunton did note that "While this is proper, I fear . . . specialism is apt to cause a narrowing of one's mental outlook. . . . The individual with a knowledge of many things has more interest in the world in general." (47, p 26)

Dunton continued to write and publish his observations, each one elaborating on a previous one. His texts became required reading for students preparing for practice. Even in his 90s, well beyond retirement from practice, he maintained an interest in our profession and continued to offer counsel.

Eleanor Clarke Slagle: Founder-Pioneer

Eleanor Clarke Slagle qualifies as both a founder and a pioneer. She was at the birth of the Association in 1917. Before that time she had received part of her education in social work and had completed one of the early Special Courses in Curative Occupations and Recreation at the Chicago School of Civics and Philanthropy. Following this, she taught in two courses for attendants of the insane; directed the occupations program at Henry Phipps Clinic, Johns Hopkins Hospital, Baltimore, under Dr. Adolf Meyer; returned to Chicago to become the Superintendent of Occupational Therapy at Hull House. Later, Mrs. Slagle moved to New York where she pioneered in developing occupational therapy in the State Department of Mental Hygiene. In addition, she served with high distinction in every elective office of the American Occupational Therapy Association, including President (1919-1920) and as a paid Executive Secretary for 14 years (48, pp 122-125); (49, pp 473-474); (50, p 18); (51).

She found occupational therapy to be ". . . an awkward term . . ." but felt ". . . it has been well defined as a form of remedial treatment consisting of various types of activities . . . which either contribute to or hasten recovery from disease or injury . . . carried on under medical supervision and that it be *consciously* motivated." Further, she emphasized that occupational therapy must be "a *consciously* planned progressive program of *rest, play, occupation and exercise.* . . ." (52, p 289) In addition, she explained it is ". . . an effort toward normalizing the lives of countless thousands who are mentally ill, . . . the normal mechanism of a fairly well-balanced day." (53, p 14) She enjoyed quoting C. Charles Burlingame, a prominent psychiatrist of her day: " 'What is an occupational therapist? She is that newer medical specialist who takes the joy out of invalidism. She is the medical specialist who carries us over the dangerous period between acute illness and return to the world of men and women as a useful member of society.' " (52, pp 290-291)

Slagle placed considerable emphasis upon the personality factor of the therapist: ". . . the proper balance of qualities, proper physical expression, a kindly voice, gentleness, patience, ability and seeming vision, adaptability . . . to meet the particular needs of the individual patient in all things. . . . Personality plus character also covers an ability to be honest and firm, with infinite kindness. . . ." (54, p 13)

The issue would constantly arise about the use of handicrafts as a therapeutic measure in the machine age. Her response is a classic: ". . . handicrafts are so generally used, not only because they are so diverse, covering a field from the most elementary to the highest grade of ability; but also, and greatly to the point, because their development is based on primitive impulses. They offer the means of contact with the patient that no other medium does or can offer. Encouragement of creative impulses also may lead to the development of large interests outside oneself and certainly leads to social contact, an important consideration with any sick or convalescent patient." (52, pp 292-293)

Habit training was first attempted at Rochester (New York) State Hospital in 1901. Slagle adopted the basic principles and developed a far greater perspective and use among mental patients who had been hospitalized from 5 to 20 years and who had steadily regressed. The functional plan was ". . . to arrange a twenty-four hour schedule . . . in which physicians, nurses, attendants and occupational therapeutists play a part. . . ." (54, p 13) It was a re-education program designed to overcome some disorganized habits, to modify others and construct new ones, with the goal that habit reaction will lead toward the restoration and maintenance of health. "In habit training, we show clearly an academic philosophy factor . . . that is, the necessity of requiring attention, of building on the habit of attention—attention thus becomes application, voluntary and, in time, agreeable."(54, p 14)

The purposes of habit training were twofold: the reclamation and rehabilitation of the patient, with the eventual goal of discharge or parole; and, if this was not reasonable, to assist the patient in becoming less of an institutional problem, that is, less destructive and untidy.

A typical habit training schedule called for the patients to arise in the morning at 6:00, wash, toilet, brush teeth, and air beds; then breakfast; return to ward and make beds, sweep; then classwork for two hours, which consisted of a variety of simple crafts and marching exercises. After lunch, there was a rest period; continued classwork and outdoor exercises, folk dancing, and lawn games. Following supper, there was music and dancing on the ward, followed by toileting, washing, brushing the teeth, and preparing for bed (55, p 29).

Once the patient had received maximum benefit from habit training, he or she was ready to progress through three phases of occupational therapy. The first was what Slagle called *the kindergarten group.* "We must show the ways and means of stimulating the special senses. The employment of color, music, simple exercises, games and storytelling, along with occupations, the gentle ways and means . . . (used) in educating the child are equally important in re-educating the adult. . . ."(54, p 14) Occupations were graded from the simple to the complex.

The next phase was *ward classes in occupational therapy,* ". . . graded to the limit of accomplishment of individual patients."(56, p 100) When able to tolerate it, the patient joined in group activities. The third and final phase was the *occupational center.* "This promotes opportunities for the more advanced projects . . . (a) complete change in environment; . . . comparative freedom; . . . actual responsibilities placed upon patients; the stimulation of seeing work produced; . . . all these carry forward the readjustment of patients."(56, p 102)

This founder, this pioneer, this distinguished member of our profession provided a summary of her own accomplishments and philosophy by stating: "Of the highest value to patients is the psychological fact that the patient is working for himself. . . . Occupational therapy recognizes the significance of the mental attitude which the sick person takes toward his illness and attempts to make that attitude more wholesome by providing activities adapted to the capacity of the individual patient and calculated to divert his attention from his own problems."(54, p 290) Further, she declared: "It is directed activity, and differs from all other forms of treatment in that it is given in increasing doses as the patient improves."(57, p 3)

Adolf Meyer: Philosophy of Occupation Therapy

Dr. Adolf Meyer is cited in this account of the evolution of occupational therapy because of his outstanding support and because his approach to clinical psychiatry was entirely consistent with the emerging occupational therapy movement.

Adolf Meyer, a Swiss physician, immigrated to the United States in 1892 and accepted a position initially as pathologist at the Eastern Illinois Hospital for the Insane in Kankakee. Over the next 14 years he held various positions in the United States and became professor of psychiatry at Johns Hopkins University in 1910. Throughout this period he developed the fundamentals of what was to become the psychobiological approach to psychiatry, a term he coined to indicate that the human is an indivisible unit of study, rather than a composite of symptoms. "Psychobiology starts not from a mind and a body or from elements, but from the fact that we deal with biologically organized units and groups and their functioning . . . the 'he's' and 'she's' of our experience—the bodies we find in action . . ."(58, p 263) Meyer took strong issue with those in medicine: ". . . who wish to reduce everything to physics and chemistry, or to anatomy, or to physiology, and within that to neurology. . . ."(58, p 262) His enlightened point of view is that one can only be studied as a total being in action and that this ". . . whole person represents an integrate of hierarchically arranged functions."(59, p 1317)

His common sense approach to the problems of psychiatry was his keynote: "The main thing is that your point of reference should always be life itself . . . . I put my emphasis upon specificity . . . . As long as there is life there are positive assets action, choice, hope, not in the imagination but in a clear understanding of the situation, goals, and possibilities . . . . To see life as it is, to tend toward objectivity is one of the fundamentals of my philosophy, my attitude, my preference. It is something that I would recommend if it can be kept free of making itself a pest to self and to others."(60, pp *vi-xi*)

From the very beginning of his work in Illinois, he was concerned with meaningful activity. In time, it became the fundamental issue in treatment. "I thought primarily of occupation therapy," he stated, "of getting the patient to do things and getting things going which did not work but which could work with proper straightening out."(60, p 45) In a report to the Governor of the State of Illinois in 1895, Meyer wrote: "Occupation is, with good right, the most essential side of hygienic treatment of most insane patients."(60, p 59)

By 1921, Meyer had become Professor of Psychiatry at Johns Hopkins University in Baltimore, and had had extensive experiences with others, such as William Rush Dunton, Jr., Eleanor Clarke Slagle, and Henrietta Price, leaders in the occupational therapy movement. At the Fifth Annual Meeting of the National Society for the Promotion of Occupational Therapy in Baltimore, October 1921, Meyer brought together his fundamental concepts of psychobiology to produce his paper, *The Philosophy of Occupation Therapy*. Through time, this has become a classic in the occupational therapy literature. It bears study by all of us.

Psychobiology is clearly visible in his statement that ". . . the newer conceptions of *mental problems* (are) *problems of living*, and not merely diseases of a structural and toxic nature. . . ."(61, p 4) The indivisibility and integration of the human are cited in this manner: "Our conception of man is that of an organism that maintains and balances itself in the world of reality and actuality by being in active life and active use. . . ."(61, p 5)

Because of the nature of his paper, *The Philosophy of Occupational Therapy*, Meyer emphasized occupation, time, and the productive use of energy. Interwoven are the elements of psychobiology. He stated, "The whole of human organization has its shape in a kind of rhythm . . . . There are many . . . rhythms which we must be attuned to: the larger rhythms of night and day, of sleep and waking hours . . . and finally the big four—work and play, and rest and sleep, which our organism must be able to balance even under difficulty. The only way to attain balance in all this is actual doing, actual practice, a program of wholesome living is the basis of wholesome feeling and thinking and fancy and interests."(61, p 6)

According to Meyer, a fundamental issue in the treatment of the mentally ill is ". . . the proper use of time in some helpful and gratifying activity. . ."(61, p 1) He expands on this precept by stating: "There is in all this a development of the *valuation of time and work*, which is not accidental. It is part of the great espousal of the *values of reality and actuality* rather than of mere thinking and reasoning. . ."(61, p 4) The introduction of activity is ". . . in giving opportunities rather than prescriptions. There must be opportunities to work, opportunities to do and to plan and create, and to learn to use material. . . . It is not a question of specific prescriptions, but of opportunities . . . to adapt opportunities."(61, p 7) He concluded his philosophic essay by returning once again to time and occupations: "The great feature of man is his new sense of time, with foresight built on a sound view of the past and present. Man learns to organize time and he does it in terms of doing things, and one of the many things he does between eating, drinking, and . . . the flights of fancy and aspiration, we call work and occupation."(61, pp 9-10)

Near the end of his working life, Meyer summed up his major efforts. He wrote of dealing with individuals and groups from the viewpoints of *good sense; of science,* ". . . with the smallest numbers of assumptions for search and research. . . ."; of *philosophy;* and of *religion,* ". . . as a way of trust and dependabilities in life."(62, p 100)

Occupational Therapy Definitions and Principles

As the founders and pioneers were experimenting with and writing their concepts, a definition of occupational therapy was emerging. It is remarkable that so early in the formation of the 20th century movement, a definition could be developed and stand for several decades and several generations of occupational therapists. In school, many of us were required to immortalize it through needlepoint, embroidery, and even printing.

H.A. Pattison, M.D., medical officer of the National Tuberculous Association, advanced his view at the annual conference of the National Society for the Promotion of Occupational Therapy in Chicago, September 1919. It was also adopted by the Federal Board of Vocational Education: "Occupational Therapy may be defined as any activity, mental or physical, definitely prescribed and guided for the distinct purpose of contributing to and hastening recovery from disease or injury."(63, p 21) Twenty-two years later, in 1931, John S. Coulter, M.D., and Henrietta McNary, OTR, added one phrase: ". . . and assisting the social and institutional adjustment of individuals requiring long and indefinite periods of hospitalization."(64, p 19) This was inserted in order to recognize occupational therapy's involvement in chronicity.

By 1925, a committee, made up of four physicians including William Rush Dunton, compiled an outline for lectures to medical students and physicians (65, pp 277-292). Though their document never received the official imprimatur of the AOTA, it nevertheless served for several years as a guide for practice (66, p 347). Fifteen principles were enunciated:

"Occupational therapy is a method of training the sick or injured by means of instruction and employment in productive occupation; . . . to arouse interest, courage, confidence; to exercise mind and body in . . . activity; to overcome disability; and to re-establish capacity for industrial and social usefulness." (65, p 280) Application called for as much system and precision as other forms of treatment; activity was to be prescribed, administered, and supervised under constant medical advice. Individual patient needs were paramount.

The outline stressed that "employment in groups is . . . advisable because it provides exercise in social adaptation and stimulating influence of example and comment . . . ." (65, p 280) In selecting an activity, the patient's interests and capabilities were to be considered and as strength and capability increased, the occupation was to be altered, regulated, and graded accordingly because "The only reliable measure of the treatment is the effect on the patient." (65, p 280)

Inferior workmanship could be tolerated, depending upon the patient's condition, but there should be consideration of ". . . standards worthy of entirely normal persons . . . for proper mental stimulation." (65, p 281) Articles made were to be useful and attractive, and meaningful tasks requiring healthful exercise of mind and body provided the greatest satisfaction. "Novelty, variety, individuality, and utility of the products enhance the value of an occupation as a treatment measure." (65, p 281) While quality, quantity, and the salability of articles made could be of benefit, these should not take precedence over the treatment objectives. As adjuncts to occupations, physical exercise, games, and music were considered beneficial and fell into two main categories: gymnastics and calisthenics, recreation and play.

One last principle spoke of the qualities of the occupational therapist: ". . . good craftsmanship, and ability to instruct are essential qualifications; . . . understanding, sincere interest in the patient, and an optimistic, cheerful outlook and manner are equally essential." (65, p 281)

Occupational Therapy's Second Generation

The die was cast. Practice rapidly expanded in a phenomenal number of settings following the establishment of the founders' principles and definition. A *second generation* of therapists emerged during the late 1920s and the 1930s. They were the practitioners and educators who elaborated, codified, and applied the initial theory upon which present-day practice is based. A chronicle of their efforts would offer a highly valuable and valued study in itself. The names of Louis Haas, Mary Alice Coombs, Winifred Kahmann, Henrietta McNary, Harriet Robeson, Marjorie Taylor, and Helen Willard would figure prominently in such an account.

For the purpose of this history, a composite of these and others is drawn into one individual who exemplifies the spirit and deeds of the *second generation* of occupational therapists—those whose efforts are lasting and ensure our present and future education and practice.

Understandably, it would be a woman. She would devote her professional career to either teaching, practicing, or administering. Quite possibly she would combine two or more of these. She would acquire an expertise in one area of practice, such as the mentally ill.

Her belief in the treatment of the total patient would guide her thoughts and actions. Occupational therapy, she would declare, "since its founding has concerned itself with the basic tenet—the treatment of the total patient. This approach is unique to occupational therapy among the . . . health disciplines . . . . There has always existed a strong component concerned with the behavior of the physically ill or disabled, as well as the mentally sick; with the entirety of man and his functioning as a patient. This occupational therapy concept," she would continue, "prevented (as has occurred in medical practice) an undesired separation of the psychiatric therapist from those who develop knowledge and skills centered in the treatment of the physically disabled."(67, p 1) Stated another way, "The major emphasis in occupational therapy is not the body *as such* but the individual *as such*. The therapist's background is strongly weighted in an understanding of personality adjustment and reactions to social situations; . . . and in the patients' attitudes toward an adjustment to acute and chronic disabilities."(68, p 9)

At some point in her work, she would be asked to serve as a consultant to one or more medical facilities, possibly a state hospital system. In time, she would produce a report and restate her definition of occupational therapy. It might well go this way: "The goal of all treatment in a modern mental hospital is the physical, social and economic rehabilitation of the patient . . . . The accepted function (of occupational therapy) . . . is the scientific utilization of mental and physical activities for the purpose of raising the patient to the highest level of integration; to assist him in making his initial adjustment to the hospital; to sustain him while his body responds to physical treatment and his mind to psychotherapy; or to assist him in making a satisfactory adjustment to chronic illness."(69, p 24)

In the report she would also call for an atmosphere as normal as possible, where a patient could be encouraged to respond in as normal a manner as possible: a balanced program of work and play, with flexibility to meet individual needs: "There must be organized a succession of steps through which the patient will be gradually led to his highest level of integration . . . . At each level . . . the patient experiences a feeling of success and self-respect. One cannot overemphasize the importance of careful planning . . . in order that there be a systematic progression up this ladder of integration."(69, p 24)

In another context, supportive care, as a vital concern to the therapist, would also be described, particularly in the care of the physically disabled: "To name only a few of its treatment objectives, occupational therapy may function as a diagnostic evaluative instrument; as corrective treatment; . . . or a design for effecting prevocational evaluation. Incorporated in each . . . is a treatment phase referred to as supportive care. This is a most fundamental and yet less definitive and indeed the least spectacular element of the total rehabilatory program. In supportive care, the occupational therapist (is concerned) with the behavioral factors which have and will affect the patient's response to the rehabilitation program . . . ." Convincingly, she would say: ". . . it can be said with conviction that successful rehabilitation can be effected only when the patient has attained a true state of rehabilitation 'readiness.' "(70)

Not just a woman of words, she would find one or more ways to activate her philosophy. She might well become active with a group of former patients and assist in organizing an association of and for individuals who have been hospitalized—for instance, the mentally ill. Such an endeavor would be the first of a kind. Through such an experience, she would conclude: "One difficulty which presented itself again and again was the need to instill in these (former) patients a philosophy toward their own rehabilitation; . . . an organized effort beyond the hospital which would offer special training, guidance and professional evaluation of their potentials."(71, p 3)

This would lead her to even greater endeavors on behalf of a whole category of patients. As an example, she would find that the 1920 Federal Vocational Rehabilitation Act excluded former psychiatric patients. In the manner of Dorothea Lynde Dix, whom she probably emulated, she would wage a relentless battle to right such a wrong. By enlisting the assistance of physicians' associations and veterans' groups she would see the legislation change. As part of her campaign she would write: "The former mental patient, in his struggle for economic rehabilitation, incurs the burden imposed on the physically handicapped 'plus' the stigmatization based on the popular misconception of mental disease. He must cast aside self-pity or the idea that the world owes him a living. The world does owe him understanding and guidance."(72, p 114) Finally, amendments to Public Law 113 were passed and signed by President Franklin Roosevelt. Psychiatric patients could now qualify for the benefits of the vocational rehabilitation act.

With such efforts the therapist's personal beliefs about emotional illness become even more strongly felt: "The majority of mentally ill are (sick) through no fault of their own . . . any more than one who has contracted a physical illness. Persons suffering from mental disease are generally ill as a result of an accumulation of unsuccessful efforts . . . to adjust to his environment."(72, p 83)

Two continuing concerns of all occupational therapists would be commented upon: the qualifications of the therapist and the use of media. One is as significant as the other. "The personality of the therapist," she would say, "must command respect, admiration, hope and confidence, . . . for no therapy is better than the therapist who directs it."(72, p 83) Therapeutic media have a number of inherent qualities, such as providing a vehicle for objectively recording patient performance, and, for the patient, affording opportunities for ". . . creative expression and evidence of accomplishment. The therapist should have a wide variety of activities (available) in accordance with the interests, aptitudes, and mental state of the patient. A craft track mind has no place in preparing such a program," she would state (72, p 103).

The accumulation of experiences as a clinician, and educator, or an administrator or possibly a combination of these, would lead this *therapist of the second generation* to arrive at a new definition of occupational therapy. It would precede by several years an altered definition by the national organization. It would incorporate the social and behavioral sciences, with a diminished emphasis upon medicine. Human development would appear for the first time as a focus for the treatment of physical and psychosocial dysfunction. She would declare, "Occupational therapy's function is to provide skilled assistance in influencing human objectives; its approach is inextricably conjoined with the behavioral factors involved. It is interested in how the process of growth and development is modified by hospitalization, chronic illness or a permanent handicap."(73, p 2)

This refocus was quite explainable and understandable to her since occupational therapy, and its ancestral emphasis, has always been the totality of the human organism. She would say, "It was inevitable, therefore, that there evolve an ever increasing emphasis in occupational therapy ... a greater understanding of the part that the developmental process plays in the preventive and therapeutic factors of this form of treatment."(74, p 3)

The foregoing has been a descriptive composite of a whole generation of therapists and assistants. The composite is actually the story of one individual; her observations alone have been cited. That individual is *Miss Beatrice D. Wade, OTR, FAOTA.*

The story is far from finished. Without a doubt, someone sometime will chronicle the lives and works of those who are still making contributions from that era to the present generation. Among them are Marjorie Fish, Virginia Kilburn, Mary Reilly, Ruth Robinson, Clare Spackman, Ruth Brunyate Wiemer, Carlotta Welles, and Wilma West. Each one, together with many others, continues to serve us well as clarifiers and definers of reasonable and reasoned alternatives. As counselors, they confirm old values and clearly point out new directions as well as our faithfulness or infidelity to those timeless principles established by our professional ancestors.

Lessons from Our History

The history of occupational therapy is the most neglected aspect of our professional endeavors. Seemingly, old values are least considered when charting new directions. On occasion we have been accused of taking leave of our historical senses. More to the point is that we have no historical sense. The problem primarily lies in not taking the time to assiduously locate our profession's diggings, to excavate what is relevant, and, then, to learn from what has been unearthed.

Archival materials from the past 200 years have been abundantly used in the development of this paper. Location and excavation has been difficult at times; however, it is reassuring to note that records and accounts still exist that are extremely relevant to today's endeavors. Lessons can be learned and they must. May I encourage each of you to determine for yourself what you have learned from this paraphrastic journey to our profession's diggings? To assist in this endeavor, may I cite a few lessons I have gained?

Mind and Body Inextricably Conjoined. No less than our professional ancestors, we must refuse to accept any alternative to the belief in the wholeness of the human—that the mind and body are inextricably conjoined. Illness, treatment, and the return to a healthful state simultaneously affect the physiological and emotional processes. Indeed, should these processes ever be separated, then occcupational therapy would be of no value. The patient has died!

The Natural Science of the Human. The inextricable union of the human leads to another lesson. The science fundamental to our practice is the natural science of the human. No amount of neurophysiology, psychology, sociology, or child development alone can determine the differential diagnosis, treatment, or prognosis of the patient undergoing occupational therapy. The current trend toward specialization, with its varying emphases upon one or another science, to the neglect of other human sciences, and indeed to the neglect of other nonscientific aspects of occupational therapy, borders on superstition and mythology. It is the continuous acquisition and scientific synthesis of the ingredients of the human organism and its surround that guarantees authentic occupational therapy.

The Human Organism's Involvement in Tasks. Occupational therapy is the only major health profession whose focus centers upon the *total* human organism's involvement in tasks—a making or doing. In spite of the many grafts we have effected, our roots remain in the subsoil of the *art*, the *craft*: a paradigm of the total activity of the human. Just as those who have come before us, we think of ourselves and others fundamentally as makers, as users, as doers, as tools. We look at: " . . . craft as a way in which man may create and cross a bridge within himself and center himself in his own essential unity." (75, p *vii*) The procedures one goes through in rearranging and reassembling the basic elements in art or craft operate upon and within the doer: " . . . his material modifies him as he modifies it, in proportion to his openness, his awareness of the exchange that is taking place." (75, p *x*)

The Differentiation of Occupational Therapy. Any definition, any description, any differentiation between ourselves and other health providers must have as its major theme occupation and leisure. Without it, we become a blurred copy, a xerography of a host of others.

Without the dynamics of human motion inherent in purposeful activity, we become quasi-physical therapists. Without the interaction between human objects and the objects of work and leisure, we become quasi-social workers, psychologists, or nurses. Without the demonstrated and proven interrelationships between healthful, normal growth and development, activity, and the pathology of illness and disabling conditions, we become quasi-physicians and psychiatrists.

The more we intermingle our fundamental philosophy and our treatment techniques with others, the more we intermarry, the more likely we will become enfeebled, the more likely we will degenerate, the more likely we will eventually disappear. Though speaking in another context, the Durants offer a lesson we must accept: "All strong characters and peoples are race conscious and are instinctively averse to marriage outside their own . . . group." (76, p 26)

A Refusal to Accept the Common Verdict. As Hugh Sidey has noted, "History is a marvelous collection of stories about men and women who refuse to accept the common verdict that certain achievements (are) impossible (77, p 18). The history of occupational therapy is the story of the ideals, deeds, hopes, and works of *individuals*. Changes and advancements came from those who eliminated inhumaneness, which prevented or discouraged the sick and disabled from achieving their potential. These same individuals were willing to assume the care and responsibility for those *who were not highly valued by the society:* the mentally ill and the retarded, the severely disabled—all those defined as "nonproducing, . . . an economic burden." (65, p 277)

In numerous places and on countless occasions these same individuals were derided, hated or, at best, ignored, because they pressed for change in the human condition. Yet, they persevered, knowing there was nothing innately unusual about themselves or what they wished to achieve. Few ever saw their names inscribed on monuments.

They were a *cast* quite diverse in character, and largely obscured because of the immensity of the saga being enacted. A few received *speaking parts*, primarily through reporting their own clinical findings. Only very few were singled out to be stars. None ever became members of the *audience*, passively observing events. All were *actors*.

The very same can be said of the present occupational therapy generation. We are actors, not observers. We continue to willingly strive on behalf of those who are not highly valued by the society. We refuse to see this as a burden. Rather, we perceive it as an obligation, as an opportunity, as a way of life.

Legacy of Experience. Too often we are disposed to think that those lessons another generation learned do not apply to the present generation. We should be remindful that there are two ways to learn: by our own experience and from those who have made discoveries, regardless of how long ago they were made. The experience of others is a magnificent heritage, and the more we learn from them, the less time we waste in the present, proving what already has been proved.

Those of us who are teachers and clinicians have a special obligation to pass on the legacy of experience, the knowledge of timeless principles and practices that do not change merely because times change.

Who They Were, What They Did. The legacy of experience suggests one more lesson. So often we are caught up in our daily activities we tend to forget what it is we owe those who came before us. All probably agree that each occupational therapy generation seemingly acquires a sense of self-sufficiency. It is true that we of the present occupy the positions that once were filled by others.

It is, however, of great import that we realize we are influenced by those who came before us more than we can truly know. Who they were and what they did has immeasurable bearing upon what we are and what we do. No generation is capable of isolating itself from its past. The past, plus what we are and what we do, greatly assists in fashioning our future.

The archives, the portraits and photographs, the published accounts, the personal memorabilia and scrapbooks are records of considerable moment. At the least, they are a profound reminder of the possibility that someday, someone may be looking back and may be wondering who we were and what we did.

Conclusion

It is altogether fitting and proper to conclude this lecture with the observations of two former Presidents of the Association, Mr. Thomas B. Kidner and Mrs. Eleanor Clarke Slagle. In 1930, Mr. Kidner offered a personal impression of the state of occupational therapy at the annual meeting of the Connecticut Occupational Therapy Society. In part, he said: "May we, therefore, look on occupational therapy—with increased faith as the years go by—as a natural means of aiding in the restoration of the sick and disabled to health and working capacity (which means happiness) because it appeals to all our human attributes."(57, p 11)

Mrs. Slagle, a year after she retired in 1937, made this observation: "The story of the profession of occupational therapy will never be fully told, nor will that of the patients who have so abundantly appreciated the opportunities of the service. There has been no fanciful crusading 'for the cause'; it has meant that a few have perhaps borne many burdens, but in the slow process that makes permanent things of great value, it can be said that there is a fine body of professional workers, experienced and well trained, coming forward and being welcomed to a really great human service, that of helping to show the way to the person with large disabilities to make the best of his incomplete self."(78, p 382) Finally, in an editorial "From the Heart," she concluded: "The integrity of your profession is in your hands. I bid you all Godspeed in your work."(79, p 345)

ACKNOWLEDGMENTS

A study of this nature and scope is not possible without the valuable and valued assistance of numerous individuals and sources. I wish to recognize the incomparable services provided by the staffs of the Moody Medical Library, The University of Texas Medical Branch at Galveston; the Quine Library, University of Illinois at the Medical Center, Chicago; the McGoogan Library of Medicine, University of Nebraska Medical Center, Omaha; and the Archives, Shapiro Developmental Center (Eastern Illinois State Hospital), Kankakee.

Lillian Hoyle Parent, OTR, was unusually helpful in locating obscure documents for me. The prior research of Kathryn Reed, OTR, greatly facilitated my search. William C. Levin, M.D., President, The University of Texas Medical Branch, was most generous with his support and consistent encouragement.

Several reviewers' comments helped to improve the manuscript: John G. Bruhn, Ph.D., a medical sociologist, Dean, The University of Texas School of Allied Health Sciences, Galveston; Chester R. Burns, M.D., Ph.D., a historian, The Institute for Medical Humanities, The University of Texas Medical Branch, Galveston; and four occupational therapists: James L. Cantwell, Ph.D.; Charles H. Christiansen, Ed.D., of The University of Texas School of Allied Health Sciences, Galveston; Suzanne Hooker, DipOT, Western Australian Institute of Technology,

Shenton Park, Western Australia; and Lillian Hoyle Parent, M.A., College of Associated Health Professions, University of Illinois at the Medical Center, Chicago. Eleanor Porter, Managing Editor, *Texas Reports on Biology and Medicine*, was a valuable adviser.

Others who provided invaluable help with ideas, documents, memorabilia, and personal remembrances were Shirley H. Carr, OTR, Tuskegee Institute; Barbara Loomis, OTR, University of Illinois at the Medical Center; Margaret Mirenda, OTR, Mount Mary College; Beatrice D. Wade, OTR, Professor Emeritus, University of Illinois at the Medical Center; and Kay B. Hudgens, OTR, Archivist, Shapiro Developmental Center, Kankakee, Illinois.

Two members of the AOTA staff were extremely helpful: James Garibaldi and Mardy Hicks. Betty Cox also provided needed assistance. Three members of the Learning Resource Center, The University of Texas School of Allied Health Sciences, Galveston, accomplished the highly effective visual presentation: Randall Rogers, W. Gregory Hunicutt, and Judy Hargett. I am indebted to them. Other individuals must be mentioned: Daniel L. Creson, M.D., Ph.D., offered his counsel and unqualified support throughout this endeavor; Lucille M. Burnworth typed several drafts and the final copy of the paper; Adele Jaco offered valuable clerical assistance; Laura Reed and Judy Grace, both occupational therapists, provided creative assistance at a much needed time. All personify the finest meanings of *friends*.

Finally, I wish to recognize Frances Sawyer, COTA, and the Board of Directors, The Texas Occupational Therapy Association, Inc., who placed my name in nomination for this exalted honor. My gratitude to them is immeasurable.

REFERENCES

1. Locke J: *An Essay Concerning Human Understanding* (Two Volumes). New York: Dover Press, 1894F
2. Frost SE: *Basic Teachings of the Great Philosophers*, New York: Barnes and Noble, Inc., 1942
3. Riese W: *The Legacy of Philippe Pinel: An Inquiry into Thought on Mental Alienation*, New York: Springer Publishing Co., 1969
4. Condillac EB de: *Oeuvres Philosophiques de Condillac*, Paris: Presse Universataires de France, 1947
5. Ackerknecht EH: *A Short History of Psychiatry*, New York: Hafner Publishing Co., 1968
6. Tuke DH: *A Dictionary of Psychological Medicine* (Vol One). Philadelphia: P Blakiston, Son & Co., 1892

7. Pinel P: *Traité Médico-Philosophique sur 'Alienation Mentale*. Paris: Richard, Caille & Rover, 1801

8. Pinel P: *A Treatise on Insanity In Which Are Contained the Principles of a New and More Practical Nosology of Maniacal Disorders*, Translated by DD Davis. London: Cadell & Davis, 1806 (Facsimile published by Hafner Publishing Co., New York, 1962)

9. Mackler B: *Philippe Pinel: Unchainer of the Insane*, New York: Franklin Watts, Inc., 1968

10. Folsom CF: *Diseases of the Mind: Notes on the Early Management, European and American Progress*, Boston: A. Williams & Co., Publishers, 1877

11. Jones K: *Lunacy, Law and Conscience: 1744-1845: The Social History of Care of the Insane*, London: Routledge & Kegan Paul, Ltd., 1955

12. Dillenberger J, Welch C: *Protestant Christianity: Interpreted Through Its Development*, New York: Charles Scribner's Sons, 1954

13. Philadelphia Yearly Meeting of the Religious Society of Friends: *Faith and Practice*, Philadelphia: Philadelphia Yearly Meeting, 1972

14. Tuke DH: *Reform in the Treatment of the Insane. Early History of the Retreat, York; Its Objects and Influence*, London, J & A Churchill, 1872

15. Tuke DH: *Reform in the Treatment of the Insane: An Early History of the Retreat, York: Its Objects and Influence*, London: J & A Churchill, 1892

16. Tuke S: *Description of the Retreat, An Institution Near York for Insane Persons of the Society of Friends: Containing an Account of Its Origins and Progress, The Modes of Treatment, and a Statement of Cases*, York, England: Alexander, 1813

17. Hunter R, Macalpine I: *Three Hundred Years of Psychiatry, 1535-1860: A History Presented in Selected English Texts*, London: Oxford University Press, 1963

18. Connolly J: *The Treatment of the Insane Without Mechanical Restraints*, London: Smith, Elder & Co., 1856 (Facsimile copy published by Dawson's of Pall Mall, London, 1973, with introduction by R Hunter, and I Macalpine)

19. Ellis WC: *A Treatise on the Nature, Symptoms, Causes, and Treatment of Insanity*, London: Holdsworth, 1838

20. Goodman N: *Benjamin Rush: Physician and Citizen, 1746-1813*, Philadelphia: University of Pennsylvania Press, 1934

21. Rush B: *Medical Inquiries and Observations Upon the Diseases of the Mind* (4th Edition). Philadelphia: J Grigg, 1830

22. Buckmaster H: *Women Who Shaped History*, New York: Macmillan Pub. Co., 1966

23. Bucknill JC, Tuke, DH: *A Manual of Psychological Medicine*, New York: Hafner Pub. Co., 1968 (Facsimile of 1858 Edition)

24. Barlow J: *Man's Power Over Himself to Prevent or Control Insanity*, London: William Pickering, 1843

25. Skultans V: *Madness and Morals: Ideas on Insanity in the Nineteenth Century*, London: Routledge & Kegan Paul, 1975

26. Tuke DH: *A Dictionary of Psychological Medicine: Volume Two*, Philadelphia: P Blakiston, Son & Co., 1892

27. Bockhoven JS: *Moral Treatment in American Psychiatry*, New York: Springer Publishing Co., Inc., 1963

28. Dain N: *Concepts of Insanity in the United States, 1789-1865*, New Brunswick, NJ: Rutgers University Press, 1964

29. Deutsch A: *The Mentally Ill in America: A History of Their Care and Treatment from Colonial Times* (2nd Edition). New York: Columbia University Press, 1949

30. Tracy SE: The development of occupational therapy in the Grace Hospital, Detroit, Michigan. *Trained Nurse Hosp Rev* 66:5, May 1921

31. Tracy SE: The place of invalid occupations in the general hospital. *Modern Hosp* 2:5, June 1914

32. Tracy SE: Twenty-five suggested mental tests derived from invalid occupations. *Maryland Psychiatr Q* 8: 1918

33. Barrows M: Susan E. Tracy, RN. *Maryland Psychiatr Q* 6: 1916-1917

34. Tracy SE: Treatment of disease by employment at St. Elizabeths Hospital. *Modern Hosp* 20:2, February 1923

35. Parsons SE: Miss Tracy's work in general hospitals. *Maryland Psychiatr Q* 6: 1916-1917

36. Tracy SE: *Studies in Invalid Occupation*, Boston: Witcomb and Barrows, 1918

37. Tracy SE: Power versus money in occupation therapy. *Trained Nurse Hosp Rev* 66:2, February 1921

38. Barton GE: A view of invalid occupation. *Trained Nurse Hosp Rev* 52:6, June 1914

39. Barton GE: Occupational nursing. *Trained Nurse Hosp Rev* 54:6, June 1915

40. Barton GE: Occupational therapy. *Trained Nurse Hosp Rev* 54:3, March 1915

41. Barton GE: The existing hospital system and reconstruction. *Trained Nurse Hosp Rev* 69:4, October 1922

42. Barton GE: What occupational therapy may mean to nursing. *Trained Nurse Hosp Rev* 64:4, April 1920

43. Barton GE: *Re-education: An Analysis of the Institutional System of the United States*, Boston: Houghton Mifflin Co., 1917

44. Sheppard Asylum: *Third Annual Report of the Sheppard Asylum*, Towson, MD: 1895

45. Dunton WR: The relationship of occupational therapy and physical therapy. *Arch Phys Ther* 16: January 1935

46. Dunton WR: The Principles of Occupational Therapy. *Proceedings of the National Society for the Promotion of Occupational Therapy: Second Annual Meeting*, Catonsville, MD: Spring Grove State Hospital, 1918

47. Dunton WR: *Occupation Therapy: A Manual for Nurses*, Philadelphia: WB Saunders, 1915

48. Komora PO: Eleanor Clarke Slagle. *Ment Hyg* 27:1, January 1943

49. Pollock HM: In memoriam: Eleanor Clarke Slagle, 1876-1942. *Am J Psychiatr* 99:3, November 1942

50. American Occupational Therapy Association: *Then and Now, 1917-1967*. New York: American Occupational Therapy Association, 1967

51. Loomis B, Wade BD: *Chicago . . . Occupational Therapy Beginnings: Hull House, The Henry B. Favill School of Occupations and Eleanor Clarke Slagle*.

52. Slagle EC: Occupational therapy. Recent methods and advances in the United States. *Occup Ther Rehab* 13:5, October 1934

53. Slagle EC: History of the development of occupation for the insane. *Maryland Psychiatr Q* 4: May 1914

54. Slagle EC: Training aides for mental patients. *Arch Occup Ther* 1:1, February 1922

55. Slagle EC, Robeson HA: *Syllabus for Training of Nurses in Occupational Therapy*, Utica, NY: State Hospital Press, date unknown

56. Slagle EC: A year's development of occupational therapy in New York State Hospitals. *Modern Hosp* 22:1, January 1924

57. Kidner TB: Occupational therapy, its development, scope and possibilities. *Occup Ther Rehab* 10:1, February 1931

58. Meyer A: The psychological point of view. In *Classics in American Psychiatry*, JP Brady, Editor. St. Louis: Warren H Green, Inc., 1975 (Also, In *The Problems of Mental Health*, M Bentley, EV Cowdey, Editors. New York: McGraw-Hill, 1934)

59. Arieti S: *American Handbook of Psychiatry* (Vol Two), New York: Basic Books, Inc., Publishers, 1959
60. Lief A: *The Commonsense Psychiatry of Dr. Adolf Meyer: Fifty-two Selected Papers*, Edited with Biographical Narrative. New York: McGraw-Hill Book Co., 1948
61. Meyer A: The philosophy of occupation therapy. *Arch Occup Ther* 1:1, February 1922 Also in *Am J Occup Ther* 31(10): 639-642, 1977
62. Meyer A: The rise to the person and the concept of wholes or integrates. *Am J Psychiatr* 100: April 1944
63. Pattison HA: The trend of occupational therapy for the tuberculous. *Arch Occup Ther* 1(1): February 1922
64. Coulter JS, McNary H: Necessity of medical supervision in occupational therapy. *Occup Ther Rehab* 10(1): February 1931
65. An outline of lectures on occupational therapy to medical students and physicians. *Occup Ther Rehab* 4(4): August 1925
66. Elwood, ES: The National Board of Medical Examiners and medical education, and the possible effect of the Board's program on the spread of occupational therapy. *Occup Ther Rehab* 6 (5): October 1927
67. Wade BD: Occupational Therapy: A History of Its Practice in the Psychiatric Field. Unpublished paper presented at 51st Annual Conference, American Occupational Therapy Association, Boston, October 19, 1967
68. Advisory Committee in Occupational Therapy: The Basic Philosophy and Function of Occupational Therapy. *University of Illinois Faculty—Alumni Newsletter of the Chicago Professional Colleges.* 6:4, January 1951
69. Wade BD: A survey of occupational and industrial therapy in the Illinois state hospitals. *Illinois Psychiatr* 2 (1): March 1942
70. Wade BD: Supportive care *Bull Rehab Inst Chicago*, date unknown
71. Wade BD: Supportive care. *Bull Rehab* Rehabilitation of the Mentally Ill. Unpublished paper presented to the Department of Public Welfare, State of Minnesota, June 26, 1958
72. Willard HS, Spackman CS: *Principles of Occupational Therapy* (First Edition). Philadelphia: JB Lippincott Co., 1947
73. Wade BD: The Development of Clinically Oriented Education in Occupational Therapy: The Illinois Plan. Unpublished paper presented at 49th Annual Conference, American Occupational Therapy Association, Miami, November 2, 1965
74. Wade BD: Introduction. *The Preparation of Occupational Therapy Students for Functioning with Aging Persons and in Comprehensive Health Care Programs: A Manual for Educators*, Chicago: University of Illinois at the Medical Center, 1969
75. Dooling EM: *A Way of Working*, Garden City, NY: Anchor Press/Doubleday, 1979
76. Durant W, Durant A: *The Lessons of History*, New York: Simon and Schuster, 1968
77. Sidey H: The presidency. *Time* 116 (22): December 1, 1980
78. Slagle EC: Occupational therapy. *Trained Nurse Hosp Rev* 100 (4): April 1938
79. Slagle EC: Editorial: From the heart. *Occup Ther Rehab* 16(5): October 1937

Clinical Reasoning: The Ethics, Science, and Art

Joan C. Rogers

A therapist, employed at a regional rehabilitation center, extracts cues from the records of acute hospitals, to judge the rehabilitation potential of patients referred for admission. Another therapist, working with persons with mental retardation, selects a treatment approach based on task analysis to teach self-care skills. A third therapist, serving on a geriatric assessment team, uses scores on a mental status examination and performance ratings in daily living activities to estimate patients' ability to continue living alone in their homes. A fourth therapist reviews patients' progress in manual dexterity to formulate a recommendation for or against hand surgery. These four therapists are using their clinical reasoning skills to collect and transform data about patients into decisions that have critical implications for the quality of life of their patients.

If we questioned the therapists about their decisions, they would probably comment on their potential fallibility. Some patients, denied occupational therapy because of a perceived lack of potential for rehabilitation, would make substantial gains in functional skills if intervention were initiated. Some patients with mental retardation will not benefit from the task breakdown approach to self-care training. Some geriatric patients admitted for institutional living could have been supported adequately in the community. Some patients undergoing hand surgery will lose functional abilities. The possibility of error in our clinical judgments and the potential ensuing negative consequences urge us to develop ways of improving our assessment and treatment decisions.

Reprinted from *The American Journal of Occupational Therapy*, Vol. 37, No. 9, 1983

Despite the obvious importance of clinical judgment in the occupational therapy process, little attention has been given to explicating the thinking that guides practice. My research, albeit with a small number of occupational therapists, suggests that our cognitive processes are regarded as intuitive and ineffable. For example, when therapists were asked how they arrived at their treatment decisions, they commonly responded by saying, "I have never really thought about it." or "I don't know how I reached that conclusion. I just know." Cognitive activity constitutes the heart of the clinical enterprise. Our failure to study the process of knowing and understanding that underlies practice precludes an adequate description of clinical reasoning. This in turn prevents the development of a methodology for systematically improving it and for teaching it.

I intend to explore here the reasoning process through which we learn about patients so that we may help them through engagement in occupation. I will construct an intellectual device for viewing clinical reasoning from the perspective of the basic questions the therapist seeks to answer through clinical inquiry. The scientific, ethical, and artistic dimensions of clinical reasoning will be elucidated as these questions are explored. The device will be useful for directing and appraising our thoughts about treating patients and for developing a clinical science of occupational therapy. In developing my thoughts, I have relied on the basic scheme of clinical judgment presented by Pellegrino (1) for medicine and have adapted it to the occupational therapy process.

The Goal of Clinical Reasoning

The goal of the clinical reasoning process has an impact on each of the steps taken to achieve the goal. Hence, an appreciation of this goal provides insight on the whole process.

Patients come to occupational therapy when they, their physicians, family members, or caregivers perceive that they are not adequately performing their daily activities. Performance in self-care, work, and leisure occupations has been compromised because of the consequences of disease, trauma, abnormal development, age-related changes, or environmental restrictions. The disruptions in occupational functions are characteristically severe and enduring as opposed to transitory. To regain a former level of performance, maintain the current level, or achieve a more optimal one, the patient enlists the aid of the therapist. The therapist's task, therefore, is to select a right therapeutic action for the patient (1). In other words, the goal of clinical reasoning is a treatment recommendation issued in the interests of a particular patient. Decision making is highly individualized.

The occupational therapy treatment plan details what a particular patient should do to enhance occupational role performance. The therapeutic action must be the right action for this individual. This implies that it must be as congruent as possible with the patient's concept of the "good life." Treatment should be in concert with the patient's needs, goals, life-style, and personal and cultural values. A therapeutic program that is right for one patient is not necessarily right for another. The ultimate question we, as clinicians, are challenged to answer is: What, among the many things that could be done for this patient, ought to be done? This is an ethical question. It involves a judgment to which facts contribute but that must be decided by weighing values. A salient criterion of an ethical action is its agreement with the patient's valued goals. The clinical reasoning process terminates in an ethical decision, rather than in a scientific one, and the ethical nature of the goal of clinical reasoning projects itself over the entire sequence.

Ethical decisions regarding treatment are not made in isolation from scientific knowledge. The patient comes to the therapist for expert advice regarding adaptation to chronic dysfunction. The factual basis for decision making is provided by the therapist. When therapists set out to solve clinical problems, they are confronted with an unknown—the patient. Scientific methodologies are used to learn about the patient. Once the patient's condition is adequately understood, scientific and empirical knowledge is applied in the efforts to enhance occupational status. Although ethical consideration can override scientific ones, they do not displace the need to secure a scientific opinion.

Clinical Questions

To ascertain the right action for each patient, clinical inquiry focuses on three questions: What is the patient's current status in occupational role performance? What could be done to enhance the patient's performance? And what ought to be done to enhance occupational competence? These are the fundamental questions that I previously alluded to as guiding the clinical process. Each question will be considered first in terms of the knowledge needed to answer it, and, subsequently, in terms of the cognitive processes used to obtain the knowledge.

What Is the Patient's Status?

The first question to be considered is the assessment question: What is the patient's occupational status? The occupational therapy assessment is a concise and accurate summary of a patient's occupational role performance that arises from an investigation of the patient. The occupational therapy assessment tells us what we need to know about the patient to plan a sound intervention or prevention program. To serve this function, the assessment includes several features: it indicates what is wrong with the patient, it indicates the patient's strengths, and it indicates the patient's motivation for occupation.

The word *assessment* is preferable to the terms *diagnosis* or *problem definition* for the evaluation of occupational status because it has much broader meaning. Diagnosis and problem definition connote the identification of pathological, abnormal, dysfunctional, or problematic processes or states. To assess means to rate the value of property for the purpose of taxation. The word *assessment*, then, with its emphasis on the evaluation of the worth of something, is an appropriate term to apply to the process of collecting information to resolve clinical problems and to the statement that summarizes the results of that process. Occupational therapy is concerned with helping disabled persons to adapt to chronic disability more effectively. This may be accomplished by enhancing abilities as well as by remediating or reducing dysfunction. The occupational therapy assessment serves as the end point for treatment planning. To serve this pivotal function, the assessment must specify both assets and liabilities. Thus, diagnosis, or the determination of what is wrong with the patient, is only a part of the assessment.

Knowledge. The assessment process usually begins with diagnosis, since knowledge of dysfunction tells us what is wrong and requires correction or amelioration. The therapist seeks to ascertain the specific problems the patient is having in performing self-care, work, and leisure occupations. Disruptions in occupational role are commonly of two major types: an inability to perform socially defined age-appropriate tasks and an inability to coordinate these tasks effectively in daily life. To the extent that a person has disruptions in occupational role, or impairments that we can predict will result in such disruptions, that person is an appropriate candidate for occupational therapy. The occupational therapy diagnosis clearly articulates the disruption in occupational role that is of concern for treatment. For example, we might state that Tom Smith is totally dependent in hygiene and dressing and requires physical assistance with feeding. This diagnosis indicates that these are the major problems at this time.

The occupational therapy diagnosis has a temporal quality. Participation in daily living tasks may change over the course of an illness or other disorder. For example, as Tom Smith gains competence in self-care, the diagnosis may switch to dysfunctions in home management. Similarly, as an individual matures and needs and interests change, the occupational therapy diagnosis changes, and intervention is refocused. Thus, the range of problems that comprise the occupational therapy diagnosis is broad and variable, and the diagnosis may change over time.

Often, the occupational therapy diagnosis indicates not only the disruption in occupational role, but also the suspected cause or causes for this disruption. This is the etiological component of the diagnostic statement and it offers an explanation of why the individual behaves or fails to behave in some way.

The most prevalent perspective for defining the etiology of occupational role dysfunctions is based on the biopsychosocial model. This enables us to pinpoint the causes of performance dysfunctions in terms of biological, psychological, and social variables. For example, we might state that Ida Cox cannot dress herself because she has contractures in her upper extremities, thus attributing the cause to a biological variable. Or, we might suggest that she cannot dress herself because of a memory problem, thus attributing the cause to a psychological variable. Or, we might conclude that the reason she is unable to dress herself is because she cannot reach her clothes from a wheelchair. In this case, the dressing dysfunction is attributed to the interaction of a biological variable, motor impairment, and a social variable, the man-made environment. Such attributions allow us to plan appropriate treatment. We can plan to remediate the contracture or memory defect or to circumvent their effects on performance. We can remove the architectural barriers.

An occupational therapy diagnosis stemming from the biopsychosocial model is so specific that it is applicable to only one patient. For instance, an occupational therapy diagnosis might state: Homemaking disability secondary to a lack of endurance for shopping to procure groceries, and postural instability in negotiating the stairs to the laundry facilities in the basement; ability is complicated by blurred vision in both eyes as a consequence of cataracts. Such a diagnosis is unlikely to be appropriate for more than one patient. Although the diagnostic statement is highly descriptive, it is also highly prescriptive. For example, the above diagnosis suggests such interventions as: employing homemaker services, scheduling and performing activities in such a way as to control fatigue, using good light with no glare, and using mobility aids or environmental supports.

In addition to a description of what the patient cannot do and why, the occupational therapy assessment includes a description of what the patient can do and how well it can be done. Although the problem is diagnosed, it is the person who is assessed. The need to acknowledge positive factors was well expressed by the little boy who reacted to the scolding he received about his report card by saying, "Daddy, I think your eyes need fixing. You only saw the D and not the four As." Knowing a person's problems or deficits tells us little about his or her strengths. The image of the patient drawn from problem behaviors is distorted. It needs to be supplemented with snapshots of the patient's occupational competencies and strengths to enable the therapist to construct a fair and valid impression of the patient.

The assessment of occupational competence requires a wide-angled lens. Occupational performance emerges from a complex network of transactions between the internal characteristics of the individual and the external properties of the surrounding environment. Just as features of a particular situation may account for a limitation of ability, so they may also allow the expression of ability. The qualities of the environment are important enablers of human performance. You cannot swim without water or play tennis without a partner. Both the physical and the social environments influence the patient's ability to occupy time productively. To assess occupational competence, the therapist evaluates the people, places, and objects associated with the patient's occupational endeavors to determine the extent to which they support occupation.

The final requirement of the occupational therapy assessment is to summarize the patient's motivation to engage in occupation. Who among us has never pondered over the patients with excellent potential who fail to achieve and those with intractable conditions who surpass all expectations. We cannot understand the patient without an appreciation of the way in which the urge toward competence has been habitually satisfied. The ontogenetic aspects of occupation have critical implications for recovery and growth. The patient's history of occupation informs us whether the present dysfunction is extenuated by a pattern of adaptive behavior or augmented by a career of maladaptive behavior. The patient's mastery of the environment is documented in occupational achievement, while exploration of the environment is recorded in the use of time. Since time is occupied by doing things of value, the patient's use of time provides insight into the varieties of occupations that are meaningful to him or her. The patient's past is reviewed to shed light on how occupational behavior is organized and to lend perspective to activities that are important and incidental to the life plan.

Historical assessment is directed toward a deeper understanding of the patient's occupational nature. The normative sequence of occupational endeavors begins in childhood play and self-care. Participation in arts and crafts, games, academics, chores, and part-time work are added to the repertoire through young adulthood. Productive occupation in the form of employment predominates in adulthood. This often changes to leisure pursuits during later maturity. The therapist thus captures the development and balance of self-care, work and leisure occupations in studying the sequence of pre-school, school age, worker, and retiree roles.

The yield of the occupational therapy assessment is a model of the patient that describes and explains his or her unique functioning in occupation. The model superimposes current functional abilities on disabilities, and relates these to environmental demands and to past performance. It is from this comprehensive model of the patient that future capacity is predicted and treatment goals are recommended.

Process. Having described the requirements of the occupational therapy assessment, I will now turn to the cognitive processes used to formulate it. What is involved in clinical inquiry? How do we go about the task of constructing a model of the patient? The approach used here for looking at the cognitive processes that undergird practice reflects on information-processing view of cognition. The human mind is thus conceptualized as a computer that has certain information processing capabilities. It can do some things better than others and uses certain labor-saving strategies to overcome its limitations. A primary limitation of the human mind is its small capacity for short-term or working memory. Because of this limitation, data must be selected judiciously, processed serially, and managed through simplifying strategies (2). In assessment, the clinician has as intake to the information-processing system cues gathered from the patient or about the patient. The output is the conclusions summarized in the occupational therapy assessment. The conversion of intake data to output conclusions is a critical feature of clinical reasoning.

The therapist begins the assessment by choosing a plan for studying the patient. We say to ourselves, "Of all things that I could consider about this patient, what am I going to think about?" We typically respond to this question by constructing an image of the patient from the preassessment data and use this image to direct our plan. Our preassessment image tells us what to include and what to exclude as we observe the patient. Thus, the first labor-saving device the therapist uses is to limit the parameters within which the patient will be studied.

The preassessment image of the patient is derived from the conceptual frame of reference or postulate system of the therapist. A conceptual frame of reference represents a therapist's unique view of occupational therapy. It consists of facts derived from research studies, empirical generalizations drawn from experience, theories and models accepted by the therapist, and principles of practice obtained from instructors and colleagues. My frame of reference represents what I believe about occupational therapy practice. A frame of reference operates largely as a nonconscious ideology in forming the preassessment image. The therapist links his or her frame of reference with the preassessment data to construct an image of the patient that furnishes the outline for the clinical investigation.

Two salient preassessment factors are the medical diagnosis and age. By knowing even these elementary facts, we can predict certain things about a patient. For example, if we know that a patient's dominant arm has been amputated, we can anticipate problems in manual dexterity and bilateral coordination. If, in addition, we know that the patient is 6 years of age, rather than 76, we can expect to direct treatment toward habilitation of hand skills as opposed to rehabilitation.

The preassessment image of the patient is used to generate a series of testable working hypotheses. The therapist reasons that, if a particular hypothesis is valid, then it should follow that such and such will be found in further study of the case. For example, a therapist learns from the occupational therapy referral that the patient is a 40-year-old woman with depression. The therapist reasons that, if this patient is depressed, she is likely to be disheveled, to have a low level of involvement in activities, and to concentrate on events associated with negative affect. In other words, by knowing that the patient is depressed, the therapist is able to view the patient as a representative of the class of depressed patients, and, thus, hypothesizes that she will exhibit characteristics of depression. The therapist then sets out to perform the procedures needed to substantiate the hypothesis.

Up to this point, the reasoning process is essentially deductive in nature. The therapist recalls some general postulates from memory and applies them to a specific patient. The open-ended question of what is wrong with the patient has now been refined to a set of better-defined problems for exploration and resolution.

The working hypotheses provide a plan for acquiring cues from the patient to test the hypotheses. A cue is any bit of information that guides or directs the assessment (3). Cues arise from the observational process that employs three general types of data-gathering methodologies: testing or measurement; questioning, including history-taking and interviewing; and observation. Accurate clinical decisions are dependent on the collection of good cues. Two tests of the goodness of cues are reliability and validity.

Cues can be used to test the working hypotheses developed from deductive reasoning. By comparing each cue to the working hypotheses, sense may be made of the data. The therapist reasons, "This is what I expect to find, now what do I find?" A cue may be interpreted as confirming a hypothesis, disconfirming a hypothesis, or noncontributory to a hypothesis. Thus, as information is collected about the patient, the therapist decides repeatedly whether or not a finding is related to the patient's problems. Confidence in each hypothesis increases or decreases, based on the interpretation of additional data. Extensive case data are reduced by eliminating, or holding in reserve, data that do not appear significant. Hypothesis testing is thus another of the mind's strategies for simplifying data management. Hypotheses direct the collection of data and determine how they are organized and filed in memory. This organization prevents the mind from becoming overloaded with irrelevant facts and assists the therapist in retrieving information from memory.

Cues may also be combined to formulate new hypotheses. As cues are collected to test the validity of the deduced hypotheses, some cues may not fit well. Some of the performance problems we had expected to find will not be found, and others that we had not anticipated will become manifest. Our thinking begins to move from the classical, textbook picture of the disorder, to the disorder as it is uniquely manifested in this patient. The reasoning process now becomes inductive, with problem definition induced from empirical study of the patient, rather than deduced from the therapist's frame of reference. Additional cues may then be collected to test the inductively derived hypotheses. Clinical reasoning proceeds by developing hypotheses that pull together several inferences into a broader pattern or model of the patient.

After gleaning a clear perception of the patient's problems, the therapist then begins to search for cues indicative of the health of the patient as avidly as the search was conducted to identify dysfunction. Inductive reasoning and hypothesis testing are the basic processes through which the clinician assesses the patient's competencies, motivation for occupational achievement, and the environments in which the patient operates or will operate. These kinds of data are highly personal and hence are less likely to be deduced from knowledge of disease or disorder.

Data collection cannot continue indefinitely, and at some point the therapist decides that adequate information has been collected. How much data constitutes adequate data is dependent on the ethical consequences of an error in judgment (2,4). A recommendation to institutionalize a patient because he or she is unable to look after his or her self-care needs would require more evidence than that required for the prescription of a rocker knife. Regardless of how many data are collected, however, the data base represents only a sampling of the patient's behavior. The therapist's task is to use this incomplete information to make a judicious decision. Decision making takes place under conditions of uncertainty.

Throughout the process of data collection, the therapist's preassessment image of the patient has been revised and elaborated, based on the accumulated cues. Once cue collection is stopped and no new information is being generated, hypothesis testing also ceases. The clinical reasoning of the therapist now resembles the dialectical process in which the therapist argues or defends the interpretation of the data in much the same way as a lawyer pleads a case in court. Does the patient have a dressing problem that is of concern? Is the cause of the patient's performance difficulties visual-perceptual problems? Is the mental status of the patient adequate for self-care? The evidence supporting or opposing each alternative is weighed with the objective of rendering one explanation more cogent than another. Inferences that are compatible are retained and others are rejected or modified as contradictions appear. Through the dialectical process the model of the individual patient is polished and repolished. In this way, the therapist arrives at a cohesive conception of the patient, and, having grasped the whole, reinterprets the parts in the light of this understanding. Once a holistic picture of the patient has been devised, the function of the assessment moves from model building to decision making.

What Are the Available Options?

The second of the three general questions guiding clinical inquiry is the therapeutic question: What can be done for this patient? Having proposed a model of the patient's occupational status, we then begin to explore the actions that could be taken to enhance occupational role performance. The intent is to generate a list of the treatment options available for the problems and assets presented by this patient. For example, suppose a patient's problems in self-care were attributed to hemiplegia subsequent to a cerebral vascular accident. To treat this problem, we might consider a neurological approach aimed at regaining controlled action in the involved arm, or a rehabilitative approach aimed at training the uninvolved arm to perform skilled activities, or a combination of these approaches. The aim, at this stage of clinical reasoning, is to foster an awareness of the range and kind of treatment possibilities. In effect, the therapist uses the model of the patient to construct a theory of practice for the patient.

Knowledge. The therapist's consideration of what could be done includes a review of the relative effectiveness of each treatment approach. If a particular treatment option is initiated, what results can be expected, and how long will it take to achieve them? Any hazards associated with the various treatments, or with no treatment, are evaluated in the light of the potential benefits.

Decision making concerning the appropriate action can approach certitude if the deleterious effects of a disorder without treatment are known, and if there is substantial evidence of how these effects can be altered by a particular treatment. We know, for instance, that if joints are not moved, contractures develop and the joints become immobile. Thus, movement becomes the scientifically acceptable treatment for preventing contractures.

For most occupational therapy approaches or procedures, however, the scientific evidence is not definitive. Rarely are the outcomes of research so specific that they allow us to know with 100% accuracy what will happen. Scientific findings generally emerge as probabilities rather than as certainties. They may, for example, tell us that 95% of the patients with right hemiplegia receiving self-care training will become independent in self-care. But when we apply this finding to Edith Jones, we do so with the recognition that her chances of becoming independent remain 50-50. The response of a patient to treatment cannot be predicted with certitude. Scientific knowledge can improve our chances of making accurate technical decisions but it cannot assure this. When the scientific evidence is inconclusive, the therapist has considerable leeway in devising treatment recommendations.

In the absence of scientific knowledge about the effectiveness of treatment options, clinicians rely on knowledge gleaned from their own clinical experience or from the experiences of others. Knowledge derived from practice rather than research indicates what works but may not indicate what works best.

Process. To draw up a list of the patient's treatment options, the therapist searches memory for relevant scientific and practice knowledge. Clinical experiences are stored and classified in memory and retrieved as needed for application to new patients. Each time a therapist treats a patient, a clinical experiment is performed in which the objective is to replicate a successful outcome of a past experiment (5). As a first step in reproducing the experiment, the therapist mentally reviews previous patients whose occupational status resembled the patient at hand. Although no two patients are exactly alike, the therapist assembles a subgroup of patients who are most similar to the patient under study (6). Treatment is selected for the new patient by analyzing and comparing the therapeutic actions and outcomes of the patients in the reference group. If there is a high degree of similarity between the patient being treated and previous patients, the therapist will select a treatment that is highly replicative. If the similarity is low, or if previous treatment was not very effective, the therapist will propose a treatment that is more inventive.

The cognitive process involved in the selection of treatment is again that of dialectical reasoning. The therapist argues one treatment option against another without recourse to new clinical data. The process of enumerating the patient's treatment alternatives relies heavily on the content of long-term memory. The more clinical experience therapists have, the more empirical data are available to guide decision making. It is impossible for therapists to consider a treatment with which they have no familiarity. Similarly, clinicians cannot debate the scientific merits of one procedure over another, unless the procedure has been scientifically investigated and the research has been assimilated.

What Ought To Be Done?

The third and final question to be considered is the ethical question: What ought to be done to enhance occupational competence? Simply because a goal appears technically feasible for the patient does not mean that it should be set as a goal. And, simply because a treatment approach can be initiated does not imply that it should be instituted. We must avoid confusing action that can be taken with action that ought to be taken. From an ethical standpoint, decisive action must take the patient's valued goals into account. It must conform to the patient's definition of health, accomplishment, and the "good life."

Knowledge. Ethical principles arise from reflection on the nature of humanity and human dignity. Respect for individuals requires that each individual be regarded as autonomous. Each individual has a definite pattern and characteristic style for mastering the environment in the pursuit of occupational competence. The life plan is guided by personal and cultural values. Values give meaning and direction to one's life by inciting future goals and sustaining involvement in activity.

The concept of respect for the individual implies that the occupational therapy treatment plan should not interfere with the patient's intentions for recovery. To develop an appropriate plan, the patient's values are distilled from the thematic continuity of the assessment of occupational status and taken into account in the review of technically feasible treatment options. When there is a range of possibilities for treatment goals and substantial lack of certitude concerning the technical merits of treatment alternatives, the therapist has considerable latitude in shaping recommendations. Expert advice is based more on opinion than fact. Ethical decision making requires the therapist to search for an understanding of the patient's life rather than to make an evaluation of it. This understanding facilitates the selection of options to be discussed with the patient.

The goal of the clinical encounter is to devise a therapeutic plan that preserves the patient's values and represents a mutual understanding between the therapist and patient. Occupational therapy involves habit training and often requires major restructuring of the way in which personal values are to be satisfied. If habits are to be developed, patients must choose the objects and processes that they want to master in occupational therapy. Worthwhile achievement is the end product of personally deliberated decision making. Occupational achievement begins with the choice to develop one's capabilities. It is the patient who restores, maintains, and enhances occupational performance. The patient, not the therapist, is the agent of change. The patient's active participation is required not only in determining and prioritizing the goals of treatment, but also in deciding on the methods to be used to achieve the goals. As a result of assuming personal responsibility for treatment decisions, the patient emerges from the assessment with an increased sense of self-determination and control, and a sense of commitment to accomplishing planned goals. In the capacity of expert adviser, the therapist guides patients through the decision-making process, and helps them fuse the intellectual and emotional aspects of decision making into choices that are right for them.

It cannot be assumed that the goals selected by a patient for himself or herself will match those the therapist would select. Each may have a different view of the "good life." Because most persons with quadriplegia secondary to a spinal cord lesion at the level of the 6th and 7th cervical vertebrae can relearn dressing skills, the therapist may reason that Tim Robbins should work toward this goal. However, Tim may conclude that he would prefer to spend his limited energy relearning how to manage his home computer.

When the therapist and patient have different goals, the potential for conflict is high, and the resolution of conflict can easily be tipped in favor of the therapist's view. Two factors contribute significantly to the therapist holding the balance of power (1). First, the therapist has the knowledge and skills to alleviate the problems facing the patient. The patient is thus dependent on the therapist for help. Second, the patient's position of dependency is compounded by the patient's vulnerability. As a result of disease or other disorders, patients sustain insults to functions regarded as integral to human life and living. The very fact that they need help may diminish their sense of autonomy. Adaptive functioning in basic life tasks, such as eating and dressing, may be impeded. Patients may even be unable to express their own values or make rational patient's moral agency at risk, and often make it easy to take advantage of the patient's right to control his or her life.

Process. The methods used to answer ethical questions differ from those used in science. While scientific questions are answered by accumulating data and testing hypotheses, ethical questions are resolved by coming to grips with values and making value judgments (7). To empower the patient to act as his or her own moral agent, the therapist provides the patient with the knowledge needed to participate effectively in decision making. The patient's choice must not only be autonomous, it must also be informed. Patients are not adequately informed to make choices, unless they can anticipate the results of their choices. The ethical and scientific dimensions of clinical reasoning are closely intermingled. The therapist presents the possible options for treatment, projects the outcomes of each option, explains how the outcomes are achieved, and outlines a time sequence for goal attainment. Together the therapist and patient consider each recommendation and evaluate the consequences of each alternative in terms of the patient's occupational potential and goals. If necessary, the therapist tempers unrealistic expectations, corrects inaccurate information, and points out any inconsistencies in rationalization. In effect, the therapist assists the patient in imagining what might occur, if treatment is to be undertaken or rejected. The strength of arguments for one action over another is assessed by dialectic. Greater weight is assigned a position according to the importance it holds for the patient. The selection of treatment becomes more difficult as the merits of one action over other actions become more ambiguous. The therapist makes known his or her preferences for the patient's treatment as well as the rationale for this decision. The patient ends the deliberation by making a choice.

Once the patient has determined the course of action, the therapist supports or confirms the decision. The therapist captures the persuasive elements of the dialectical argument and uses them to instill in the patient a belief that treatment X is the best course of action and should be undertaken. At the same time, the therapist strives to bolster the patient's belief that he or she can carry out the treatment and achieve the goals. The reasoning process ends, therefore, in persuasive rhetoric, which we call "motivating the patient." In situations where therapists judge that they cannot lend support to the patient's choice, responsibility for providing occupational therapy services is terminated.

The therapist is privileged to help the patient select from the available opportunities those that are to be brought to fruition. As the patient executes and fulfills his or her choice, the therapist learns about the healing power of occupation. Occupational choice rekindles the will to live, and mobilizes the mind to discipline the body, in enacting the creative processes associated with reversing disability.

The subtle wisdom of participation in self-initiated and self-directed occupation becomes apparent as confidence is rebuilt and hope is restored. Choices are not confined to the outset of treatment. Assessment and planning are ongoing processes and there are repeated occasions to consider if treatment should be continued, terminated, modified, or supplemented.

This discussion of the ethical dimension of clinical reasoning has been based on three cogent assumptions: 1. that patients can serve as their own moral agents; 2. that the patient's choice is the ultimate one, and 3. that the therapist acts independently. None of these conditions may be met in a particular situation, which introduces further complications into the already complex process of ethical decision making. Surrogates may substitute for patients in the planning process because patients are too young, too impaired mentally, or too emotionally disturbed to participate in decision making. The rights of family members and the values and resources of society may limit the choices patients can make. The conjoint decision of therapist and patient may be modified or set aside by the health care team. These are vital issues that cannot be avoided in clinical decisions.

In summary, the data collected in clinical inquiry play three roles in clinical reasoning. First, clinical data are used to describe the patient's occupational status. This description includes an indication of the patient's adaptive skills, performance dysfunctions and their presumed causes, and competency motivation. Second, clinical data are used to conjure up a group of patients who have an occupational status and history comparable to the patient under consideration. These patients serve as a reference group for the identification of treatment options and prediction of treatment outcomes. Third, clinical data are used to identify therapeutic options appropriate to the specific needs of the patient, and to recommend a course of action consistent with the patient's values. As the clinical reasoning process moves from an assessment of occupational status, to a review of treatment options, to a selection of the right action, the scientific mode of reasoning gives way to nonscientific intellectual processes. Choosing a course of action involves many value considerations. The closer we come to making a clinical judgment, the less use is made of facts and hypothesis testing, and the more reliance is placed on the dialectical process, option, and persuasion.

Perfecting Clinical Inquiry

Now that what is involved in clinical study has been considered, it seems appropriate to ponder how our habits of inquiry can be improved. My suggestions are intended to be directional rather than comprehensive.

Model of the Patient. The therapist's understanding of the patient is highly dependent on the development of a model of the patient. It is pertinent to point out that studies conducted with counseling professionals have consistently supported the value of inductive theory building for practice, as opposed to the application of deductive theory. McArthur (8), for example, found that psychologists who applied existing theories in a doctrinary fashion turned out to be the poorest appraisers of personality. The critical element in devising a model of the patient is meticulous attention to the cues obtained from the patient. The ability to use assessment-related data to develop hypotheses is a vital professional skill.

Although hypotheses have adaptive value for organizing and managing data, they represent strong conceptual biases. In collecting and interpreting data, we have a tendency to overlook evidence that does not support our hypotheses. This is accompanied by an inclination to overemphasize positive evidence. In other words, we are psychologically prone to confirm our ideas and feel less compelled to refute them (4,9). Agnew and Pyke (10) drew a salient comparison between the blindness imposed by hypotheses and that generated by love. They commented: "The rejection of a theory once accepted is like the rejection of a girlfriend or boyfriend once loved—it takes more than a bit of negative evidence. In fact, the rest of the community can shake their collective heads in amazement at your blindness, your utter failure to recognize the glaring array of differences between your picture of the girl or boy, and the data." (p 128) The rigid application of a conceptual bias emerged as a major concern in my study of occupational therapists' thinking (11). The medical diagnosis was used to formulate the preassessment image of the patient and that image remained stable, even in the face of cues portending a revision.

Once cognizant of the pitfalls involved in hypothesis use, the therapist can initiate steps to avoid them. Obtaining a second opinion through consultation is one method commonly used to check the validity of one's interpretation. Consultants should perform their own assessments without reference to the patient's data base. Objectivity will be destroyed if consultants read reports or participate in discussions about the patient before conducting their own evaluations. The consultant's final opinion, however, should be based on the total available data (5).

A fixed data collection schedule is another mechanism used to prevent premature closure of hypothesis generation. The Occupational Therapy Uniform Evaluation Checklist (12) is an example of a fixed data collection schedule. It specifies the boundaries of occupational therapy practice and lists the variables to be reviewed for assessment. The Checklist forces the therapist to examine occupational performance from a panoramic view rather than microscopically. In so doing, it fosters the search for information that might suggest hypotheses the therapist might not otherwise have entertained. Adherence to a fixed routine assures the therapist that observations will be conducted that afford a fair and adequate opportunity to disprove as well as to confirm favorite hypotheses (13).

Research on the assessment processes suggests that practitioners' "favorite" hypotheses concentrate on the dysfunctional aspects of patient performance (14,15). We seem to be more interested in exploring why Alice Thompson falls so often than in ascertaining why she maintains her balance for so long. This preoccupation with problematic behaviors probably stems from the fact that they are the reason for the patient's referral to occupational therapy and constitute the focus of interventive efforts. Our first response to the question concerning the patient's occupational status is that it is dysfunctional. Our image of the patient changes as we collect additional cues and make adjustments in the initial picture. However, once our thoughts are anchored in dysfunction, it becomes difficult to switch our focus and too few modifications may be made in the image (16). Wright and Fletcher (14) point out that the perception of strengths and weaknesses as a unit, that is, as belonging to one person, requires the therapist to integrate two dissimilar qualities and that such synthesis is difficult. The same rationale may also be used to explain why practitioners are prone to see more pathology in their patients than the patients themselves perceive. Patients live with disability and adapt to it. Professionals regard disability as something to be eliminated. From this vantage point it is hard for professionals to see how disability can have any positive implications. Unfortunately, an emphasis on negative perceptions results in a skewed image of the patient. Dysfunctions are overestimated and abilities are underestimated (14).

Research also indicates that practitioners are more likely to hypothesize that a patient's problems are caused by factors within the patient as opposed to factors in the patient's physical and social milieu (14,15). For instance, we are more apt to attribute a patient's distress to an inability to deal with authority figures than to an unreasonable supervisor. One reason for this tendency is that we generally have a clearer picture of patients than we do of the situations in which they live, work, and play. We generally see patients in health care settings and rarely sample their behaviors in natural settings. Thus, the patient's environment has a quality of vagueness about it compared to the patient, who appears more real. Another explanation for our neglect of the environment is that it is often impossible or very difficult to change the environment. Even if the patient's supervisor is irrational, the patient still has to learn to manage the situation or to find another job. Nevertheless, it should be recognized that our "clinic-bound" view of the patient may lead us to ignore or underestimate impediments to occupational performance residing in the environment. Furthermore, since patients often attribute their difficulties to situations rather than to themselves, there is a potential conflict between the therapist's and patient's perceptions of causation. The validity of the patient's causal attribution should not be dismissed lightly by the therapist because patients are attuned to situational exigencies by their struggle for occupational competence.

Recognizing the distortion that may occur because of the exploration of hypotheses oriented toward dysfunction rather than function, and emphasis on the person as opposed to the environment, the therapist can take steps to countermand these biases. The data collection schedule can be arranged to include both assets and liabilities for every aspect of occupational performance evaluated. Since a patient's self-perceptions of competence are as important for participation in activity as is competence itself, the checklist should also highlight the patient's subjective impressions of occupational status. The schedule can also be extended to include the physical and social environments. These additions will serve to remind us of the significance of these variables for occupation and to foster the habit of routinely evaluating them.

Integration of Data. The challenge presented to the mind by the occupational therapy assessment is intensified by the need to integrate the wide variety of information gathered about the patient. Although we may isolate aspects of human functioning for the purposes of data management, humans function as unities or wholes. Competence requires the individual to function as an integrated organism, with the physical, mental, emotional, and social dimensions of occupational behavior interacting with the surrounding human and nonhuman environment. The selection of treatment proceeds from a holistic conception of the patient. If the therapist is to manage the array of complex clinical data required to understand occupational behavior, a simplifying strategy is needed to ward off chaos in the information processing capabilities of the human mind. Clinical judgments are not made on the basis of one or two test scores. And, although the statistical integration of clinical data may be possible in some situations, it is impractical in most. We need a labor-saving device to assist the mind in integrating data. General systems theory provides such assistance.

According to the systems metaphor, data are framed in terms of relationships between systems and systems are ordered hierarchically based on increasing levels of complexity. In the assessment of a patient with a traumatic spinal cord injury, for example, we would look at the effects of disorder on other biological systems, such as the musculoskeletal and integumentary. At the same time, the rules of systems hierarchy would direct our attention to factors in the psychological system, such as competency motivation, which will strongly influence the recovery of the biological system as well as the social reintegration of the patient. Although the assessment checklist is useful for reminding us of the spectrum of occupational performance, general systems theory provides rules for organizing the list so that the assessment data can be meaningfully related and stored in memory.

Occupational Therapy Assessment. Once an occupational therapy assessment has been made, viable therapeutic approaches are selected. The selection of treatment rests on a comparison between the patient under consideration and similar patients previously treated. Thus, the effective application of treatment requires that patients be accurately identified and grouped together according to characteristics that are salient for occupation. If the results of a clinical experiment are to be replicated, we must begin with a patient who closely resembles those used in the original experiment.

At the present time, occupational therapy has no meaningful way of systematically describing occupational role performance and of differentiating homogeneous subgroups based on occupational characteristics. The medical diagnosis is inadequate for delineating the diverse levels of occupational performance that occur in patients with the same diagnosis. It also lacks utility for identifying the similar levels of occupational performance that occur in patients with different medical diagnoses. Occupational therapy lacks a standardized way of classifying the functional disabilities that result from disease and other disorders. In the absence of an agreed upon system for thinking about, remembering, and expressing our clinical observations, each therapist develops his or her own idiosyncratic system for describing occupational performance. To the extent that these informal descriptions facilitate a comparison of patients, based on salient occupational characteristics, the inferences resulting from the comparison will be valid. However, until a systematic scheme for describing and organizing clinical data is developed, we will not be able to communicate meaningfully with each other, either in informal exchanges in the clinic, or in more scientific dialogue in our journals.

Selection of Treatment. We have seen that a treatment recommendation is largely based on the therapist's recall of similar cases. Some memories are more easily recalled than others (6). We are more likely to think of patients treated recently than those treated in the past. It is easier to remember patients who are seen frequently than those treated less often. Exceptional cases, either of success or failure, make strong impressions. Inferences gleaned from patients who happen to come to mind are likely to be less accurate than those derived from systematic analysis. Although we can all recount our brilliant successes, how many of us know what our batting average is? How good are we as judges of occupational potential? By keeping a score of the accuracy of our clinical predictions, our judgmental abilities can be improved. Checking our initial predictions against discharge data is something that can be readily incorporated into the clinic routine. Did the patient accomplish what I predicted he or she would? If not, why not? Since the ultimate test of treatment is what happens after discharge, mechanisms should also be sought for testing the accuracy of our discharge predictions with follow-up data.

A common error made by therapists in arriving at a clinical judgment is to assume that the patient is like oneself (17). This assumption enables us to know the patient through ourselves. In using the self as a referent, one rationalizes, "I will treat the patient as I would wish to be treated if I were in this situation." This kind of reasoning risks denying the validity of the patient's values. The therapist ascribes meaning to the patient's situation according to his or her own criteria. The patient is presented with a decision, rather than a list of options, and the choice of occupation is denied. Respect for the individual implies giving the patient the same opportunity to express and achieve what the patient sees as worthwhile as one would desire for oneself. We must be sensitive to the human spirit and curb the offering of pseudo choices of activity that have little meaning for the patient.

Instrumentation. The validity of clinical reasoning is grounded in the collection of good cues. This is a critical point to consider as we concentrate our energies on developing assessment instruments for practice. The nature of the phenomena we are interested in evaluating dictates the appropriate kind of instrumentation. As clinicians, our primary interest lies in evaluating performance in self-care, work, and leisure occupations. Our concern is with the ability to do and that doing is observable. You do not need to infer that I can dress from my grip strength, or mental acuity. You can observe my ability. Performance is not an abstract construct as is intelligence, anxiety, or sensory integration. We can see performance. Furthermore, we know that performance in occupation depends on the environment or situation as much as it does on the patient. Recognizing the interplay between the patient and the environment leaves us with two fundamental ways of evaluating occupational performance. First, we can go into the environments where our patients live, work, play, and observe their performance. Second, we can simulate the occupational environments of our patients by providing test stimuli, such as beds, chairs, games, arts and crafts, and work and collect a series of behavior samples in our clinics. In this case, the validity of our evaluation depends on how well we approximate the places where function is to occur.

There is inherently little uniformity in the occupational environments of our patients and, if we try to establish that uniformity, we will obscure the validity of our evaluation. The strength of occupational therapy assessment lies not in placing patients in contrived and standardized situations and recording their responses, but rather, in observing them in real life settings and evaluating their adaptive competence. Thus, development of occupational therapy instrumentation depends on conceptualization of the task environment, since this constitutes the test stimulus that evokes behavior. Our description of occupational behavior will be incomplete until we can mesh it with a description of the task environment.

The Art

Our exploration of the intellectual technology of clinical reasoning has focused on the scientific and ethical aspects. We have not considered the art except by implication and innuendo. In the peroration, I return to the therapist who says, "I don't know how I know, I just know that I know." While the scientific dimension of clinical reasoning is directed toward specifying the correct treatment from a technical standpoint, and the ethical dimension is geared toward selecting the treatment that meets the patient's criteria of right occupational role performance, the artistic dimension pursues excellence in achieving a right action—and it does this in the face of individuality, indeterminacy, and complexity (6). Artistry involves the orchestration of broad strategies for grappling effectively with the uncertainties inherent in clinical practice.

Skill in Thinking. Artistry is knowing as it is revealed in our actions (6). It is exhibited in knowing what to do and how to do it, rather than in knowing about something. In the early stages of acquiring a skill, such as dressing or piano playing, our actions are slow and clumsy. We have to think a lot about what we are doing and we make a lot of errors. But as skill develops, our actions become smooth, flexible, and spontaneous, and our thinking becomes automatic. We get a feel for the skill and that feeling allows us to repeat our performance. You know how to touch the piano keys to play a Mozart piano concerto, and your artistry is apparent in your music. If you were to describe your "knowing how to" play the piano, you would find this difficult if not impossible, just as someone else would find it difficult to acquire the skill of piano playing by following your instructions.

Clinical reasoning may be viewed as a skill akin to piano playing. The skill consists of reducing the ambiguities inherent in clinical practice to manageable risks, and by so doing, enabling the formulation of prudent decisions (6). In each clinical transaction, the therapist is challenged to apply the theories and techniques of occupational therapy to a particular patient. Our textbooks inform us of the implications of blindness, hemiplegia, and age-related changes, but the hiatus between theory and practice becomes readily apparent when 90-year-old John Green, accompanied by his loving wife and devoted daughter, stands before us with hemiplegia, blindness, and the beginning signs of brain failure.

Who among us has not experienced the gap between what we learned in school and what we need to know in the clinic.

Clinical problems are not neat. They are messy and complex. Everything that could be known about the patient is known and much of the data collected are flawed and imperfect. Clinical problems deal with the uniqueness of patients rather than with their similarities. And, as Gordon Allport (18) reminds us, uniqueness is not equivalent to the sum of the ways in which a person deviates from the hypothetical average human. Unlike the simple cause and effect problems associated with basic science, clinical problems involve a complex interplay of multiple variables, the effects of which are largely unpredictable. The outcomes of occupational therapy treatment cannot be guaranteed. Clinical problems change as patient's progress and regress and as the occupational opportunities provided by the environment fluctuate.

No one can provide "cookbook" recipes for dealing with situations in which uniqueness, uncertainty, complexity, and instability are the chief characteristics. There are no formulas or algorithms that tell us how to use the interneuronal processes associated with perception, memory, reasoning, and argument. In the clinical situation, the therapist is under pressure to act and to act now. One cannot interrupt an assessment to go to the library and read up on a critical point. In handling the uncertainties contained in clinical practice, therapists rely on their accumulated experience, conceptual and judgmental heuristics, intuition, and insight to "apply their knowledge" and make clinical judgments. In spite of defective data and incomplete information, artistic inquiry enables the therapist to make prudent decisions and to know why a treatment will work for a particular patient.

The artistry of clinical reasoning is exhibited in the craftsmanship with which the therapist executes the series of steps that culminates in a clinical decision. It is expressed in the interpersonal skills through which the therapist invites involvement in decision making, builds trust, explains treatment alternatives, and offers encouragement. Artistry manifests itself in the adeptness with which the therapist gathers cues: by selecting questions, probing for information not volunteered, clarifying discrepancies, administering tests, and observing performance. The degree of perfection with which the data to be processed are obtained influences the reliability and validity of the data, and hence sets limits on the quality of the final judgment. The art extends to grouping cues effectively, recognizing patterns, and depositing in memory organized reference images. The knowing derived from perceptual acuity, such as that needed to discern spasticity and achievement motivation, is also contained in the art of clinical reasoning. Linking the model of the patient with the appropriate memory structures to build a theory of practice for the patient requires considerable acumen. Artistic insight reaches its peak in combining evidence and opinion to support arguments convincingly, thus bringing closure to the decision-making process. Although each of these processes is difficult to master in and of itself, getting them coordinated and "on line" so that one can think "on one's feet" is an even vaster task.

Experts and Novices. The automation of clinical reasoning is not merely a matter of thinking faster. Experts think differently from novices. Because of the limited capacity of short-term memory, the human mind can only consider five to nine units of information at a time (16). This is why we find it difficult to remember telephone numbers. If I asked you to remember 9 1 9 9 6 6 2 4 5 1, chances are you would have forgotten the number long before you arrived at a telephone to dial it. However, if you knew that the area code for Chapel Hill is 919, and that all university numbers begin with the prefix 966, it is likely that you would have remembered the number 919-966-2451 correctly. Memory is aided by organizing and chunking information into larger units. By chunking telephone digits into familiar patterns, the number of units to be remembered is reduced and falls within the capacity of working memory.

Evidence is accumulating that expert and novice problem solvers differ in their use of problem-solving strategies, such as chunking (19). The expert sees and stores cues in patterns and configurations, whereas the novice records individual cues. Experts chunk data into larger information units than novices do. The expert creates memory structures by classifying data according to how they are to be applied in practice. The novice's memory structures, on the other hand, arise from features more peripheral to functional usage. The novice relies on conceptual principles to get things out of memory. The expert retrieves knowledge on the basis of situational cues as well as on conceptual stimuli. As the reasoning process unfolds, experts monitor their own thinking and understanding, which enables them to curtail errors and omissions. The ability to think faster is thus a result of thinking more efficiently, more functionally, and more critically.

Simply because our knowledge is in our action does not mean that we cannot think about it. When skill breaks down, and we strike a discordant note, drop a stitch, or fall off a bicycle, we step back, slow down our pace, and reflect on our actions. In clinical reasoning, skill breakdown occurs when clinical data are incongruous with our expectations and experience. Artistic inquiry is spurred by perplexity. As long as we are assessing patients whom we perceive as highly similar to those we have treated in the past, the clinical encounter presents no challenges, our intuitive understanding of the situation remains tacit. However, when we are no longer able to see things as we previously saw them, our curiosity is engaged, our anxiety is aroused, and we become inquisitive practitioners.

Expert clinicians are those who are competent in action and, simultaneously, reflect on this action to learn from it (6). They create opportunities for introspection by critically examining their reasoning to disclose bias and inconsistency. Artistic inquiry is also initiated through reframing, that is, by looking at the clinical situation from a new perspective. For example, a therapist might reason, "What would happen if this patient with low back pain were treated by diverting attention from back pain to pleasurable activity, instead of with exercises to improve body mechanics?"

As thinking becomes less automatic and more conscious, through self-criticism and reframing, it also becomes more accessible to explanation. Although our explanations and descriptions of clinical reasoning may never be complete, they can become progressively more adequate through reflection, and the artistic dimension can be better understood. The conversion of our practice into theory revolves around a cycle of concrete experience, reflective thinking, conceptual integration, and active experimentation.

In conclusion, the clinician functions as a scientist, ethicist, and artist. The scientific, ethical, and artistic dimensions of clinical reasoning are inextricably intertwined, and each strand is needed to strengthen the line of thought leading to understanding. Without science, clinical inquiry is not systematic; without ethics, it is not responsible; without art, it is not convincing. The intentions and potentials of chronically disabled patients are difficult to discern, but a therapist of understanding will elicit them, and use them to help patients discover health within themselves.

ACKNOWLEDGMENTS

Sincere appreciation is expressed to the following individuals for their critical review of the ideas presented in this paper: Anne Blakeney, David Hollingsworth, Teena Snow, and Joyce Sparling.

REFERENCES

1. Pellegrino ED, Thomasma DC: *A Philosophical Basis of Medical Practice*, New York: Oxford University Press, 1981
2. Scriven M: Clinical judgment. In *Clinical Judgment: A Critical Appraisal*, HT Engelhardt, SF Spicker, B Towers, Editors. Dordrecht, Holland: D. Reidel Publishing Co., 1979, pp 3-16
3. Cutler P: *Problem Solving in Clinical Medicine: From Data to Diagnosis*, New York: Basic Books, Inc., 1979
4. Sober E: The art of science of clinical judgment: An informational approach. In *Clinical Judgment; A Critical Appraisal*, HT Engelhardt, SF Spicker, B Towers, Editors, Dordrecht, Holland: D. Reidel Publishing Co., 1979, pp 29-44
5. Feinstein AR: Scientific methodology in clinical medicine, III. The evaluation of therapeutic response. *Ann Intern Med* 61: 944-966, 1964
6. Schön DA: *The Reflective Practitioner: How Professionals Think in Action*, New York: Basic Books, Inc., 1983
7. Brody H: *Ethical Decisions in Medicine*, Boston: Little, Brown, and Co., 1981
8. McArthur C: Analyzing the clinical process. *J Counseling Psychol* 1: 203-208, 1954
9. Koester GA: A study of diagnostic reasoning. *Educ Psychol Measurement* 14: 473-486, 1954
10. Agnew NM, Pyke SW: *The Science Game*, Englewood Cliffs, NJ: Prentice-Hall, 1969
11. Rogers JC, Masagatani G: Clinical reasoning of occupational therapists during the initial assessment of physically disabled patients. *Occup Ther Res* 2: 195-219, 1982
12. Shriver D, Mitcham M, Schwartzberg S, Ranucci M: Uniform occupational therapy evaluation checklist. In *Reference Manual of the Official Documents of the American Occupational Therapy Association*, Rockville, MD: AOTA, 1983
13. Elstein AS, Shulman LS, Sprafka SA: *Problem Solving: An Analysis of Clinical Reasoning*, Cambridge, MA: Harvard University Press, 1978
14. Wright BA, Fletcher BL: Uncovering hidden resources; A challenge in assessment. *Prof Psychol* 13: 229-235, 1982
15. Bateson CD, O'Quinn K, Pych V: An attribution theory analysis of trained helpers' inferences about clients' needs. In *Basic Processes in Helping Relationships*, TA Wills, Editor. New York: Academic Press 1982, pp 59-80
16. Matlin M: *Cognition*, New York: Holt, Rinehart and Winston, 1983
17. Sarbin TR, Taft R, Bailey DE: *Clinical Inference and Cognitive Theory*, New York: Holt, Rinehart, and Winston, 1960
18. Allport GW: *Pattern and Growth in Personality*, New York: Holt, Rinehart, and Winston, 1961
19. Feltovich PJ: Expertise: reorganizing and refining knowledge for use. *Professional Education Researcher Notes*, December 1982/January 1983, pp 5-9

Transformation of a Profession

Elnora M. Gilfoyle

During the past few decades occupational therapy has been in a state of identity crisis where the reality of occupational therapy and its proper place within health care systems is being questioned. Our profession must also question its value system, dimensions of practice, and educational requirements. In examining our place within health care systems, the profession must consider the current biomedical model, future trends for medicine, and the renaissance of the feminist movement. Our crisis should be recognized as a necessary impetus for the evolution that is underway. This crisis is our opportunity, not our pathology (1, p 25).

Occupational therapy is in a period of transformation, a period of paradigm shift, which is a shift in ways of thinking about old concepts. Paradigm shifts are similar to upward spirals that transform perceptions of the present into new perspectives. During a paradigm shift, an evolution takes place, a move from one form of unity through a phase of disunity and on to reintegration at a higher level (2, p 28). The disunity phase of an identity crisis can become positive in an emerging culture by shifting perspectives from static structures to perceptions of dynamic change. When we view evolution from the perspective of dynamic change, crisis becomes transformation (1, p 71).

For example, as we question our philosophical base from a perspective of dynamic change, crisis over therapeutic media and methods will lead to new perspectives of occupation and occupational. As we question our allegiance to medicine, new perspectives regarding practice

Reprinted from *The American Journal of Occupational Therapy*, Vol. 38, No. 9, 1984

dimensions will be transformed from the medical model to a model of healthfulness where patients influence their own state of health. As we question competencies needed to enter professional practice, requirements and organization of our educational process will be transformed to prepare independent health professionals. Occupational therapy's paradigm shift, as a transformation process, will evolve into new understandings of the value of occupation and the patients' occupational process in promoting their own health. Our practices and education will be organized around our evolving value system.

Our present transformation is dramatic and stressful because the rate of change in society is too rapid for us to have time to react. Our current transformation is not just a paradigm change of occupational therapy, but a crisis of multiple dimensions. Occupational therapy is involved in a crisis affecting our professionals, profession, culture, health care systems, communities, states, nation, and world.

Through this transformation period, if occupational therapists operate within a closed system, we are doomed to regress. If we enlarge our awareness to include social, economic, and political factors; admit new information from a variety of sources; and take advantage of the capacity to integrate past and present perceptions and concepts, we will leap forward. Although dramatic and stressful, crisis can bring about a positive evolution in which we come to a new understanding of the present.

Transformation directs itself to the present and the future; however, occupational therapy's history cannot be ignored. To view our present as if there were no past would make a caricature of our profession. Our present achievements are not a museum of finished products but an ongoing progress that is threefold: past, present, and future integrated into the upward spiral of our profession's evolution (3, p 20).

To prepare for this upward spiral, we need a new recognition of some of the values we previously discarded. Two such values are the idea of patients' "doing" as the occupational process and our mission to provide services for severely and chronically disabled. We need to reexamine those conceptual models and professional principles that dominate our present, such as our allegiance to the biomedical model, physical disabilities and psychosocial disorders as a framework for education and practice, and principles of media and methods based on activity as an extrinsic force. We need to prepare ourselves for changes that go beyond educational readjustments that are based on physical and psychosocial disabilities and acute care. We need to go beyond the debate over particular theoretical orientations and models of practice to show how occupational therapists' attitudes and behaviors reflect a value system that underlies our culture. Also, we must acknowledge that our current changes are manifestations of a much broader cultural transformation that includes the impact of the feminist movement, transition from medical care to holistic health, and change from institutional care to self-care, and of an adjustment of our allegiance to rational knowledge to include the value of intuitive knowledge (2, p 42). Through integration and examination of occupational therapy's past, present, and future, our profession's activities will show a constant flow of transformation and change.

In our past, conflict and struggle brought about important progress in our scientific foundations. Scientific progress will continue to be an essential part of the dynamics of change. However, research and science are not the only sources for paradigm change. Cultural aspects of our professional nature will also provide impetus for the profession's evolution. Additionally, social economic, and political environments external to occupational therapy have boundless capacities for influencing our transformation. Among the many factors that affect change, three merit attention: 1. the shift in our values, dimensions of practice, and educational focus that forms the reality of occupational therapy; 2. the decline of our allegiance to the biomedical model; and 3. the slow, reluctant, but inevitable decline of patriarchy (2, p 30).

Value System

Occupational therapy's reality lies in its culture. Culture is a synthesis of the objective and subjective contributions that make us a profession. Culture integrates our activities and behaviors, and provides a sense of direction for our practice. Culture has a powerful influence on what we do as occupational therapists because it is the driving force behind the development and success of our profession. Central to occupational therapy's culture is the science and art of the occupational process that facilitates meaning and order in the lives of persons with disabilities. Our culture, based on the use of occupation, includes the basic concepts and beliefs of our profession. Thus, values underlie our culture and form the heart of our profession.

In our day-to-day practices, "choices must be made and values are an indispensable guide in making them." (4, p 22) Values become the essence of occupational therapy's philosophy because they describe what we do along with what is unique about our profession. Occupational therapy's values are reflected in the profession's belief in a person's ability to influence his or her own state of health through the use of occupation. Our value system emerges from our rational knowledge of occupation and our intuitive knowledge of the purposefulness of the occupational process. Because our profession's values have profound influence on what we do, they must be a matter of great concern for our profession and Association (4, p 22).

During our transformation, our value system will change; however, we must not let external demands dictate those changes. Rather, *we should change because we continue to seek the truth of our values.* Professional values grow from the search for truth, and during our transformation we must act on the values of our history, and we must continue to seek the meaning and truth of our present (5, p 211).

Occupational therapy had its roots in the belief that the health of individuals could be influenced by "the use of muscles and mind together in games, exercise and handicraft as well as in work."(6, p 3) During the 1920s, Meyer's philosophy of occupational therapy proclaimed that human beings could maintain and balance themselves by being in active life and use. Meyer stated that the use humans make of themselves gives the ultimate stamp to their being (7).

Our early ideas of occupation and action were modified by the demands of both World Wars I and II, with wounded soldiers needing rehabilitation (8). Following the impact of the World Wars, occupational therapists' patient population changed and increased. Our early belief in games, exercise, handicrafts, and work (9,10) evolved into beliefs in constructive activities, activities of daily living, work simplification, and training in the use of adaptive equipment, and prosthetic and orthotic devices. During the 1950s and 1960s our culture was based on senso-rimotor rehabilitation techniques for physical dysfunction that were borrowed from physical therapy and on the concept of the therapeutic use of self in the treatment of psychiatric disorders, which was borrowed from psychology. In the 1960s and 1970s the idea of purposeful activity emerged. The value of activity was based on a neurobehavioral or an occupational behavior orientation, or on the biopsychosocial model underlying our practice (6, p 4-6). During the past decade, the concept of adaptation as the unifying theory for occupational therapy began to appear in our literature (11,12).

Recently, our Association adopted an official statement that proclaims our philosophy and directs our practice (13). In the statement our belief in activity is presented, including its interpersonal and environmental components; as a means to prevent and mediate dysfunction; as a means to elicit adaptation; and as having intrinsic and therapeutic purpose.

We offered this philosophy to describe our belief system and to declare what we do that makes us unique. However, in our day-to-day practices, occupational therapists frequently find themselves without convincing responses. Our proclaimed philosophy does not appear to provide us with a certainty about the sense of direction for our practices. Our literature communicates an internal debate: We have supported our values in activity, but have questioned the efficacy and credibility of activity as a therapeutic medium.

We, in occupational therapy, suffer from a pervasive uncertainty about our values, an uncertainty that undermines our commitment and leadership. Uncertainty about our therapeutic media and methods along with the interrelatedness of our science and art are central to our identity crisis. Therefore, our uncertainty must be recognized as an opportunity for us to transform traditional knowledge of activity into new perspectives of occupation and occupational. To maintain our upward spiral, our profession must re-examine the scientific view and value system that has been the basis of present concepts regarding activity and focus on future concepts based on a science of occupation and an art of purposefulness.

Re-examination of past concepts of occupation and a patient's action, together with integration of past ideas with our present concepts of activity, will direct our paradigm shift. Our paradigm shift will transform our concepts of purposeful activity into new dimensions of the concepts of occupation and occupational.

In 1909, C. Floyd Haveland said, "The therapeutic value of occupation for the insane is axiomatic and is based upon sound psychological laws." (8, p 8) Treatment by means of occupation was termed *humane treatment* or *ergotherapy* or *moral treatment* or *habit training* (8, p 6–7). In 1914, the term *occupational therapy* was first used by George Barton at a conference of hospital workers in Massachusetts. The term ran like a contagion, and earlier terms were dropped (14). By 1917, the objectives of the Association were formed, and statements of principles adopted occupational therapy as a method of treatment by means of purposeful occupation (8, p 8).

Although the term *occupational* has been used since the early 1900s, we have not defined it. We have instead discussed terms such as activity, work, play, self-care, and most recently, human occupations, but we have neglected to examine the concept of occupational. Through re-examination of our early ideas, a value system based on the dimension of occupational will emerge.

Occupational is defined as a process of action in which a person is the action agent or the "doer." Our philosophy will be based on occupation as action with the events of the environment and occupational as the action process. Values of "doing" or "action" and the "doer" or "action agent" are the integrating force that will bring the science and art of the therapeutic purposefulness of occupation into focus.

Values are not rules of conduct, but concepts that group together certain modes of behavior (4, p 14). Therefore, occupational therapists' scientific activities generate values that unite our practice and practitioners. Values provide unity and become the unifying force in our philosophy.

Our profession has been pleading for a generic or unifying theory. However, we must realize that unity may not mean a single theory, but rather a system of theories. Because theories are approximations of reality, occupational therapy needs a variety of scientific theorems, because each would be valid for a specific range of phenomena (2, p 10). There cannot be a unified or universal description of occupational therapy in a single closed theory. During our transformation, we must not expend our resources developing a generic or single theory of occupational therapy, rather we must synthesize our concepts into a unifying system of values.

In the science of occupation no concept or belief can be considered final; concepts have been made and will be remade with new ideas becoming part of a broader understanding. Thus, the science of occupational therapy becomes an endless process of analysis. Also, although science analyzes experiences, scientific analysis does not provide the total picture of the world of therapy. It provides the materials for the picture. Human imagination synthesizes the materials to provide a more coherent picture of the world. Thus, through scientific activity and human imagination, the value system of occupational therapy will evolve (15).

Imagination is the common quality in both science and art. In science, imagination organizes experiences into concepts, and in art imagination allows us to enter into human experiences (5, p 18-20). Science offers explanations and rational knowledge, whereas art carries an awareness or intuitive knowledge. Science of therapy is a creation to explain, and the art of therapy is a creation to relate, one where the patient receives and re-creates in his or her own image.

Therapeutic art is not an external giving by the therapist; it is an internal receiving by the patient. *It is through internal receiving that occupational experiences become purposeful.* Through science, the therapeutic value of occupation can be predicted and explained, but purposefulness of an occupational process cannot be measured and explained through research. Thus, the purposefulness of occupation will always remain as our art.

Society judges occupational therapists by the outcomes of our activities and behaviors. Therefore, our day-to-day practices must reflect our value system. Our lifelong learning process must also be designed to facilitate learning of and belief in our values. Study of values continually clarifies the power of our profession, and at the same time recognizes that the profession and society are in a continual interactive process. As occupational therapists we can view ourselves as professionals, freely controlling our own practice, or as adaptive therapists "at the beck and call of others."(16, p 20)

A system of values is our key to professionalism. Without a value system we will continue to be dependent on others. Conformity, the need for external approval and reliance on directions from others, characterizes an adaptive therapist. Independence, creativity, and self-directiveness characterize an integrated professional.

As an independent profession we must promote an integrative approach to our practice. Occupational therapists who argue against the effectiveness of activity are being forced to be adaptive. Arguments against the use of activity have appeared in our literature. West (17) has summarized these arguments:

1. Length of stay in acute settings is insufficient to show progress through activities.
2. There is pressure from physicians, administrators, and third-party payers to demonstrate cost-effective and objective measurable improvements.

3. Use of activities jeopardizes reimbursements.
4. Requirements for quality assurance reduce the use of crafts for substitutions that are reliable standardizations.
5. Crafts can be negative reinforcers to a patient who has lost skills.
6. Use of activities limits practice in the area of physical dysfunction.
7. Activities may be too complex for many of our low functioning patients (p 16).

These arguments are worthy of our attention, but we must also be aware that they reflect the reality of external forces, the profession's conformity to external approval, reliance on directions from others, and our need for survival and immediate recognition. Arguments presented also subscribe to a narrow perspective of activity. Through transformation, a broader perspective of occupation and occupational will emerge, and declaration of our value system will promote an integrative approach to practice.

Scientific knowledge of occupational therapy is not a notebook of facts about occupation or therapy; rather, our rational knowledge is an imaginative arrangement of concepts that are a creation of the human mind. Our scientific knowledge is a responsibility for the integrity of what we are, primarily of what it is we value. Our values come from our experiences, from testing what does and does not work; values are modified through the development of our profession and the environment and culture of our time. As occupational therapists, we cannot maintain our professional integrity if we let others direct our values while we continue to live out of a "ragbag of morals that come from past beliefs."(3, p 436).

Dimensions of Practice

Within the changing milieu of the 1980s, there are two environments for which occupational therapy must focus its actions, medical and educational. Medical and educational arenas will have a direct impact on the dimensions of our practice. Occupational therapy's allegiance to the medical model has historic roots dating back to our beginnings. Our need for acceptance and survival within the medical world, our orientation to short-term gains, and society's acceptance of patriarchal authority have been major factors in our development as an allied medical field. However, legislation in the 1970s delineated one aspect of occupational therapy services as an education-related service, not a medical service (18). The term *related service* has had important influences upon the changing concepts of our profession and the implementation of educational services. Introduction of the term *related service* has been a major impetus for change in both definition and concept of occupational therapy and education.

Implementation of related services has been a problem for our traditionally endowed public educational systems and our medically based practitioners. Factors that present problems within educational systems include

1. Occupational therapy services have traditionally been available from medical systems and therefore should not be offered through educational systems.
2. Educational personnel have neither been trained, nor do they consider themselves qualified, to deliver related services. School personnel should not supervise and have legal responsibilities for occupational therapists.
3. Problems of interagency coordination have too often been compounded with traditional health agencies refusing to assume responsibility for health care services that are now defined as educationally related.
4. Services are costly, which puts pressure on local school budgets that have been only partially funded by federal reimbursements. Thus, the ratio of therapist to students has been too large to provide services.

These factors are real. Thus, it is not surprising that educational systems have tried to protect their limited resources by searching for appropriate limits on related services. Educational organizations have tried to do this by attempting to define various services as not being educationally related at all; that is, they claimed that occupational therapy provided care to persons with conditions not educationally related but medically related.

Education's attempt to limit related services led to critical judicial decisions. Most notable was the expansion of the term *education* to encompass those self-care areas important for children with handicaps. Federal courts emphasized that education for handicapped children may be directed to achievement of "self-sufficiency or to some degree of self-care."(19, Connecticut, 1977) Thus, basic skills such as eating, walking, talking, and dressing, which come easily to nonhandicapped children, represent a high level of educational gains for some children. In effect, education is no longer defined as what schools have traditionally done; rather, education may include programs that have the capacity "to equip a child with the tools needed in life."(19, *Fialowski vs. Shapp,* Pennsylvania, 1975) As summarized in the Delaware Supreme Court in 1980: ". . . education is concerned with much more than simply the 3 R's—the definition would include instruction to teach one to dress oneself, toilet training, eating skills and other self-help skills."(19, p 26) The net result is that federal laws, expanded by federal court decisions, have adopted broad definitions of both "education" and "relatedness," and as such the laws have defined occupational therapy as an education-related service. Efforts to limit the extent of related services run counter to legal precedent. In fact, the major limitation to the concept of "relatedness" is not in the law or courts, not in regulations or policies, not with educational administrators, but within ourselves. Occupational therapists' concept of related services appears limited to direct treatment programs. Our need to hang on to our traditional medical model service delivery patterns not only presents education with questions of our medical relationships, but introduces a further dilemma with our own professional identity.

Educators and occupational therapists continue to argue that the specific services provided by and described as occupational therapy should be properly considered medical in nature and thus should be delivered in medical settings. However, medical services is a specific legal term in P.L. 94-142, the Education for All Handicapped Children Act. Despite common usage of the word *medical,* the law defines medical as only those services "provided by a licensed physician." Thus, any service that is education-related and provided by a nonphysician is not a medical service under P.L. 94-142.

Although most handicapped conditions served by an occupational therapist can be described as medical in their origin, the effect and amelioration of the conditions are often educational, particularly under the broad concept of education. Thus, related services such as occupational therapy are an educational responsibility.

Through our transformation, occupational therapy services will continue to expand within educational systems. Federal courts and federal laws will continue to mandate related services. Educational and health care systems will need to collaborate in programs for children and youth. The concept of occupational therapy as an education-related service will be accepted by our professionals, the profession, our Association, and society.

Expanding related services within public school systems will inevitably tax existing resources. However, as a legal and, perhaps even more important, as a practical matter, efforts to limit related services seem destined to fail. Public schools are becoming a lead agency in services for handicapped children and youth; thus efforts to minimize legal interpretations of related services run counter to expanding concepts of education entitlement. Our energies must be expended in optimizing interagency cooperation, developing more efficient service delivery systems, reallocating funds and staffing resources, and generating additional resources whenever possible. Regardless of the direction of the future, legal, political, economic, professional, and organizational issues will influence our transformation. By recognizing both external and internal issues and by identifying strategies, we can influence our own future.

One of the major external forces to affect education-related services of occupational therapy will be the future of health care delivery systems. Because health care industries will influence our services, we must identify issues related to health so our profession can develop appropriate strategies for action.

Health care, now the third largest category of the gross national product, represents more than $2 billion a year in costs (1). Health care has become too large, too complex, and too expensive for our practices to depend on traditional or conventional systems of providing services for persons with special needs. Health care professionals can no longer practice solo; solo practices of the past decades are too expensive. Health care services depend on collaborative efforts. Health care and educational agencies will collaboratively service children and youth, and health care and community agencies will service adults. Also, occupational therapists will find themselves practicing and providing services in collaboration with a variety of professionals.

In 1980, federal, state, and local public funds represented approximately 65 percent of medical payment, with 30 percent coming from third-party providers such as insurance companies. Less than 5 percent of health costs come from private individuals. Thus, third parties and taxpayers pay for medical care. Although the majority of the health care dollar goes to hospitals, physicians continue to decide how the dollar will be spent. However, as we move to a system of prospective payment, one that gives the hospital an economic incentive to be more efficient and less expensive in its management of patients, the incentives for physicians and health care providers may be in direct opposition to the incentives of hospitals. Prospective payment will influence the concept of acute medical care within medical establishments, and a transition to personal responsibility or self-care and home health programs will occur. Transition from institutional care to self-care will have a direct impact on service delivery patterns of occupational therapists.

Predictions for delivery modalities for the upcoming decade include: increased outpatient care; increased home health services as an alternative to hospital care; increased quality and quantity of long-term care for the severe and chronically disabled; increased sensitivity to physical and emotional suffering of the aged; an increase in multi-institutional systems that provide cost-effective services and enhance use of personnel; and increased interaction and cooperation among systems, with increased competition for personnel, new markets, and access to capital and technology.

If these predictions prove correct, the following five assumptions seem appropriate for the delivery of occupational therapy services:

1. Occupational therapy will continue to be practiced through organizational structures with increased pressures to make these organizations cost effective.
2. New and more effective communicative networks must be developed to ensure continuity of care among the various health professionals.
3. Demands for interagency collaboration will be imperative.
4. Power and political issues operating within health and educational organizations will increase rather than decrease.
5. New service delivery patterns involving consultation and monitoring and collaborative programming will be imperative.

Our literature suggests that many occupational therapists are frustrated because management concepts are not being used in practice and because students are not being taught management concepts and skills. Occupational therapists will have to learn skills associated with effective consultation, supervision, leadership, and communication. It is not enough to learn the theory and practice of occupational therapy. Obviously a problem occurs; predictions for the future suggest multidisciplinary interagency collaboration, which requires management, consultation, communication, and leadership skills. Our literature suggests we are not providing these skills for our practitioners. Thus, occupational therapy curricula must modify traditional approaches to course content to prepare professionals for the changing health care systems.

Educational Focus

The nature of our education determines essential aspects of occupational therapy practices. Attempts for paradigm change or transformation must include changes in our educational focus and certification requirements. Accreditation with the American Medical Association has established a link between medicine and occupational therapy, and this link has dominated our educational system ever since. The biomedical model's influence on education is reflected in our academic and fieldwork divisions of physical dysfunction (treatment of the body), psychosocial dysfunction (healing of the mind), and pediatric and geriatric age groups (facilitation of development). We promote an artificial division within our profession by educator's attention to a particular age group or to the body or mind. Certification to practice ensures successful mastery of knowledge of physical dysfunction and psychosocial dysfunction, not the ability to promote a patient's care of self and meaningful life through the use of occupation. Our educators must begin to base curricula on our value system of occupation and the occupational process, and on the science of occupation and the art of purposefulness. We must also address our allegiance to holistic and ecological concepts of health, and our relationship to education. In addition, management, leadership, and consultation skills need to be included in our curricula.

Transformation of our educational focus, together with our re-examination of concepts, will provide impetus to solve our identity crisis. Along with these activities, we must also examine our entry-level requirements for professional practice. Currently our entry-level requirements are inadequate for dealing with the major problems of our times and predicted demands for future practices. Predicted increases in home health practices, transition from medical to holistic health care, declaration of our profession as an education-related service, new dimensions of service delivery, and an increase in our scientific activities are but a few of the many aspects of transformation that need to be addressed by our entry-level preparation and requirements.

Decisions and recommendations related to our educational focus and requirements must be based on careful study, but they must begin immediately. Transformation of our profession is underway; our emerging culture with its new perspectives must be reflected in our educational preparation processes. Official bodies of our Association, particularly the Commission on Education, Executive Board, and Representative Assembly, must recognize the crisis in our education preparation and determine resolutions.

Occupational therapy reality will include transformations of our value system, dimensions of practice, and educational focus. Crisis of our reality will evolve into new perspectives of our profession. Although our paradigm shift occurs within, society's decline of allegiance to the biomedical model and to patriarchal authority have significance to occupational therapy's practice within health care systems.

Decline of Patriarchy

In *The Aquarian Conspiracy*, Ferguson proclaimed: "The power of women is the powderkeg of our time."(1, p 221) Feminism has become a major force in our culture. Because 95 percent of our professionals are women, it is imminent that the women's movement shall play a pivotal role in the transformation of occupational therapy. A renaissance of feminist ideals is creating new images of women and men. New modes of thinking and value systems are emerging. Role shifts and sharing of responsibilities are bringing about far-reaching changes in society's attitudes and behaviors. Our culture has been based on the belief that self-assertive behavior is ideal for men and submissive behavior is expected from women. Self-assertion was manifested through power, control, and domination of others. Competitive behaviors characteristic of self-assertion have been highly regarded and promoted in our society. Women have been expected to be submissive and to fulfill the needs of others, and to perform those services that make life more comfortable. Society has expected women to "create the atmosphere for the competitors to succeed."(2, p 45).

In the past, science and technology have been based on the belief of male supremacy and dominance. Medical societies in particular have not respected women's contributions to science and technology; rather, the culture of medicine has expected women to provide the caring, not the knowledge to understand the cure or the process to heal. Masculine supremacy has led to a medical high-tech dissonance. We are going from forced masculine technology to a balancing of "high tech/high touch." As Naisbitt (20) pointed out, high-tech dissonance is being transformed to balance with high touch. High tech/high touch is part of the balancing of feminist and masculine values. With this balancing, more respect for women's contributions to medicine, health, and education will occur. The allied health fields, dominated by women, will be recognized not as allied but as independent health professions. Transformation to an integrative power of technology and touch within medicine will further shake the foundations of occupational therapy.

Decline of Allegiance to the Biomedical Model

As medicine transforms to be in keeping with society's demands, our allegiance to the current biomedical model will decline. Modern scientific medicine has been based on a biomedical model that views the body as a machine. Disease, illness, and handicapping conditions represent malfunctions of the body machine's mechanisms. Only the physician knows how to correct malfunctioning, because he or she has been the one with scientific knowledge and technology. Authority and responsibility have been delegated to the physician who intervened and fixed the machine. Society has been spellbound by the mystique of medicine (2, p 158).

Americans are losing faith in medical establishments and physicians because the increase in medical costs far exceeds the effectiveness of care. Although human life expectancy has increased and many types of illnesses have been controlled, the health of our population has not improved. For example, there are increases in learning disabilities, child and adult abuse, mental illnesses, and suicide among youths. Medicine's dependence on high technology has increased problems of health, with biomedical interventions having little impact on the health of entire populations (2, p 138).

Current medical therapy is based on principles of intervention. The medical profession has relied on outside forces such as drugs and surgery without viewing the patient as a responsible individual who has a healing potential within and who can initiate the process of getting well (2, p 152). Principles of intervention have also dominated the practice of occupational therapy. For example, we have based our philosophy and research on the outside force of activity or the effects of adaptive equipment or devices. Although these are important, we must not forget the values that are inherent to our profession: the patient's intrinsic motivation to "do" and the "doing" aspect of healing.

Transformation of the biomedical model is underway with the paradigm shift based on an awareness of the "essential interrelatedness and interdependence of all phenomena—physical, biological, psychological, social, and cultural."(2, p 265) Concepts of prevention, relationships of physical and social environments, and the interplay of body, mind, and environment in the healing process are beginning to influence medicine. Medicine's paradigm shift is opening up new areas in search of a health orientation. Medical science now acknowledges that the art of healing is essential to all health care. With new emphasis on the human aspects of health, there will be an increased move from the medical establishment (institution) to personal responsibility (self-care and home health).

Occupational therapy has been a profession that has based its values on a paradigm of wellness. We consider patients active participants in their own care. We believe people are able to influence their own health and recognize the interplay of body, mind, and environment. With transformation of the biomedical model to a holistic health model, our profession must proclaim these values and communicate our philosophy. Medicine and society are catching up with us, but we must not let them pass us by.

Summary

Professional evolution includes a period of disunity, a phase when old values and concepts are being examined, and new perspectives emerge. Disunity can be a positive impetus for dynamic change. Transformation provides a higher level reintegration through which new understanding and progress unfold. Occupational therapy's transformation is now; it is time for careful analysis and creative synthesis.

Transformation is a three-fold process of integration of past, present, and future into an upward spiral of professional development. Transformation is a constant flow of activities influenced by both internal and external factors. Although there are multidimensions that influence occupational therapy's transformation, three major components are inherent in the profession's paradigm shift: 1. society's decline in patriarchal authority; 2. decline in allegiance to a biomedical model; and 3. shift in values, dimensions of practice, and education that form the reality of occupational therapy.

Transformation of our profession will be a paradigm shift in our value system of purposeful activity to a new perspective of occupation and occupational; in our quest to develop a unifying theory for recognition of the unifying force of values; in our concepts and theories to include the science of occupation and the art of purposefulness; from total allegiance to scientific knowledge to include intuitive knowledge; from being an allied medical field to an independent health profession that is both educationally and medically related; from a biomedical model to a paradigm of wellness; in balancing of feminine and masculine values of human nature; and in organizing educational curricula and entry-level requirements that reflect our value system and predicted practice dimensions.

As Naisbitt said, "We are living in the time of parenthesis, the time between eras."(20, p 249) Occupational therapy has not left the past behind, but it has not quite embraced the future either. Thus, our profession is in a time of parenthesis that brings us many uncertainties. Uncertainties, however, can be our opportunity. We need only make use of the challenge and possibilities that are part of our dynamic present. Transformation is a time to direct our own future. "We stand on the brink of a new age, the age of an open world, a time of renewal when a fresh release of spiritual energy in the world culture may unleash new possibilities. The sum of all our days is just our beginning."(1, p 42)

We have reached our turning point. We have the means to solve our crisis and continue our transition to higher dimensions. However, we must choose to do so.

REFERENCES

1. Ferguson M: *The Aquarian Conspiracy: Personal and Social Transformation in the 1980's.* Los Angeles: JP Tarcher, Inc., 1980
2. Capra F: *The Turning Point: Science, Society, and the Rising Culture.* Toronto: Bantam Books, 1983
3. Bronowski J: *The Ascent of Man,* Boston: Little, Brown & Co., 1973
4. Deal TE, Kennedy AA: *Corporate Cultures: The Rites and Rituals of Corporate Life.* Reading, MA: Addison-Wesley Pub. Co., 1982
5. Bronowski J: *A Sense of the Future.* Cambridge, MA: MIT Press, 1977
6. Hopkins H, Smith H: *Willard and Spackman's Occupational Therapy,* 6th Edition. Philadelphia: JB Lippincott, 1983
7. Meyer A: The Philosophy of Occupational Therapy. *Archives of Occupational Therapy* 1(1): 1-10, 1922
8. Kidner TB: *Occupational Therapy, The Science of Prescribed Work for Invalids.* Stuttgart, Germany: W Kohlhanne, 1930
9. Slagle EC: Training aids for mental patients. *Archives of Occupational Therapy* 1(1): 1-10, 1922
10. Hall HJ, Back M: *Handicraft for the Handicapped.* New York: Moffact, Yard & Co., 1916
11. King LJ: Toward a science of adaptive responses. *Am J Occup Ther* 32:429-430, 1978

12. Gilfoyle E, Grady A, Moore J: *Children Adapt.* Thorofare, NJ: Charles B. Slack, 1980, Chapter 3
13. The Philosophical Base of Occupational Therapy. American Occupational Therapy Association Resolution #531, April 1979
14. Barton GE: *Teaching the Sick: A Manual of Occupational Therapy and Re-education.* Philadelphia: W.B. Saunders, 1914, p 4
15. Bronowski J: *The Visionary Eye: Essays in the Arts, Literature and Science.* PE Ariotti, Editor. Cambridge, MA: MIT Press, 1978, pp 20,21,31
16. Hall Bryan P: *The Development of Consciousness: A Confluent Theory of Values.* New York: Paulast Press, 1976, p 20
17. West W: A reaffirmed philosophy and practice of occupational therapy for the 1980's. *Am J Occup Ther* 38:15-23, 1984
18. Education for All Handicapped Children Act, 1975, P.L. 94-142, *Federal Register,* Tuesday, Aug. 23, 1977, Sec. 121A 13
19. Related services and medical services requirements under current legal standards. *Focus* 1(2): 1981. Reprinted in Information Packet, Occupational Therapy in the School Systems. Rockville, MD: AOTA, 1982, pp 25-29.
20. Naisbitt J: *Megatrends.* New York: Warner Books, 1982, Chapter 2

Biographies and Bibliographies of the Eleanor Clarke Slagle Lecturers, 1955–1984

The following biographies and bibliographies are offered to give an overview of the professional careers and to demonstrate the achievements of each of the Eleanor Clarke Slagle lecturers. Each of the bibliographies is arranged in chronological order. Coauthors are named and all journal titles are written in full except for The American Journal of Occupational Therapy, *which is abbreviated:* AJOT.

Most of the information that follows was provided by the lecturers themselves. We acknowledge the assistance of the American Physical Therapy Association in providing a photograph of Margaret Rood, and of Ralph A. Rood and Helen Ziler for their assistance in our search for information regarding Margaret Rood, who died in September 1984.

We also acknowledge the assistance of the Wellesley College Alumnae Association in providing a biography and photograph of Alice Jantzen; and of the Hartford Easter Seal Rehabilitation Center in providing a biography and photograph of June Sokolov. Both Jantzen and Sokolov died in October 1983.

Florence M. Stattel, MA, OTR, FAOTA   1955

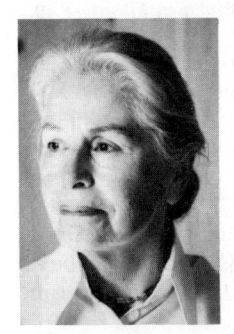

Florence M. Stattel is a former associate professor and coordinator of the occupational therapy program on the Dallas campus of the Institute of Health Sciences, Texas Woman's University, Denton.

She has served as associate professor of occupational therapy at the University of Florida and as the rehabilitation services coordinator for the Regional Interdepartmental Rehabilitation Committee of the New York City Medical and Health Research Association, Inc. She also has been associated with the National Society for Crippled Children and Adults, Inc.; New York University School of Education; Kessler Institute for Rehabilitation, West Orange, New Jersey; American Public Health Professional Examination Service, Inc., New York City; B.S. Pollack Hospital for Chest Disease, Jersey City, New Jersey; Rehabilitation Shops, Bridgeport, Connecticut; and King's County Hospital, Brooklyn, New York.

Stattel was graduated from New York University with a bachelor's degree in occupational therapy and a master's degree in vocational rehabilitation. She holds a certificate in occupational therapy from the University of Pennsylvania. She is a charter member of the World Federation of Occupational Therapists, a member of the American Public Health Association, the New York Occupational Therapy Association, and the AOTA. Stattel was an AOTA Vice-President from 1954 to 1958. She served on the AOTA Government and Legal Affairs, Occupational Therapy Assistance, Curriculum Advisory, and Finance Committees, and was named a Fellow of the AOTA in 1973. Stattel was listed in *Who's Who of American Women* in 1955.

BIBLIOGRAPHY

The student occupational therapist. *AJOT* 2:6, 162, 1948

Occupational therapy—Kessler Institute. *AJOT* 6:1, 29, 1952

The painful phantom limb. *AJOT* 8:4, 156, 1954

Frances L. Shuff, a biographical sketch. *AJOT* 9:2, 71, 1955

Equipment designed for occupational therapy. *AJOT* 10:4, 194-198, 1956

Treatment of the (congenital) arm amputee. *Proceedings of the First International Congress, World Federation of Occupational Therapists, Scotland*

Equipment designed for occupational therapy. *AJOT* 10:4, 194, 1956

The occupational therapist in rehabilitation: Projections toward the future. *AJOT* 20:3, 144, 1966

The occupational therapy consultant. *Proceedings*, Manpower Conference for Health-Related Professions, State University of New York, School of Health-Related Professions, Buffalo, 1967

———, Koestler FA: Regional planning in an urban setting. *Rehabilitation Literature* 29: 1968

A profile of state-designated comprehensive rehabilitation centers in New York City. Report to the New York State Commissioner of Health, December 1969

June Sokolov, MA, OTR, FAOTA, DHL (Hon.)   1956

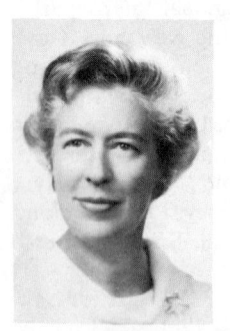

June Sokolov was founding director of the Hartford Easter Seal Rehabilitation Center in Connecticut, where she served as director from 1949 until her retirement in 1977.

She received her bachelor of science degree, magna cum laude, from New York University (NYU). During this period, she received her clinical training at various institutions, including Bellevue Hospital; Sheppard and Enoch Pratt Hospital, Baltimore, Maryland; and Bridgeport Rehabilitation Center, Connecticut. She earned her master's degree at NYU while serving as acting director of the School of Occupational Therapy.

During her early years, Sokolov danced professionally with the Martha Graham and Agnes DeMille companies. She also conducted dance classes for children. After graduation from college, she joined the Connecticut Society for Crippled Children and Adults for two years as chief occupational therapist.

Sokolov was active in both state and national occupational therapy associations. She served on the AOTA Executive Board, the Committee on Student Affiliation, and the Advisory Panel for the Office of Vocational Rehabilitation. She was Program Chairman of the 1956 Annual Conference.

Sokolov was awarded an honorary doctor of humane letters degree from the University of Hartford in 1978. She was named to the AOTA Roster of Fellows in 1973.

From her retirement until her death in October 1983, Sokolov managed the Grist Mill Gallery in Hartford and taught English to illiterates with the Hartford Literacy Volunteer Program.

BIBLIOGRAPHY

Working as a team: The occupational therapist in a rehabilitation center. *AJOT* 9:6, 270, 1955

Therapist into administrator: Ten inspiring years. *AJOT* 11:1, 13, 1956

The occupational therapist of the future, planning for. *AJOT* 19:1, 1, 1965

Ruth W. Brunyate Wiemer, MEd, LHD, OTR/L, FAOTA 1957

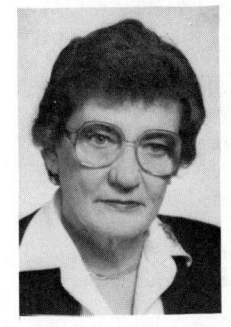

Ruth Brunyate Wiemer holds a bachelor's degree in sociology from Hollins College (1938), a certificate from the Philadelphia School of Occupational Therapy (1940), and an M.Ed from Johns Hopkins University (1967). She was awarded an L.H.D. by Towson State University (1980).

Associated with Dr. Winthrop M. Phelps' pioneer work in cerebral palsy at Children's Rehabilitation Institute in Maryland (1941-1961), she held various positions, including staff therapist, director of occupational therapy, administrative assistant to the executive director, and acting executive director (1957). She became assistant professor and acting director of the Department of Occupational Therapy at Milwaukee-Downer College in 1961.

Wiemer joined the Maryland State Department of Health as a consultant in 1962 and was named chief of the Division of Occupational Therapy in 1966. She continued as chief when the agency became the Department of Health and Mental Hygiene in 1970. She retired in 1980 and lives on Maryland's Eastern Shore.

Wiemer held many appointed and elected positions in the Maryland Occupational Therapy Association (MOTA), including the presidency, and in AOTA. She was AOTA's First Vice-President (1961-1963) and President the following three years. As Chair of the Legislation Committee and then the Government Affairs Committee, she provided the impetus for establishment of the AOTA Government Affairs Division. She was an incorporator and Board Member of the American Occupational Therapy Foundation and serves on its Research Development Committee.

Her honors include the AOTA Award of Merit, Roster of Fellows, Certificate of Appreciation of the Commission on Education, and Lindy Boggs Award; the MOTA's Roster of Merit and Presidential Commendation; the Community College of Baltimore's Brunyate Lectureship; the University of Texas School of Allied Health Sciences Class Dedication; *Who's Who In America, Who's Who In American Women, Who's Who in Health Care*; the State of Maryland's Governor's Citation, and the Department of Health and Mental Hygiene's Certificate of Appreciation.

BIBLIOGRAPHY

Occupational therapy in cerebral palsy clinics. *Canadian Journal of Occupational Therapy* 13: 27-33, 1946

Occupational therapy for patients with cerebral palsy. In *Principles of Occupational Therapy*, Willard HS, Spackman CS, Editors. Philadelphia: JB Lippincott, 1947

Occupational therapy means freedom for parents. *Crippled Child* 26:11, National Society for Crippled Children and Adults, Inc, Chicago, 1949

———, Phelps WM: Occupational therapy in the treatment of cerebral palsy. In *Occupational Therapy Principles and Practice*, Dunton WR, Licht S, Editors. Springfield: Charles C Thomas, 1950

Mrs. Elizabeth Martin Wagner, a biographical sketch. *AJOT* 5:5, 213, 1951

The importance of pre-skill activities in occupational therapy for the cerebral palsied. *Proceedings of the Second Cerebral Palsy Institute*, New York: The Coordinating Council for Cerebral Palsy, Inc, 1952

Occupational therapy department, The Children's Rehabilitation Institute, Cockeysville, Maryland. The featured occupational therapy department. *AJOT* 6:5, 219, 1952

Occupational therapy for patients with cerebral palsy. In *Principles of Occupational Therapy*, Willard HS, Spackman CS, Editors. Philadelphia: JB Lippincott, 1954

A study of the use of magnetic toys in the treatment of cerebral palsied children. *AJOT* 8:4, 151, 1954

———, Phelps WM: Occupational therapy in the treatment of cerebral palsy. In *Occupational Therapy Principles and Practice*, Dunton WR, Licht S, Editors. Springfield: Charles C Thomas, 1957

Powerful levers in little common things. *AJOT* 12:4, 193, 1958

The clinical center—An integral part of the education program. *AJOT* 16:2, 61, 1962

Graphs: Their value as a record form in the management of the cerebral palsied. *AJOT* 16:1, 13, 1962

The student in pre-clinical education: Impressions of a clinically-oriented therapist. *AJOT* 17:5, 181, 1963

Occupational therapy for patients with cerebral palsy. In *Occupational Therapy*, Willard HS, Spackman CS, Editors, Philadelphia: JB Lippincott, 1963

Nationally speaking. *AJOT* 18:2, 69, 1964

Keynote Address. *AJOT* 20:1, 9, 1966

After fifty years, what stature do we hold? *AJOT* 21:5, 262, 1967

Guidelines for establishing services and recommended standards for occupational therapy and activity programs. Baltimore: Maryland State Department of Health, 1968

———, West WL: Occupational therapy in community health. *AJOT* 24:5, 323, 1970

Some concepts of prevention as an aspect of community health: A foundation for development of the occupational therapist's role. *AJOT* 26:1, 1, 1972
What is the National Health Council? Is AOTA's membership in it worthy of budget priority? Nationally speaking. *AJOT* 26:1, 3a, 1972
Traditional and nontraditional practice arenas. In *Occupational Therapy: 2001 AD*, Rockville, MD: AOTA, 1979
Student transition from academic to fieldwork. In *Fieldwork Manual*, Rockville, MD: AOTA, 1984

Margaret S. Rood, OTR, RPT, MA, FAOTA 1958

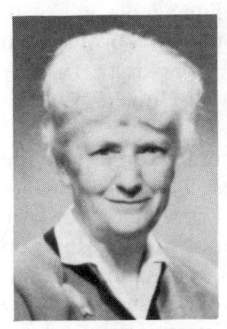

Margaret S. Rood, Professor Emeritus, University of Southern California (USC), was best known for her development of a neurophysiological approach in the treatment of central nervous system disorders, which has been used internationally by various therapy professions and medical fields. She has presented numerous workshops, lectures, and symposia on this treatment approach.

Registered as both an occupational therapist and a physical therapist, Rood was chair of the Department of Physical Therapy at USC from 1959 until 1966 where she initiated the second physical therapy master's degree program in the United States. She established the Department of Occupational Therapy at USC in 1943 and served as professor and department chairperson and director of programs until 1952. While at USC, she developed a method of therapeutic exercise known as the Rood System.

Rood also worked with the Elks Major Project at Riverside County, California from 1952 until 1955 and spent the next year investigating swallowing and speech procedures with bulbar poliomyelitis patients at Rancho Los Amigos Hospital, Hondo, California. She was staff occupational therapist for the Asylum for Chronic Insane, Wauwatosa, Wisconsin (1933-36) and therapy supervisor in the Cerebral Palsy Clinic, Indiana University Medical Center, Indianapolis (1937-43).

Rood received a bachelor's degree (1932) and a diploma in occupational therapy (1933) from Downer College, Milwaukee, Wisconsin. She earned a master's degree and a certificate in physical therapy from Stanford University.

She received the Mary McMillan Lectureship Award from the American Physical Therapy Association in 1969. She was elected a Fellow of the AOTA in 1973. She received the Distinguished Emeriti Award from USC in March 1984, six months before her death in September 1984.

BIBLIOGRAPHY

A program for paraplegics. *AJOT* 1:1, 22, 1947
University of Southern California, Los Angeles, California (School Section). *AJOT* 1:4, 258, 1947
Occupational therapy in the treatment of the cerebral palsied. *Physical Therapy* 32: 76, 1952

Neurophysiological reactions as a basis for physical therapy. *Physical Therapy* 34: 444, 1954
Neurophysiological mechanisms utilized in the treatment of neuromuscular dysfunction. *AJOT* 10:4, Part II, 220, 1956
Every one counts. *AJOT* 12:6, 326, 1958
Neurophysiology in the Treatment of Neuromuscular Dysfunction. In a seminar sponsored by the Wyoming Valley Crippled Children's Association, Inc., Moyer and Davis, Editors, National Society for Crippled Children and Adults, 1959

Lilian S. Wegg, OTR, FAOTA   1959

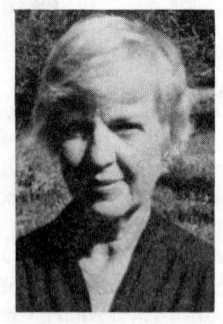

Lilian S. Wegg is a vocational counselor with Work-Wise, a private rehabilitation counseling agency in Cotati, California. A graduate of the University of Toronto with a degree in occupational therapy, Wegg holds a certificate in rehabilitation administration from the University of San Francisco.

Wegg began her occupational therapy career with the Workmen's Compensation Convalescent Centre in Toronto, Canada. In 1948, she moved to San Francisco, where she was the chief occupational therapist for the Morrison Rehabilitation Center until 1954 and work sample administrator from 1954 to 1959. After attending the University of San Francisco, she held several positions as rehabilitation counselor and administrator of workshops and agencies for the developmentally disabled. She was named to the AOTA Roster of Fellows in 1973.

BIBLIOGRAPHY

The role of the occupational therapist in vocational rehabilitation. *AJOT* 11:4, Part II, 252, 1957
The essentials of work evaluation. *AJOT* 14:2, 65, 1960
The essentials of work evaluation. *AJOT* 31:10, 651, 1977

Muriel E. Zimmerman, MA, OTR, FAOTA   1960

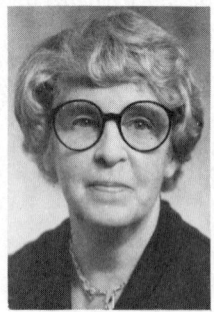

Muriel E. Zimmerman has been with the Institute of Rehabilitation Medicine (IRM), New York University (NYU) Medical Center since 1950, where she currently is associate director of occupational therapy and assistant professor of clinical rehabilitation medicine at the NYU School of Medicine.

A 1939 graduate of the Philadelphia School of Occupational Therapy, Zimmerman received a bachelor of science degree in 1960 and a master of arts degree in 1966 from NYU. From 1956 to 1974 she was an instructor of occupational therapy at NYU in the area of adaptive equipment. She has participated in all in-service and special courses at IRM.

Zimmerman has completed and directed extensive research on self-help devices. She has also prepared and contributed to numerous exhibits of self-help devices and equipment in the U.S. and abroad, and she has produced several films in this area.

Zimmerman has chaired many international and national committees since 1957, and has been a member of the International Society for Rehabilitation of the Disabled's advisory committee to the International Center on Technical Aids, Transportation, and Housing. She directed the research committee of the Clothing Research and Development Foundation.

Zimmerman has served the AOTA as Chairman of the Special Studies Committee and as contributing editor to *AJOT*. She was named an AOTA Fellow in 1973. She is listed in *International Who's Who in Education* and in *International Who's Who of Intellectuals*.

BIBLIOGRAPHY

Rusk HA, Taylor EJ, ———, Judson J: *Living with a Disability.* New York: McGraw-Hill, 1953

Morrisey AB, ———: Helps for the handicapped. *American Journal of Nursing* 53:316-318 and 454-456, 1953

Adapted equipment for rehabilitation, Part 6. In *Principles of Occupational Therapy*, 2nd Edition, Willard HS, Spackman C, Editors. Philadelphia: JB Lippincott, 1954

Accent on progress. *IPMR* 1:3, 19-23, 1955

Analysis of adapted equipment, Part 2. *AJOT* 4:2, 229-237, 1957

Self-Help Devices for Rehabilitation: Part 1. Dubuque, Iowa: William C Brown, 1958

Principles of orthotics. Principles in the training of the disabled homemaker. In *Rehabilitation Medicine*, 1st Edition, Rusk HA, et al. St. Louis: CV Mosby, 177-196, 1958

———, Hicks T: Clamp device to aid in placement of tunnel pin of bilateral amputee with cineplastic operated prosthesis. *American Orthotic and Prosthetic Journal* 13:4, 55-58, 1959

Modern materials and methods for splinting. Self-help devices. In *Arthritis: General Principles, Physical Medicine and Rehabilitation*, Lowman EW, et al. Boston: Little, Brown, 135-164, 1959

Rusk HA, Lawton E, Elvin F, Judson J, ———: *The Functional Home for Easier Living*, Institute of Rehabilitation Medicine, NYU Medical Center, 1960

Devices: Development and direction. In *Proceedings of the Annual Conference*, AOTA, 17-24, 1960

Independence through equipment. *Orthopedic and Prosthetic Appliance Journal* 4: 71-77, 1960

Cookman H, ———: Functional fashions for the physically handicapped. In *Patient Publication III*, Institute of Rehabilitation Medicine, NYU Medical Center, 1961

Rusk HA, Kristeller EL, Judson JS, Hunt GM, ———: Rehabilitation Monograph No. VIII, *A Manual for Training the Disabled Homemaker.* Institute of Rehabilitation Medicine, NYU Medical Center, 1961

A model home for the disabled. In *Rehabilitation Record* 2:6, 17-20, 1961

The disabled homemaker and their problems: Summary of conference. *The Physically Disabled and Their Environment.* Report Proceedings, ISRD Conference, Stockholm, Sweden, 1961

Judson J, Wagner EM, ———: Homemaking and Housing for the Disabled in the USA. Monograph XX, NYU Medical Center, 1962

Current concepts and use of self-help devices (1-3). Architectural planning (38-40). Problems on clothing and dressing and their solutions (63-64). In *Approaches to Independent Living, Post Congress Study Course IV*, World Federation of Occupational Therapists, Wagner E, Zimmerman ME, Editors. New York, 1962

Occupational Therapy in the ADL Program. In *Occupational Therapy*, 3rd Edition, Willard HS, Spackman C, Editors. Philadelphia: JB Lippincott, 320-357, 1963

Clothing for the disabled. In Section III, *Proceedings of a Workshop, Rehabilitation of the Physically Handicapped in Homemaking Activities*, US Department of HEW, Vocational Rehabilitation Administration and American Home Economics Association, 69-74, 1963

Principles of orthotics. Principles of homemaking and housing. In *Rehabilitation Medicine*, 2nd Edition, Rusk HA, et al. Editors. St. Louis: CV Mosby, 189-228, 1964

Self-help devices for rehabilitation, Part II. Dubuque, Iowa: William C Brown, 1965

Homemaking training units for rehabilitation centers. *AJOT* 10:5, 226-235, 1966

Overcoming architectural barriers in the USA. *Through Youth to Age, Proceedings of the Fourth International Congress of the World Federation of Occupational Therapists*, London, 330-333, 1966

The tasks of an information center of technical aids. *International Program Development Series*, No. D-6 ISRD, 1967

Bibliography on self-help devices and orthotics. *Rehabilitation Monograph XXXV*, 1950-1967, Institute of Rehabilitation Medicine, NYU Medical Center, 1968

Functional motion test as an evaluation tool for patients with lower motor neuron disturbances. *AJOT* 23:1, 49-56, 1969

A learning experience in occupational therapy using 8mm loop films. In *Methods & Media for Academic and Clinical Teaching*, AOTA Workshop, University of Utah, 55-60, 1969

Occupational Therapy in the ADL Program. In *Occupational Therapy*, 4th Edition, Willard HS, Spackman C, Editors. Philadelphia: Lippincott, 217-256, 1971

Principles of self-help devices. Principles of homemaking. Principles of housing. In *Rehabilitation Medicine*, 3rd Edition, Rusk H, et al. Editors. St. Louis: CV Mosby, 152-198, 1971

Technical aids for developing countries. In *Proceedings Preview, Wednesday and Thursday, Twelfth World Congress of Rehabilitation International*, Sydney, Australia, 1972

———, Stratford C: Interim report: Evaluation of various electronic devices to increase mobility and independence of very high level quadriplegic patients. In *Proceedings of the 1976 Conference on Systems and Devices for the Severely Disabled*, 86-88, 1976

Principles of self-help devices. Principles of homemaking. Principles of housing. In *Rehabilitation Medicine*, 4th Edition, Rusk H, et al. Editors. St. Louis: CV Mosby, 1976

Role of special equipment in the rehabilitation of the spinal cord-injured. In *Physical Medicine and Rehabilitation Medicine Approaches in Spinal Cord Injury*, Cull J, Hardy, Editors. Springfield, IL: Charles C Thomas, 224-278, 1977

———, Stratford C, Sell GH: A continuing program of development and evaluation of a breath and of voice control for a powered wheelchair for the severely disabled, Part 1: Evaluation and testing. In *Proceedings of Conference on Systems and Devices for the Disabled*, Seattle, Washington: 1977

Youdin M, Sell GH, Clagnaz M, Louie H, Stratford C, ———: Initial evaluation of the IRM-NYU voice controlled powered wheelchair and environmental control system for the severely disabled. In *Proceedings of the Fifth Annual Conference on Systems and Devices for the Disabled*, Houston, Texas: 177-182, 1978

Sell H, Stratford C, ———, Youdin M, Milner D: Environmental and typewriter control systems for the high level quadriplegic patient: Evaluation and prescription. *Archives of Physical Medicine and Rehabilitation*: 1979

———, Kuo T, Sell GH, Sarno M, Reidel K, Feder C, Youdin M, Stratford C, Greenspan L, Diller L, Louie H: Application of voice and/or breath controls for powered wheelchairs and environmental equipment for the cerebral palsied. In *Research Report*, Institute of Rehabilitation Medicine, 1979

Stratford CD, Dickey R, ———, Sell GH, Youdin M: Voice control: Clinical evaluation by persons with severe physical disabilities with and without speech impairments. In *Proceedings of International Conference on Rehabilitation Engineering*, Toronto, Canada, 98-101, 1980

Mary Reilly, EdD, OTR 1961

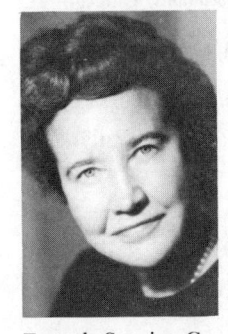

Mary Reilly retired in 1977 as professor and graduate coordinator of occupational therapy at the University of Southern California (USC), Los Angeles. She is Professor Emeritus at USC. Reilly holds an Ed.D. degree from the University of California at Los Angeles, a master's degree from San Francisco State College, a B.S. degree from USC, and a certificate in occupational therapy from Boston School of Occupational Therapy.

Reilly was occupational therapy consultant, Service Command Surgeon's Office, Fourth Service Command, Atlanta, Georgia, from 1944 to 1946. Her work in the Fourth Service Command included supervising occupational therapy programs in 11 general, 2 convalescent, and 6 regional and station hospitals, for which she received the Meritorious Civilian Service Award. Before World War II she was director of occupational therapy in the Sigma Gamma Hospital School, Detroit, Michigan.

Reilly has been named a charter member of the American Occupational Therapy Foundation Academy of Research. She is also on the AOTA Roster of Fellows (1973).

Since her retirement, Reilly has served as a consultant for USC programs at Oxford and Kent Universities, England, and at the University of Madrid. She was guest lecturer at selected tutorial sessions at Oxford.

BIBLIOGRAPHY

Organization of an occupational therapy section in an army or navy hospital. *War Medicine* 3: 512-531, May 1943

Correlation of physical and occupational therapy. *Occupational Therapy and Rehabilitation* 28: 171-175, August 1943

Technical Manual 8-291 Occupational Therapy. (coauthor) War Department, 1944

(Editor) Army issue. *Occupational Therapy and Rehabilitation* 25: 163-187, October 1946

Ruth A. Robinson, a biographical sketch. *AJOT* 3:6, 316, 1949

The role of the therapist in protective and functional devices. *AJOT* 10:3, 118, 1956

Therapeutically influenced recovery. *AJOT* 10:4, Part II, 229-232, 1956

An occupational therapy curriculum for 1965. *AJOT* 12:6, 293-299, 1958

Occupational therapy, report of coordinated training in rehabilitation. *Western Interstate Commission for Higher Education*, 1959

Research potentiality of occupational therapy. *AJOT* 14:4, 206, 1960

Planning curriculum revisions in physical therapy. *Physical Therapy Review*, 1961

Occupational therapy can be one of the great ideas of 20th century medicine. *AJOT* 16:1, 1, 1962

The Eleanor Clarke Slagle. *Canadian Journal of Occupational Therapy* 30:1, 1963

Medical information in the occupational therapy curriculum. In *Studies in Rehabilitation Counselor Training*, Monograph 4, 1965

Role of parent as model for child as future wage earner. *Today's Child*, April 1966

A psychiatric occupational therapy program as a teaching model. *AJOT* 20:2, 61, 1966

The challenge of the future to an occupational therapist. *AJOT* 20:5, 221, 1966

The mental health team—Occupational therapy. In *Proceedings, AMA 13th Annual Conference of State Mental Health Representatives of State Medical Associations*, Chicago, IL: February 1967

Needed: A revolution in the care of chronic patients. Tufts Alumni, Medford, MA: Tufts Univ., March 1968

Introduction of scientific method into clinical practice. In *Proceedings of the Northern and Southern California Joint Occupational Therapy Association Conference*, Morro Bay, CA: March 1968

The educational process. *AJOT* 23:4, 299, 1969

Occupational therapy—A historical perspective: The modernization of occupational therapy. *AJOT* 25:5, 243, 1971

Play as Exploratory Behavior: A Study of Curiosity Behavior, Beverly Hills, CA: Sage, 1974

The issue is—The importance of the client versus patient issue for occupational therapy. *AJOT* 38:6, 404-406, 1984

Naida Ackley, OTR, FAOTA   1962

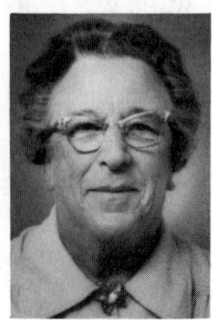

Naida Ackley retired in 1972 as director, occupational therapy, Trenton Psychiatric Hospital, New Jersey. She is a graduate of Sargent College (Boston University) and the Philadelphia School of Occupational Therapy (University of Pennsylvania), where she received an advanced standing certificate.

Named a Fellow of the AOTA in 1973, Ackley also holds an honorary life membership in the AOTA and a life membership in the New Jersey Occupational Therapy Association. She has been active in both state and national professional associations and has held offices and committee assignments in both.

BIBLIOGRAPHY

Elizabeth P. Ridgeway, a biographical sketch. *AJOT* 7:3, 138, 1953

Accreditation of occupational therapy departments. *AJOT* 15:2, 68, 1961

The challenge of the sixties. *AJOT* 16:6, 273, 1962

(Editor): *Basic Services and Equipment for Rehabilitation Centres, Occupational Therapy Department in a Mental Hospital*. United Nations Monograph, 1970

A. Jean Ayres, PhD, OTR, FAOTA 1963

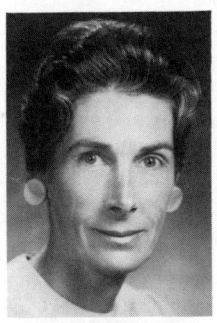

A. Jean Ayres has been in private practice since 1977. Except for three years of doctoral and postdoctoral study, she served on the faculty at the University of Southern California from 1955. Before joining the USC faculty, she held occupational therapy positions with United Cerebral Palsy, California Rehabilitation Center, Braewood Sanitarium, and the Veteran's Administration.

Ayres holds bachelor's and master's degrees in occupational therapy and a doctorate in educational psychology—all from the University of Southern California. Her postdoctoral traineeship was at the Brain Research Institute, University of California, Los Angeles.

In addition to her main profession of occupational therapy, she holds a California state license in psychology. She is a member of the AOTA, the American Psychological Association, and a life member of the Occupational Therapy Association of California. Her awards include the AOTA Award of Merit, 1965; Roster of Fellows, 1973; and charter membership in the Academy of Research from the American Occupational Therapy Foundation, 1983.

BIBLIOGRAPHY

An analysis of crafts in the treatment of electroshock patients. *AJOT* 3:4, 195-198, 1949

A form used to evaluate the work behavior of patients: A preliminary report. *AJOT* 8:2, 73-74, 1954

Ontogenetic principles in the development of arm and hand functions. *AJOT* 8:3, 95-99, 1954

Proprioceptive facilitation elicited through the upper extremities. Part I, Background. *AJOT* 9:1, 1-9; Part II, Application. *AJOT* 9:2, 57-58; Part III, Specific Application. *AJOT* 9:3, 121-126, 1955

A pilot study on the relationship between work habits and workshop production. *AJOT* 9:6, 264-276, 1955

A study of the manual dexterity and workshop wages of thirty-nine cerebral palsied trainees. *American Journal of Physical Medicine* 36: 6-10, 1957

The visual-motor function. *AJOT* 12:3, 130-138, 1958

Basic concepts of clinical practice in physical disabilities. *AJOT* 12:6, 300-302, 311, 1958

Hemiplegia. Occupational Therapy Reference Manual for Physicians, New York: AOTA, 1960

Occupational therapy for motor disorders resulting from impairment of the central nervous system. *Rehabilitation Literature* 21: 302-310, 1960

Research for therapists. *Proceedings of the American Occupational Therapy Association 1960 Conference*, New York: AOTA, 79-82, 1960

Development of the body scheme in children. *AJOT* 15:3, 99-102, 1961

The role of gross motor activities in the training of children with visual motor retardation. *Journal of the American Optometric Association* 33: 121-125, September 1961

Perception of space of adult hemiplegic patients. *Physical Medicine and Rehabilitation* 43: 552-555, November 1962

Integration of information. *Approaches to the Treatment of Patients with Neuromuscular Dys-function*, Study Course VI, Third International Congress, World Federation of Oc-cupational Therapists, Dubuque, IA: William C Brown, 1962

The development of perceptual-motor abilities. A theoretical basis for treatment of dys-function. *AJOT* 17:6, 221-225, 1963

Occupational therapy directed toward neuromuscular integration. In *Occupational Therapy*, 3rd Edition, Willard HS, Spackman CS, Editors. Philadelphia: JB Lippincott, 358-466, 1963

Perceptual-motor dysfunction in children. Offset Monograph from the Greater Cincinnati District, Ohio Occupational Therapy Association Conference, Cincinnati: 1964

Perceptual-motor training for children. *Approaches to the Treatment of Patients with Neuro-muscular Dysfunction*, Study Course VI, Third International Congress, World Feder-ation of Occupational Therapists, 1962, World Federation of Occupational Therapists, 1964, pp 17-22

Perspectives on neurological bases of reading. Claremont Reading Conference, 28th Year-book, 1964, Douglass MP, Editor. Claremont, CA: Claremont Graduate School Cur-riculum Laboratory, 113-118, 1964

Tactile functions: Their relation to hyperactivity and perceptual-motor behavior. *AJOT* 18:1, 6-11, 1964

A method of measurement of degree of sensorimotor integration. *Archives of Physical Medicine and Rehabilitation* 46: 433-435, 1965

Patterns of perceptual-motor dysfunction in children: A factor analytic study. *Perceptual and Motor Skills* 20: 335-368, 1965

Interrelation of perception, function, and treatment. *Journal of the American Physical Therapy Association* 46: 741-744, 1966

————, Reid W: The self-drawing as an expression of perceptual-motor dysfunction. *Cortex* 2: 254-265, 1966

Interrelationships among perceptual-motor functions in children. *AJOT* 20:2, 68-71, 1966

Interrelations among perceptual-motor abilities in a group of normal children. *AJOT* 20:6, 288-292, 1966

Remedial procedures based on neurobehavioral constructs. In Proceedings, 1967 Inter-national Convocation on Children and Young Adults with Learning Disabilities, Pitts-burgh, PA: 1967

Sensory integrative processes and neuropsychological learning disability. In Learning Dis-orders. Vol III, Special Child Publications, Seattle, WA: 1968

Reading—A product of sensory integrative process. In *Perception and Reading*, Smith HK, Editor. Proceedings of the Twelfth Annual Convention International Reading As-sociation, Newark, DE: 1968

Relation between Gesell developmental quotients and later perceptual-motor performance. *AJOT* 23:1, 11-17, 1969

Deficits in sensory integration in educationally handicapped children. *Journal of Learning Disabilities* 2: 160-168, 1969

Characteristics of types of sensory integrative dysfunction. *AJOT* 25:7, 329-334, 1971

The challenge of the brain. Perceptual Motor Conference, sponsored by the Physical Education Division of the American Association for Health, Physical Education, and Recreation. Sparks, NV: August 26, 1971

Types of sensory integrative dysfunction among disabled learners. *AJOT* 26:1, 13-18, 1972

Basic concepts of occupational therapy for children with perceptual-motor dysfunction. Proceedings of the Twelfth World Congress of Rehabilitation International. Sydney, Australia: August 27-September 1, 1972

Sensory Integration and Learning Disorders. Los Angeles: Western Psychological Services, 1972. Also published in Japanese

————, Heskett WM: Sensory integrative dysfunction in a young schizophrenic girl. *Journal of Autism and Childhood Schizophrenia* 2: 174-181, 1972

Sensory integrative process: Implications for deaf-blind from learning disability children. In Proceedings of the National Symposium for Deaf-Blind, Blea WA, Editor. Pacific Grove, CA: 81-89, July 1972

Improving academic scores through sensory integration. *Journal of Learning Disabilities* 5: 338-343, 1972

An interpretation of the role of the brain stem in intersensory integration. In *The Body Senses and Perceptual Deficit*, Henderson A, Coryell J, Editors. Proceedings of the Occupational Therapy Symposium on Somatosensory Aspects of Perceptual Deficit, Boston University, 1973

Sensorimotor foundations of academic ability. In *Perceptual and Learning Disabilities in Children* 2, Cruickshank WM, Hallahan DP, Editors. Syracuse University Press, 1975

Effect of sensory integrative therapy on the coordination of children with choreoathetoid movements. *AJOT* 31:5, 291-293, 1977

Cluster analyses of measures of sensory integration. *AJOT* 31:6, 362-366, 1977

Learning disabilities and the vestibular system. *Journal of Learning Disabilities* 11: 18-29, 1978

Dichotic listening performance in learning disabled children. *AJOT* 31:7, 441-446, 1977

A response to defensive medicine. *Academic Therapy* 13: 149-152, 1977

The sensory registration function in autistic and aphasic/apraxic children. In Piagetian Theory and Its Implications for the Helping Professions. Proceedings of the Ninth Interdisciplinary Conference, 1979. Univ of Southern California

Sensory Integration and the Child. Los Angeles: Western Psychological Services, 1979. (Written with assistance of Jeff Robbins)

————, Tickle LS: Hyper-responsivity to touch and vestibular stimuli predict positive response to sensory integration procedures in autistic children. *AJOT* 34:6, 375-381, 1980

————, Mailloux Z: Influence of sensory integration procedures on language development. *AJOT* 35:6, 383-390, 1981

————, Mailloux Z: Possible pubertal effects on therapeutic gains in an autistic girl. *AJOT* 37:8, 535-540, 1983

Cermak SA, ————: Crossing the body midline in learning-disabled and normal children. *AJOT* 38:1, 35-39, 1984

Slavik BA, Kitsuwa-Lowe J, Danner PT, Green J, ————: Vestibular Stimulation and Eye Contact in Autistic Children. *Neuropediatrics*, In press.

Republished Articles

Proprioceptive erleichterungsmethoden. *Krankengymnastic*, 11: 181-185, 196-200, 220-225, October, November, December 1959. Translated from English by Susanne Klein-Vogelbach

Types of perceptual motor deficits in children with learning difficulties. In *Readings in Learning Disability*, Bilovsky, Attwell, Jamison, Editors. New York: Selected Academic Readings, 1967

Interrelations among perceptual-motor abilities in a group of normal children. In *Readings in Early Development for Occupational and Physical Therapy Students*, Kopp C, Editor. Springfield, IL: Charles C Thomas, 1971

The Development of Sensory Integrative Theory and Practice: A Collection of Works of A. Jean Ayres. Compiled by A Henderson, L Llorens, E Gilfoyle, C Myers, and S Prevel. Dubuque, IA: Kendall-Hunt, 1974

Professional Films

Perceptual-motor Evaluation of a Perceptually Normal Child, 1966, Los Angeles: Univ of California
Perceptual-motor Evaluation of a Child with Dysfunction, 1966, Los Angeles: Univ of California
———, Heskett WM: Clinical Observations of Dysfunction in Postural and Bilateral Integration. 1969, Univ of Southern California
———, Heskett WM: A Therapeutic Activity for Perceptual-motor Dysfunction. 1969, Univ of Southern California

Gail S. Fidler, OTR, FAOTA   1965

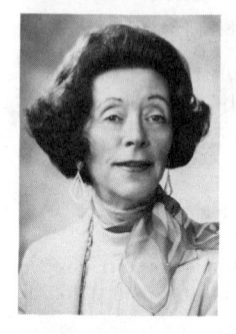

Gail S. Fidler is rehabilitation consultant, New Jersey Division of Mental Health and Hospitals; and consultant, New York University Occupational Therapy Curriculum. She has held appointments at Columbia University, New York University, San Jose State University, and the University of Pennsylvania. She has been a clinician and administrator in both public and private psychiatric centers, including consultant, Maryland State Department of Health and Mental Hygiene; assistant hospital administrator, Greystone Park Psychiatric Hospital, New Jersey; director, activities therapy, Hillside Hospital, New York; director of professional education, Department of Occupational Therapy, New York State Psychiatric Institute; director of occupational therapy, Veteran's Administration Hospital; and staff therapist, Norristown State Hospital.

From 1971 to 1975, Fidler served as Associate Executive Director for the AOTA. She has served on the AOTA Board of Management and Executive Committee at various intervals for many years, and has chaired and been active in numerous National and State Association Committees. She was named an AOTA Fellow in 1983, and she earned the Award of Merit in 1980.

Fidler holds a certificate in occupational therapy from the University of Pennsylvania, and a bachelor's degree from Lebanon Valley College.

BIBLIOGRAPHY

Psychological evaluation of occupational therapy activities. *AJOT* 2:5, 284-287, 1948
———, Fidler JW: *Introduction to Psychiatric Occupational Therapy*, New York: Macmillan, 1954
———, Ridgway EP: Occupational therapy: Laboratory for living. *Public Health Views* 3: 1955
The role of occupational therapy in a multi-discipline approach to psychiatric illness. *AJOT* 11:1, 8-12, 1957

Some unique contributions of occupational therapy in the treatment of the schizophrenic. *AJOT* 12:1, 9-12, 1958

Educational experiences for the occupational therapist. *South African Journal of OT*, 1958

(Contributing author). In *Changing Concepts and Practices in Psychiatric Occupational Therapy*, West WL, Editor. New York: AOTA, 1959

————, Fidler JW: *Occupational Therapy: A Communication Process in Psychiatry*, New York: Macmillan, 1963

A guide to planning and measuring growth experiences in clinical affiliation. *AJOT* 18:6, 240-243, 1964

————, Fine SB: The occupational therapist and psychotherapy. In *Transitional Program in Psychiatric Occupational Therapy*, IA: William C Brown, 1964

Learning as a growth process: A conceptual framework for professional education. *AJOT* 20:1, 1-8, 1966

A second look at work as a primary force in rehabilitation and treatment. *AJOT* 20:2, 72, 1966

The task-oriented group as a context for treatment. *AJOT* 23:1, 43-48, 1969

Mazer, J, ————, et al: *Exploring How a Think Feels*. Rockville, MD: AOTA, 1969

From plea to mandate. *AJOT* 31:10, 653, 1977

————, Fidler JW: Doing and becoming: Purposeful action and self-actualization. *AJOT* 32:5, 305-310, 1978

Specialization. *AJOT* 31:1, 34-35, 1979

Professional or non-professional. In *Occupational Therapy: 2001*, Rockville, MD: AOTA, 1979

————, et al: Overview of occupational therapy in mental health. Rockville, MD: AOTA, 1981

From crafts to competence. *AJOT* 35:9, 567-573, 1981

The activity laboratory: A structure for observing and assessing perceptual, integrative, and behavioral strategies. The lifestyle performance profile: An organizing frame. In *The Evaluative Process in Psychiatric Occupational Therapy*, Hemphill B, Editor. Thorofare, NJ: Charles B Slack, 1982

————, Fidler JW: Doing and Becoming: The Occupational Therapy Experience. In *Health Through Occupation*, Kielhofner G. Philadelphia: FA Davis, 1983

Design of Rehabilitation Services in Psychiatric Hospital Settings. Laurel, MD: RAMSCO, 1984

Elizabeth June Yerxa, EdD, OTR, FAOTA   1966

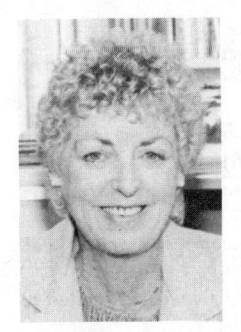

Elizabeth J. Yerxa is professor and chairperson, Department of Occupational Therapy, University of Southern California, Los Angeles.

A graduate of the University of Southern California with a degree in occupational therapy, she holds master's and doctoral degrees in educational psychology from Boston University. Before her academic appointment, she worked 15 years as an instructor, educational coordinator, and research coordinator in the Occupational Therapy Department of Rancho Los Amigos Hospital.

Yerxa was named a Fellow of the AOTA in 1973 and a Charter Member of the Academy of Research of the American Occupational Therapy Foundation in 1983.

BIBLIOGRAPHY

Authentic occupational therapy. *AJOT* 21:1, 1, 1966

The American Occupational Therapy Foundation is born. *AJOT* 21:5, 299, 1967

Human Interaction and Physical Differences, Volumes I and II. Costa Mesa, CA: Concept Media, 1974

Occupational therapy research 1974: Models of enlightenment. *Proceedings of the World Foundation of Occupational Therapy Sixth International Congress*, Vancouver, 674-681, 1975

On being a member of a feminine profession. *AJOT* 30: 597-598, 1976

The profession of occupational therapy: Today and tomorrow. In *Willard and Spackman's Occupational Therapy*, 5th Edition. JB Lippincott, 697-703, 1978

The occupational therapist as consultant and researcher: Autonomous change agentry. In *Willard and Spackman's Occupational Therapy*, 5th Edition. Lippincott, 689-693, 1978

Mazur H, Beeston J, ———: Clinical interdisciplinary health team care: An educational experiment. *Journal of Medical Education* 54: 703-713, 1979

Furgang N, ———: Expectations of teachers for physically handicapped and normal first grade students. *AJOT* 33:3, 697-704, 1979

The philosophical base of occupational therapy. In *Occupational Therapy: 2001 AD*, 26-30, Rockville, MD: AOTA, 1979

Burnett S, ———: Community-based and college-based needs assessment of physically disabled persons, *AJOT* 34:3, 201-207, 1980

Occupational therapy's role in creating a future climate of caring, *AJOT* 34:8, 529-534, 1980

Chaparro CJ, ———, Nelson J, Wilson L: The incidence of sensory integrative dysfunction among children with oro-facial cleft, *AJOT* 35:2, 96-100, 1981

Tickle L, ———: Need satisfaction of older persons living in the community and in institutions: Part I, The environment. *AJOT* 35:10, 644-649, 1981

Tickle L, ———: Need satisfaction of older persons living in the community and in institutions: Part II, Role of activity. *AJOT* 35:10, 650-655, 1981

Basic or applied? A "developmental assessment" of occupational therapy research in 1981. *AJOT* 35:62, 820-821, 1981

Review of *Children Adapt*. *Occupational Therapy Journal of Research* 1: 99-101, 1981

A response to testing and measurement in occupational therapy: A review of current practice with special emphasis on the Southern California Sensory Integration Tests. *AJOT* 36:6, 399-404, 1982

Research priorities. *AJOT* 37:10, 699, 1983

Audacious values, the energy source for occupational therapy practice. In *Health Through Occupation: Theory and Practice in Occupational Therapy*, Kielhofner G, Editor. Philadelphia: FA Davis, 149-162, 1983

Barber LM, Diaz O, Black W, Azen SP: Development of a hand sensitivity test for use in desensitization of the hypersensitive hand. *AJOT* 37:3, 176-181, 1983

Gregory JL, ———: Standardization of the prone extension postural test on children ages four through eight. *AJOT* 38:3, 187-194, 1984

The role of the occupational therapist. In *Rheumatic Diseases: Rehabilitation and Management*, Riggs GK, Gall, Editors. Boston: Butterworth, 19-21, 1984

Cooper-Fraps C, ———: Denial: Implications of a pilot study on activity level related to sexual competence in burned adults. *AJOT* 38:8, 529-534, 1984

———, Baum S: Occupational therapy in rehabilitation: Reduction of patient incapacity across the lifespan. In *Annual Review of Rehabilitation*, in press, 1984

Su, RV, ———: Comparison of the test-retest reliability between the motor tests of the Southern California Sensory Integration Tests (SCSIT) and the Luria-Nebraska Neuropsychological Battery: Children's version (L-NNBC) in 30 dysfunctional children aged 8 years, *Occupational Therapy Journal of Research* 4:2, 1984

Wilma L. West, MA, OTR, FAOTA   1967

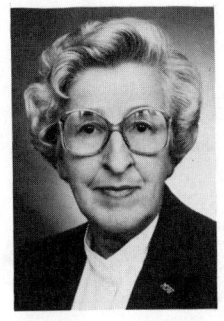

Wilma L. West, a retired occupational therapist, is a 1939 graduate of Mount Holyoke College. She also has a certificate in occupational therapy from Tufts University and a master's degree from the University of Southern California.

Long active in the AOTA, West's roles included Educational Field Secretary, Executive Director, Treasurer, and President. She also served as President, American Occupational Therapy Foundation, from 1972 to 1982, and was named President Emeritus in 1982. Her major clinical interests have been in physical disabilities and pediatrics, while her experience includes positions in administration, education, research, and consultation. In 1977, she retired from the United States Department of Health, Education, and Welfare (HEW) after 10 years as consultant in occupational therapy with the agency's Children's Bureau and Maternal and Child Health Service. West also served four years as Chief, Health Services Research and Training, HEW.

Her honors include the Bernard Baruch Fellowship for Graduate Study, 1946; the AOTA Award of Merit, 1951; the AOTA Roster of Fellows, 1973; and the HEW Superior Service Award, 1972. West received the Army Surgeon General's Meritorious Civilian Service Award in 1946 and served as consultant to the Surgeon General from 1958 to 1964. She has served on the Professional Advisory Council of the National Easter Seal Society for Crippled Children and Adults and on the Advisory Council on Physical Therapy Education, American Physical Therapy Association.

BIBLIOGRAPHY

The future of occupational therapy in the army. *AJOT* 1:2, 89; and 1:3, 155, 1947
———, Winifred C. Kahmann: Occupational therapy in the United States Army hospitals, World War II. In *Principles of Occupational Therapy*, Willard HS and Spackman CS, Editors. Philadelphia: Lippincott, 1947
Report of the executive director. *AJOT* 2:5, 303, 1948
Report on the performance of War Emergency Course graduates. *AJOT* 4:4, 199, 1949
Annual report of the executive director. *AJOT* 3:5, 252, 1949
The need for graduate study in occupational therapy. *AJOT* 3:6, 309, 1949
The need for an international association of OTs. *AJOT* 4:1, 23, 1950
Annual report of the executive director. *AJOT* 4:6, 274, 1950
Report of the mid-century White House Conference on children and youth. *AJOT* 5:1, 31, 1951

The profession's stand against licensure of OTs. *AJOT* 5:2, 60, 1951

Annual report of the executive director. *AJOT* 5:6, 258, 1951

Hyman Brandt, a biographical sketch. *AJOT* 4:2, 75, 1950

The principles of occupational therapy in the rehabilitation of the physically handicapped. In *Principles and Practices of Rehabilitation* (chapter 7), Kessler H. Philadelphia: Lea and Febiger, 1950

————, Clark AW: Planning the complete occupational therapy service. *Hospitals*, October 1951

Evaluation of the institute. In *Proceedings of the Occupational Therapy Institute: A Reassessment of Professional Education and Practice in Occupational Therapy as Related to Rehabilitation.* New York: AOTA, 1955

————, McNary H: The present and potential role of occupational therapy in rehabilitation. *AJOT* 10:3, 103; and 10:4, 150, 1956

Essentials of treatment. In *Proceedings of the 1956 Regional Occupational Therapy Institutes and Annual Institute.* New York: AOTA, 165-169, 1958

The specific role of the occupational therapist in implementing group goals. Keynote address. Traditional versus prevocational media in occupational therapy. In *Proceedings of the 1956 Regional Occupational Therapy Institutes and Annual Institute.* New York: AOTA, 16-22, 121-126, 136-138, 1958

Synthesis (of AOTA's 40th Anniversary Conference). *AJOT* 12:4, 225 1958

The present status of graduate education in occupational therapy. *AJOT* 12:6, 291, 1958

(Editor); *Changing Concepts and Practice in Psychiatric Occupational Therapy.* New York: AOTA, 1958

The President's address, 1962 Annual Conference. *AJOT* 17:1, 26, 1963

The President's address, 1963 Annual Conference. *AJOT* 17:6, 250, 1963

Graduate education as a requisite for status and advancement. *AJOT* 18:2, 68, 1964

The role of occupational therapy in work adjustment. In *Work Adjustment as a Function of Occupational Therapy.* Study Course V, Third International Congress, World Federation of Occupational Therapists. Dubuque, IA: William C Brown, 1964

(Editor): *Occupational Therapy for the Multiply Handicapped Child.* Chicago: University of Illinois, 1965

The President's address. *AJOT* 19:1, 31, 1965

Occupational therapy in neuropsychiatry. In *Neuropsychiatry in World War II*, Vol 1, Part IV, Chap XXII, Washington, DC: Office of the Surgeon General, Department of the Army, 1966

The occupational therapist's changing responsibility to the community. *AJOT* 21:5, 312, 1967

Professional responsibility in times of change. *AJOT* 22:1, 9, 1968

Statement to the committee on health manpower, American Medical Association. Chicago, September 15, 1967. *AJOT* 22:2, 89, 1968

Occupational therapy: Philosophy and perspective. *American Journal of Nursing* 68:8, 1968

Professional services of occupational therapists, World War II (chapter IX) (with Vogel, Manchester and Gearin); Wartime organization and administration (chapter V); Training in World War II (chapter VII). In *Army Medical Specialist Corps.* Washington, DC: Office of the Surgeon General, 1968

The growing importance of prevention. *AJOT* 23:3, 226, 1969

————, Wiemer RB: Occupational therapy in community health care. *AJOT* 24:5, 323, 1970

(Editor): *Occupational Therapy Functions in Interdisciplinary Programs for Children.* Los Angeles: University of Southern California, 1970

The emerging health model of occupational therapy practice. In *Occupational Therapy Today—Tomorrow.* Basel, Switzerland: S Karger, 1971

The principles and process of consultation. In *Consultation in the Community: Occupational Therapy in Child Health*. Llorens L, Editor, Dubuque, IA: Kendall-Hunt, 1973
The foundation: The first decade. *AJOT* 29:10, 636, 1975
Problems and policies in the licensure of occupational therapists. *AJOT* 30:1, 40, 1976
Research seminar. *AJOT* 30:8, 477, 1976
Reflections at retirement. Address of AOTF President at AOTA's 60th Anniversary Conference. *AJOT* 32:1, 9-12, 1978
Professional unity. *AJOT* 33:1, 40-49, 1979
Historical perspectives. In *Occupational Therapy: 2001 AD*. Rockville, MD: AOTA, 1979
Fifteenth anniversary celebration: American Occupational Therapy Foundation. *AJOT* 34:10, 683-685, 1980
————, Cox RC: *Fundamentals of Research for Health Professionals*. Laurel, MD: RAMSCO, 1982
In Memoriam—Winifred Conrick Kahmann. *AJOT* 36:7, 472-475, 1982
A reaffirmed philosophy and practice of occupational therapy for the 1980s. *AJOT* 38:1, 15-23, 1984

Lela A. Llorens, PhD, OTR, FAOTA 1969

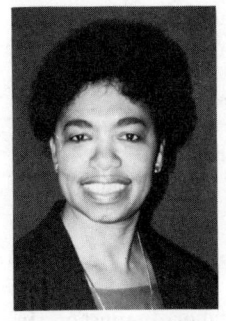

Lela A. Llorens is professor, chair, and graduate coordinator, Department of Occupational Therapy, School of Applied Arts and Sciences, San Jose State University, California.

A graduate of Western Michigan University with a bachelor's degree in occupational therapy, she holds a master's degree in vocational rehabilitation and a doctorate from Walden University. Llorens worked as a staff therapist at Wayne County General Hospital, Northville State Hospital and Lafayette Clinic, Michigan. During this period, she also served as instructor, Department of Occupational Therapy at Wayne State University. In 1968 Llorens held the position of consultant, occupational therapy, at Mount Zion Hospital. She later served as professor, chair, and graduate coordinator at the University of Florida. Llorens returned to the West Coast in 1982.

Llorens was named to the AOTA Roster of Fellows in 1973 and received the Award of Excellence from the Florida Occupational Therapy Association (FOTA) in 1977. She received AOTF's Certificate of Appreciation and Honorary Life Membership, FOTA. Among her honors is the Sadie Philcox Lecture (1981), University of Queensland, Brisbane, Australia. Llorens was also elected to Outstanding Young Women of America in 1966; Outstanding Educators of America; Wall of Distinction, Western Michigan University; and Mentor, Class of 1976, University of Texas Medical Branch.

BIBLIOGRAPHY

Psychological tests in planning therapy goals. *AJOT* 14:5, 243-246, 1960

————, Young GG: Fingerpainting for the hostile child: case history. *AJOT* 14:6, 306-307, 1960

Bridging the gap: Vocational rehabilitation counseling in a psychiatric setting. *Michigan Rehabilitation Associate Digest* 2: 24-26, 1961

————, Rubin EZ: Occupational therapy is therapeutic: A research study with emotionally disturbed children. *Proceedings of 1961 AOTA National Conference*, Rockville, MD: AOTA, 1962

————, Rubin EZ: A directed activity program: For disturbed children. *AJOT* 16:6, 287-290, 1962

————, Bernstein SP: Fingerpainting: With an obsessive-compulsive organically-damaged child. *AJOT* 17:3, 120-121, 1963

————, Levy R, Rubin EZ: Work adjustment program: A pre-vocational experience. *AJOT* 18:1, 15-19, 1964

————, Rubin EZ, Braun J, Beck G, Mottley N, Beall D: Cognitive-perceptual-motor functions. A preliminary report on training. *AJOT* 18:5, 202-208, 1964

Beck GR, Rubin EZ, Braun JS, ————, Beal D, Mottley N: Educational aspects of cognitive-perceptual-motor deficit in emotionally disturbed children. *Psychology in the Schools* 2: 233-238, 1965

Braun JS, Rubin EZ, ————, Beck GR, Beall D, Mottley N: Cognitive-perceptual-motor functions in children: A suggested change in approach. *Journal of School Psychology* 3: 3, 1965

————, Rubin EZ, A directed activity program for emotionally disturbed children. In *The Guidance of Exceptional Children*, Gowan JC and Demos GD. New York: David McKay, 1965

Aspects of pre-vocational evaluation with psychiatric patients. *Canadian Journal of Occupational Therapy* 33: 1-8, 1966

————, Johnson PA: Occupational therapy in an ego-oriented milieu. *AJOT* 20:4, 178-181, 1966

————, Rubin EZ: *Developing Ego Functions in Disturbed Children: Occupational Therapy in Milieu*, Detroit, MI: Wayne State Univ Press, 1967

An evaluation procedure for children 6 to 10 years of age. *AJOT* 21:2, 64-69, 1967

Projective technique in occupational therapy. *AJOT* 21:4, 226-229, 1967

————, Beck GR: Treatment methods for cognitive-perceptual-motor dysfunction. In *Normal Growth and Development with Deviations in the Perceptual Motor and Emotional Areas, Proceedings of O.T. Seminar*, St. Louis: Washington Univ School of Medicine, 1966

Cognitive-perceptual-motor dysfunction in disturbed children. In *Perceptual-Motor Dysfunction, Evaluation and Training, Proceedings of O.T. Seminar*, Madison: Univ of Wisconsin, 1966

Braun JS, Rubin EZ, ————, Beck GR: Cognitive-motor deficits: Definition and intervention. In *Proceedings of the International Convocation on Learning Disabilities*, Pittsburgh: Crippled Children's Home of Pittsburgh, 1967

Gauging emotional, intellectual and professional growth in students. *Education Newsletter*, AOTA 2: 2, 1967

Cognitive-perceptual-motor dysfunction and training. In *Selected Papers from Professional Program Segments of United Cerebral Palsy's Annual Conference*, New Orleans: United Cerebral Palsy Associations, 1967

Changing methods in treatment of psychological dysfunction. *AJOT* 22:1, 26-29, 1968

Identification of the Ayres' syndromes in children with behavior maladjustment. *AJOT* 22:4, 286-288, 1968

Rubin EZ, Braun JS, ———, Beck GR: *Testing for Cognitive-Perceptual-Motor Dysfunction*. Eric Document Reproduction Service, The National Cash Register Co, Bethesda, MD, 1968

Rubin EZ, Braun JS, ———, Beck GR, Beall CD: *An Investigation of an Evaluation Method and Retraining Procedures for Emotionally Handicapped Children with Cognitive-Motor Deficits: Final Report*, Project #7-0319, Grant No. 32-32-7545-5017, U.S. Department of Health, Education and Welfare, Washington, DC, 1969

———, Rubin EZ, Braun JS, Beck GR, Beall CD: The effects of cognitive-perceptual-motor training approach on children with behavior maladjustment. *AJOT* 23:6, 502, 1969

The occupational therapist in a community health program. In *Proceedings of SOTA Annual Conference, Mandate for Change*, Morro Bay: SOTA, 1969

The role of the occupational therapist in a children and youth project. In *Proceedings of the National Conference of Children and Youth Projects*, New York: New York Univ Medical Center, 1969

Facilitating growth and development: The promise of occupational therapy. *AJOT* 24:2, 93-101, 1970

Black culture and child development. *AJOT* 25:3, 144-148, 1971

Occupational therapy in community child health. *AJOT* 25:7, 335-339, 1971

Rubin EZ, Braun JS, Beck GR, ———: *Cognitive Perceptual Motor Dysfunction: From Research to Practice*, Detroit: Wayne State Univ Press, 1972

Problem-solving the role of occupational therapy in a new environment. *AJOT* 26:5, 234-238, 1972

Activity analysis for cognitive-perceptual-motor dysfunction. *AJOT* 27:8, 453-456, 1973

(Editor): *Consultation in the Community: Occupational Therapy in Child Health*, Dubuque, IA: Kendall-Hunt Publishers, 1973

A case presentation: Billy. In *The Effects of Hospitalization on Children*, Oremland EK and JD, Springfield, IA: Charles C Thomas, 1973

Canfield AA, Williams MR, ———, Wroe MC: Competencies for Allied Health educators. *Journal of Allied Health* Fall: 180-186, 1973

What journal editors want. In *Publishing in the Health Related Professions*, Morgan MK, Filson DM, Canfield AA, Gainesville, FL: Center for Allied Health Personnel

The effects of stress on growth and development. *AJOT* 28:2, 82, 1974

———, Gilfoyle E, Myers C, Prevel S: *Ayres AJ: The Development of Sensory Integrative Theory and Practice*. Dubuque, IA: Kendall-Hunt, 1974

———, Sieg KW: A profile for managing sensory integrative test data. *AJOT* 29:4, 205-208, 1975

Consultation in occupational therapy programs for children. *Canadian Journal of Occupational Therapy* 41: 114-117, 1975

Occupational therapy consultation in community programs for children. *Canadian Journal of Occupational Therapy* 41: 114-117, 1975

Occupational therapy consultation in community programs for children. In *Proceedings from Consultation in the Community: A Conference for Occupational Therapists*, Gainesville: Univ of Florida, 1975

———, Adams SP: Student learning styles. In *Allied Health Teacher Preparation*, Morgan M, Ford C, St. Louis: Mosby, 1976

Application of a Developmental Theory for Health and Rehabilitation. Rockville, MD: AOTA, 1976

Evaluation of a Client Care Record for Occupational Therapy, Doctoral dissertation, Walden University, Naples, FL, 1976 and University Microfilms, 300 North Zeeb Road, Ann

Arbor, Michigan 48106, 1980. Abstract in *In Progress: A Journal of Studies in Occupational Therapy*, Western Michigan Univ, Kalamazoo, Michigan, 1980

———, Schuster JJ: Occupational therapy sequential client care recording system: A comparative study. *AJOT* 31:6, 367-371, 1977

A developmental theory revisited. *AJOT* 31:10, 656-657, 1977

———, Adams SP: Learning style preferences of occupational therapy students. *AJOT* 32:3, 161-164, 1978

Thinking research in occupational therapy. *Developmental Disabilities Specialty Section Newsletter*, AOTA 2: 1, 1979

———, Burris BB: Development of sensory integration in learning disabled children. In *Developmental Theories and Research in Learning Disabilities*, Baltimore: Univ Park, 1981

Research in occupational therapy: The need, the response. An editorial. *Occupational Therapy Journal of Research* 1: 3-6, 1981

On the meaning of activity in occupational therapy. *Journal of the New Zealand Association of Occupational Therapy* 32: 3-6, 1981

Maintaining credibility: The academic occupational therapist. *Education Newsletter*, AOTA, Fall, 1981

The role of occupational therapy in vocational rehabilitation. *Mental Health Special Interest Section Newsletter*, AOTA 4: 1-2, 1981

Occupational therapy: State of the art-potential for development. In *Proceedings of the New Zealand Occupational Therapy Association Annual Conference*, Auckland, New Zealand, 1981

Occupational Therapy Sequential Client Care Record Manual, Laurel, MD: RAMSCO, 1982

Facilitating achievement of higher level behaviors. In *Readings in Clinical Education: A Resource Manual for Clinical Instructors*, Henry JH, Editor. Augusta: Medical College of Georgia (Department of Occupational Therapy), 1982

The DSM III, Sensory integration and child psychiatry: Implications for treatment and research. *Sensory Integration Special Interest Section Newsletter*, AOTA 6: 2, 1983

Continuing clinical competency for the occupational therapy educator. *Journal of the New Zealand Association of Occupational Therapy* 33: 13-14, 1982/3

Theoretical conceptualizations of occupational therapy: 1960-1982. *Occupational Therapy in Mental Health*, Summer, 1984

Educating for professional competency—Accountability theory in practice. *Journal of the New Zealand Association of Occupational Therapy* 34: 22, 24, 1983

———, Donaldson K: Documentation of occupational therapy: A process model. Accepted for publication, *Canadian Journal of Occupational Therapy* 50:5, 171-175, 1983

———, Ward JM, Still JA, Eyler RK: The role of professional education for occupational therapy. Accepted for publication, *Occupational Therapy Education Newsletter*, AOTA, Spring 1984

Geraldine L. Finn, MS, OTR 1971

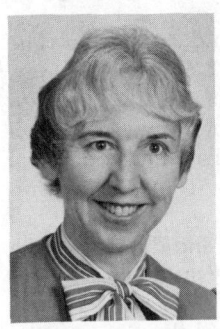

Geraldine Finn is a psychotherapist at the House of Affirmation, Inc., in Hopedale, Massachusetts. A 1955 graduate of Tufts University with a certificate in occupational therapy, Finn holds a bachelor of arts degree from Regis College, Weston, Massachusetts; and a master of science degree from Simmons College, Boston, where her studies concentrated on the family with special interest in family relationships.

Finn worked as a staff therapist at Boston State Hospital and the Fernald State School before moving to Cleveland as an occupational therapy supervisor and later, director of the Occupational Therapy Department at the Cleveland Psychiatric Institute. In 1964 she established the Occupational Therapy Department in the Day Treatment Center at the Cleveland State Hospital. She returned to New England to become an occupational therapy consultant at the Hartford Rehabilitation Center in Connecticut.

In 1969 she became director of the Occupational Therapy Department at Boston State Hospital. She also was a clinical instructor in psychiatric occupational therapy at Boston University and a lecturer in psychiatric occupational therapy at Tufts University.

With a grant from the Virginia Scullen Fund, the American Occupational Therapy Foundation, Finn established an early intervention program for preschool inner city children and expanded the role of the occupational therapist into community prevention programs. In 1976 she became director of the Occupational Therapy Department at Middlesex County Hospital in Waltham, Massachusetts. She was named an AOTA Fellow in 1973.

BIBLIOGRAPHY

Severe character disorders: Treatment through occupational therapy. *AJOT* 18:5, 185-190, 1964

The occupational therapist in prevention programs. *AJOT* 26:2, 59-66, 1972

Children's development workshop. In *Consultation in the Community: Occupational Therapy in Child Health*, Dubuque, IA: Kendall-Hunt, 1973

Gardos G, Orzach MH, Cole JO, ———: High and low dose thiothixene treatment in chronic schizophrenia. *Diseases of the Nervous System*, February 1974

Jerry A. Johnson, MBA, EdD, OTR, FAOTA 1972

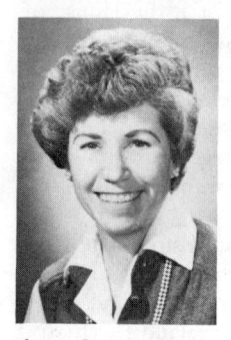

Jerry A. Johnson is president and director of The Resource Center for Health and Well-Being, Inc., Denver, Colorado. A graduate of Texas Woman's University with a B.S. degree in occupational therapy, Johnson holds a M.B.A. degree from Harvard University and a doctoral degree in educational administration from Boston University.

Johnson was founder, professor, and director of the Department of Occupational Therapy at Boston University from 1967 to 1972. From 1972 to 1973, she served as chairman of the Graduate Division and then as associate dean for academic affairs. Later, Johnson served as director of graduate education and research in the Occupational Therapy Department at Colorado State University.

In 1976 she assumed the chairmanship and also served as a professor in occupational therapy at Washington University in St. Louis until 1982, when she moved to Colorado.

Johnson's awards include serving as a visiting professor at Queensland University, Brisbane, Australia, and the AOTA Award of Merit and Roster of Fellows. She is the recipient of the Spirit of Sargent College Award from Boston University. Most recently, Johnson was named a Distinguished Alumna of 1984 by Texas Woman's University.

BIBLIOGRAPHY

Guest editorial on the emerging role of occupational therapy in psychiatry. *AJOT* 19:4, 215-218, 1965

———, Smith M: Changing concepts of occupational therapy in a community rehabilitation center. *AJOT* 20:6, 267-273, 1966

Occupational therapy techniques applicable to the stroke patient in the rehabilitation center and general hospital. *Journal of Medical Science*, 1969

Consideration of work as therapy in the rehabilitation process. *AJOT* 25:6, 303-308, 1971

Report of task force on social issues. *AJOT* 26:7, 332-359, 1972

Occupational therapy: A model for the future. *AJOT* 27:1, 1-7, 1973

Annual review of occupational therapy education. *Annual Review of Allied Health Education*, 1974

Allied health professions—Proliferation or restraint. *Israel Journal of Medical Science* 10: 96-102, 1974

Nationally speaking. No more waiting. *AJOT* 29:9, 519-532, 1975

Nationally speaking. Commitment to action. *AJOT* 30:3, 135-148, 1976

Nationally speaking. *AJOT* 30:10, 619-621, 1976

Nationally speaking. Mission alpha: A new beginning. *AJOT* 31:3, 143-149, 1977

Challenges confronting occupational therapy. *Canadian Journal of Occupational Therapy* 44: 113-117, 1977

Nationally speaking. Humanitarianism and accountability: A challenge for occupational therapy on its 60th anniversary. *AJOT* 31:10, 631-637, 1977
Nationally speaking. Issues in education. *AJOT* 32:6, 355-358, 1978
Nationally speaking. Sixty years of progress: Questions for the future. *AJOT* 32:4, 209-213, 1978
Reorganization in relation to the issues. In *Occupational Therapy: 2001 AD*, Rockville, MD: AOTA, 1979
Old values—New directions: Competence, adaptation, integration. *AJOT* 35:9, 589-598, 1981
Occupational therapy and the patient with pain. *Occupational Therapy in Health Care* 1:3, 1984

Alice C. Jantzen, PhD, OTR, FAOTA 1973

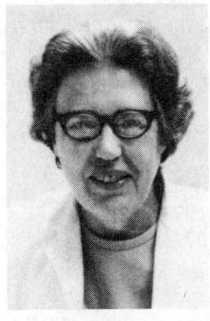

During her 31 years as an occupational therapist, Alice C. Jantzen had a distinguished career in health care, both as a practitioner and as an educator. She began her occupational therapy career in 1952 as a staff therapist in the Cerebral Palsy Department of New York State Rehabilitation Hospital; her career in education came two years later with an assistant professorship at Western Michigan University.

Two years later, Jantzen became a National Foundation Teaching Fellow and instructor at the University of Pennsylvania. She spent more than 18 years at the University of Florida in various positions, including director of occupational therapy services, Shands Teaching Hospital and Clinics; and professor and chairman, Department of Occupational Therapy, College of Health Related Professions, before she retired in 1978.

Jantzen served on many AOTA committees and was a Vice-President; she was also the first President of the AOTF, and past vice-president and president of the Florida Occupational Therapy Association. Her honors include AOTA's Roster of Fellows and Award of Merit; and listings in *Who's Who in America*; *Who's Who of American Women*, and *Leaders in American Science*.

Jantzen graduated with honors from Wellesley College and the Boston School of Occupational Therapy, where she received her certificate. She received a master's degree in education from the University of Pennsylvania and a doctorate in counseling psychology from Boston College. She died in October 1983.

BIBLIOGRAPHY

Miller AS, ———: An evaluation method for cerebral palsy. *AJOT* 9:3, 105, 1955
Proposed revision of the professional education of occupational therapists. *AJOT* 12:6, 314, 1958
The contribution of occupational therapy to patient care. *Journal of the Florida Medical Association*: 46, 1360-1362, 1960
Some strengths of occupational therapy. *AJOT* 16:3, 124, 1962; *Canadian Journal of Occupational Therapy* 30:1, 1963
———, et al: Graduate degrees held by occupational therapists. *AJOT* 28:4, 152, 1963

The role of research in occupational therapy. In *Proceedings*, AOTA Annual Conference, New York: AOTA, 1964

———, Anderson HE: Patient evaluation of occupational therapy programs. *AJOT* 19:1, 19, 1965

Anderson HE, ———: A prediction of clinical performance. *AJOT* 19:2, 76, 1965

Anderson HE, ———, et al: The effects of response sets in questionnaire studies. *AJOT* 19:6, 348, 1965

Objectives of the clinical experience—A university viewpoint. Evaluation of the clinical center by a curriculum director. In *The Clinical Experiences*, Massachusetts Association of Occupational Therapy, 1966

Theses and dissertations 1963-1966. *AJOT* 21:3, 166, 1967

Bailey JP, ———, Dunteman GH: Relative effectiveness of personality, achievement and interest measures in the prediction of a performance criterion. *AJOT* 23:1, 27, 1969

Definitions of mental health and mental illness. *AJOT* 23:3, 249, 1969

Some characteristics of female occupational therapists. Part I: Descriptive study. *AJOT* 26:1, 19, 1972

Some characteristics of female occupational therapists. Part II: Employment patterns of female occupational therapists. *AJOT* 26:2, 67, 1972

Some characteristics of female occupational therapists. Part III: A comparison: Faculty and clinical practitioners. *AJOT* 26:3, 150, 1972

Some characteristics of male occupational therapists. *AJOT* 27:7, 388, 1973

Academic occupational therapy: A career specialty. *AJOT* 28:2, 73, 1974

A proposal for occupational therapy education. *AJOT* 31:10, 660, 1977

Mary R. Fiorentino, OTR, FAOTA   1974

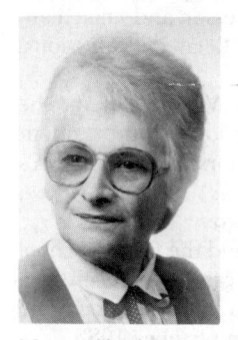

Mary R. Fiorentino, a self-employed occupational therapist, organizes educational workshops in health-related fields in Hartford, Connecticut. A graduate of Tufts University School of Occupational Therapy with a post-graduate certificate in occupational therapy, she received her bachelor of music degree from Boston University.

Fiorentino worked as a staff therapist, assistant director, and director of occupational therapy at the Newington Children's Hospital, Connecticut. She retired from the Children's Hospital in 1978. Since her retirement, Fiorentino has been on the consultant teaching staff at Mount Sinai Hospital, Hartford, Connecticut, and consultant to the rehabilitation services of St. Francis Hospital and Medical Center and the Oakhill School for the Blind.

Her awards include *Who's Who of American Women*, 1968; and the Award of Merit, Connecticut Occupational Therapy Association, 1975. Fiorentino was named a Fellow of the AOTA in 1973.

BIBLIOGRAPHY

Mysak ED, ———: Neurophysiological considerations in occupational therapy for the cerebral palsied. *AJOT* 15:3, 112, 1961

————, Nathan C: Visual aid board. *AJOT* 17:5, 198, 1963

Reflex Testing Methods for Evaluating CNS Development, Springfield, IL: Charles C Thomas, 1963 (Translated into Japanese, 1967; into French, 1974; into Italian, 1978; into Spanish, 1979)

The changing dimension of occupational therapy. *AJOT* 20:5, 251, 1966

Normal and Abnormal Development: The Influence of Primitive Reflexes on Motor Development. Springfield, IL: Charles C Thomas, 1972

Occupational therapy: Realization to Activation. *AJOT* 29:1, 15-21, 1975

A Basis of Motor Development: Normal & Abnormal. Springfield, IL: Charles C Thomas, 1981

Josephine C. Moore, PhD, OTR, DSc   1975

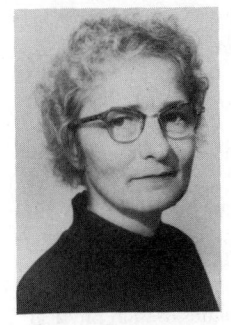

Josephine C. Moore holds a bachelor's degree in geology, and master's and doctoral degrees in anatomy from the University of Michigan. Her bachelor's degree in occupational therapy is from Michigan State Normal College (now Eastern Michigan University).

After six years as an associate professor of anatomy, University of South Dakota Medical School, Moore is now a professor of anatomy. She stepped down in June 1984 as head of the neuroanatomy section, and vice-chairman of anatomy at the school.

Moore served as consultant to the U.S. Consumer Product Safety Commission; the Post-Professional Graduate Education in the Physical Therapy program at the Chicago Medical School; and the Center for the Developmentally Disabled, University of South Dakota.

Active in the field since 1955, Moore's membership in professional organizations include the AOTA, where she has served on the *AJOT* editorial board; the American Association of Anatomists; American Women in Science; World Federation of Occupational Therapists; American Association for the Advancement of Science; and the South Dakota Occupational Therapy Association.

Moore is listed in *American Men and Women of Science*: Medical and Health Services, 13th and 15th editions; *Dictionary of International Biography*: A biographical record of contemporary achievement; *Men of Achievement*, 6th edition; *The World's Who's Who of Women in Education*, 1st edition; and *Who's Who in American Women*, 13th edition.

Moore has received certificates of appreciation from the Occupational Therapy Associations of South Dakota and New Hampshire. She also received an honorary doctor of science degree from Eastern Michigan University's College of Health and Human Services in 1982. She was named an AOTA Fellow in 1973.

BIBLIOGRAPHY

Adjustable reading rack for the visually handicapped. Part II. *AJOT* 10:2, 82, 1956
Reading aids for a quadriplegic patient. *AJOT* 10:3, 119-120, 1956
The Occupational Therapy Glossary. Ypsilanti: Eastern Michigan Univ, 1956

Simplified Neurological Review for Students and Therapists. Ann Arbor, MI: Overbeck, 1956

Adaptive Equipment and Appliances. Ann Arbor, MI: Overbeck, 1957

Rehabilitation Equipment and Supplies Directory. Ann Arbor, MI: Cushing-Malloy, 1958

———, Champaign I: The wheelchair side-board. *AJOT* 13:2, 66, 1959

Bending jigs and dies. *AJOT* 13:1, 13-15, 1959

Dura-foam pre-fabricated sheets: A new fabricating material for occupational therapists. *AJOT* 14:5, 256, 1960

———, et al: *Medical Abbreviations: A Cross Reference Dictionary.* Michigan Occupational Therapy Association, 1961

Are we half-breeds? *AJOT* 10:8, 1963

Utilization of Active Resistive Stretch to Obtain an Improved Response in the Forearm Flexors of Normal Adults. Ann Arbor: Univ of Michigan Press, 1964

Neuroanatomy simplified: Part I. *AJOT* 19:4, 208-212, 1965

Neuroanatomical and neurophysiological factors basic to the use of neuromuscular facilitation techniques. In *Occupational Therapy for the Multiply Handicapped Child*, West W, Editor. Univ of Illinois, 1965

Facilitation of a forearm flexor response. Utilization of active resistive stretch in normal adults. *Journal of Applied Physiology* 21:2, 649-654, 1966

Fabrication of suction-cup electrodes for electromyography. *Journal of Electroencephalography and Clinical Neurophysiology* 20: 405-406, March 1966

Neuroanatomy simplified, Part II, Section A: Introduction to the neuron. *AJOT* 20:2, 80, 1966

Neuroanatomy simplified, Part II, Section B: The neuron. *AJOT* 20:3, 130, 1966

Perceptual motor dysfunction in rehabilitation personnel. (editorial) *AJOT* 20:1, 1966

Part I, The developing nervous system in relation to treatment techniques used in physical disabilities. Part II, Structure and function of the nervous system in relation to treatment techniques. Confusion and controversy concerning treatment techniques utilized in physical disabilities. *Cleveland Symposium*, Western Reserve Univ, 1967

Changing methods in the treatment of physical dysfunction. *AJOT* 21:1, 18, 1967

Basic research in occupational therapy. In *Proceedings of the Occupational and Physical Therapy Conference on Research*, Puerto Rico, Department of Health, Education, and Welfare, 42, 1967

Medical Abbreviations, 2nd edition. Chairman of Committee of MOTA-MSSC. Published by Michigan Occupational Therapy Association, 1967

A new look at the nervous system in relation to rehabilitation techniques. *AJOT* 22:6, 489, 1968

The neuron, Part II, Section C: The location of cell bodies in the central nervous system. *AJOT* 23:3, 232, 1969

The developing nervous system in relationship to techniques in treating physical dysfunction. Structure and function of the nervous system in relation to treatment techniques. Confusion and controversy concerning treatment techniques utilized in physical dysfunction. In *Expanding Dimensions in Rehabilitation*. Chapters 1-3, Zamir L, Editor. Baltimore, Charles C Thomas, 3-51, 1969

Neuroanatomy Simplified. Some Basic Concepts for Understanding Rehabilitation Techniques. Dubuque, IA: Kendall-Hunt, 1969

Active resistive stretch and isometric exercise in strengthening wrist flexion in normal adults. *Archives of Physical Medicine and Rehabilitation* 52:6, 264-269, 1971

Differences in electrical activity of the biceps brachii and brachioradialis muscles performing isometric-like supination and pronation exercises. *AJOT* 25:8, 391-397, 1971

Physiological properties of nerve fibers. *AJOT* 26:5, 244-248, 1972

A review of the nervous system in chart form. *AJOT* 26:6, 305-308, 1972

Terminology today. *AJOT* 27:3, 149-155, 1973

Concepts from the Neurobehavioral Sciences in Relation to the Mentally/Physically Handicapped. Dubuque, IA: Kendall-Hunt, 1973

Cranial nerves and their importance in current rehabilitation techniques. In *The Body Senses and Perceptual Deficit.* Henderson A, Coryell J, Editors. Sargent College of Allied Health Professions, Boston Univ, 102-120, 1973

Excitation overflow. An EMG investigation. *Archives of Physical Medicine and Rehabilitation* 56:3, 115-119, 1975

Behavior, bias and the limbic system. *AJOT* 30:1, 11-19, 1976

Individual differences and the art of therapy. *AJOT* 31:10, 663-665, 1977

———, Bunger PC: Brain-stem manual and guidelines for neuroanatomy. Univ of South Dakota School of Medicine, 1978

Neuroanatomical considerations relation to recovery of function following brain injury. In *Recovery of Function Following Brain Injury: Theoretical Considerations.* Bach-y-rita P, Editor. Verlag Hans Huber, 1980

Oral and related vital functions. In Syllabus, Eighth Annual Sensorimotor Symposium. Office of Continuing Education in the Health Sciences, San Diego: Univ of California School of Medicine, 5-38, 1981

Grady A, Gilfoyle E, ———: Nervous system development in relation to pediatric rehabilitation. We hold these truths to be self-evident re adaptation and the spiraling continuum. In *Children Adapt,* New York: Charles B Slack, 1981

Foreword. In Fiorentino MR, *A Basis for Sensorimotor Development—Normal and Abnormal,* Springfield, IL: Charles C Thomas, 1981

Hemispheric specialization and integration. In Syllabus, Ninth Annual Sensorimotor Symposium. San Diego: Univ of California School of Medicine, 1-38, July 1981

Bunger PC, Neufeld DA, ———, Carter GA: Persistent left superior vena cava and associated structural and functional considerations. *Journal of Angiology* 32:9, 601-608, 1981

Sensory Systems Influence on Movement and Tone. In Syllabus. Tenth Annual Sensorimotor Integration Symposium. San Diego, July 1982, 1-41, Office of Continuing Education in Health Sciences, Univ of California, San Diego School of Medicine

Apraxia: Developmental and Acquired. In Syllabus. Eleventh Annual Sensorimotor Integration Symposium. San Diego, July 1983, 1-34, San Diego District, California Chapters of APTA/OTAC and CSSID

The golgi tendon organ: A review and update. *AJOT* 38:4, 227-236, 1984

The Ventricular System: A Focal Point of Dysfunction. In Syllabus. Twelfth Annual Sensorimotor Integration Symposium. San Diego, July 1984, 1-48, San Diego District, California Chapters of APTA/OTAC and CSSID.

A. Joy Huss, MS, OTR, RPT, FAOTA 1976

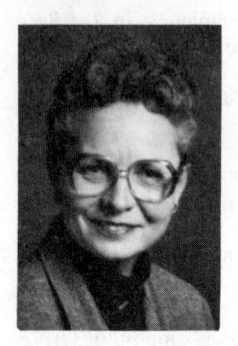

A. Joy Huss is an associate professor, Occupational Therapy Program, at the University of Minnesota, Minneapolis. A graduate of Whittier College with a degree in sociology, Huss holds a certificate in occupational therapy from the University of Southern California, a certificate in physical therapy from the University of Michigan, and a master of science degree in educational psychology from Butler University.

Huss has served as staff occupational therapist at Crippled Children's Hospital School, Sioux Falls, South Dakota, and at the Cerebral Palsy Clinic, Indiana University. She was occupational therapy and physical therapy consultant for Crippled Children's Services, Indiana; supervisor of occupational therapy at Riley Children's Hospital, Indiana; and on the occupational therapy faculties at Indiana University, University of Wisconsin-Eau Claire, and, since 1972, at the University of Minnesota.

Since 1962 Huss has conducted 200 workshops on a neurophysiological approach to CNS dysfunction throughout the United States and Canada. Her awards include Fellow of the AOTA; Mentor, Occupational Therapy Class of 1983 at the University of Texas Medical Branch; *Who's Who of American Women* and World's *Who's Who of Women*.

BIBLIOGRAPHY

Application of Rood techniques to the treatment of the cerebral palsied. In *Occupational Therapy for the Multiply Handicapped Child*, West W, Editor. Chicago: Univ of Illinois Press, 1965

Clinical application of sensorimotor treatment techniques in physical dysfunction, and clinical aspects of controversy and confusions in physical dysfunction treatment techniques. In *Expanding Dimensions in Rehabilitation: A Guide for Therapists, Counselors and Rehabilitation Specialists*, Zamir L, Editor. Springfield, IL: Charles C Thomas, 1969

An introduction to treatment techniques developed by Margaret Rood. In *Neuroanatomy and Neurophysiology Underlying Current Treatment Techniques for Sensorimotor Dysfunction*, Perlmutter S, Editor. Chicago: Univ of Illinois Press, 1971

Sensorimotor treatment approaches. In *Occupational Therapy*, 4th Edition, Willard H, Spackman C, Editors. Philadelphia: Lippincott, 1971

Farber S, ———: *Sensorimotor Evaluation and Treatment Procedures for Allied Health Personnel*, 2nd Edition. Indianapolis: Indiana Univ Foundation, 1974

Touch with care or a caring touch? *AJOT* 31:1, 11-18, 1977

Neuroanatomy and neurophysiology; and sensorimotor approaches. In *Willard and Spackman's Occupational Therapy*, 5th Edition, Smith H, Hopkins H, Editors. Philadelphia: Lippincott, 1978

From kinesiology to adaptation. *AJOT* 35:9, 574-580, 1981

Basis for sensorimotor approaches—Neuroanatomy and neurophysiology. Overview of sensorimotor approaches. In *Willard and Spackman's Occupational Therapy*, 6th Edition, Smith H, Hopkins H, Editors. Philadelphia: Lippincott, 1983
Whither thou goest? *AJOT* 38:2, 81-84, 1984

Lorna Jean King, OTR, FAOTA 1978

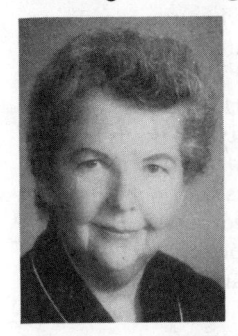

Lorna Jean King, president of the Center for Neurodevelopmental Studies, Inc. in Phoenix, Arizona, specializes in programs for autistic and developmentally delayed children and for schizophrenic adolescents and adults. She is a graduate of Milwaukee-Downer College and has taken graduate courses in juvenile delinquency, criminology, and education at the University of Southern California, the University of California at Los Angeles, and the University of Arizona.

King began her professional career as instructor in the Occupational Therapy Department at the University of Southern California. She has worked with psychiatric programs in the Veteran's Administration Medical Center, Los Angeles, and with delinquent and emotionally disturbed adolescents for the Los Angeles County Juvenile Courts. From 1966 to 1974, King was director of Rehabilitative Therapies at Arizona State Hospital. Since 1974 she has been a consultant and lecturer in the United States, Canada, Australia, New Zealand, and South Africa.

King was elected to the AOTA Roster of Fellows in 1973.

BIBLIOGRAPHY

A sensory-integrative approach to schizophrenia. *AJOT* 28:9, 529-536, 1974
Occupational therapy research in psychiatry: A perspective. *AJOT* 32:1, 15-18, 1978
Toward a science of adaptive responses. *AJOT* 32:7, 429-437, 1978
Theory and Application of Sensory Integrative Treatment for Residents of Long Term Care Facilities with Histories of Chronic Schizophrenia. Phoenix, AZ: Greenroom Publications, 1978
Creative caring. *AJOT* 34:8, 522-528, 1980
The person symbol as an assessment tool. In *The Evaluative Process in Psychiatric Occupational Therapy*, Hemphill B, Editor. Thorofare, NJ: Charles B Slack, 1982
Parachek, JF, ———: *Parachek Geriatric Rating Scale and Treatment Manual*. Phoenix, AZ: 1974, Second Edition, 1982

L. Irene Hollis, OTR   1979

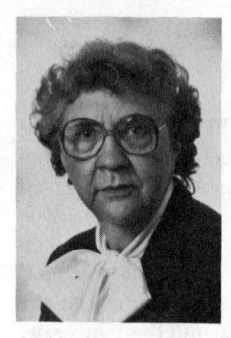

Lucy Irene Hollis entered the field of occupational therapy after working nine years as a high school home economics teacher. She served as a weekend volunteer at an Army Hospital in Texas in 1944 when the War Emergency Courses were initiated. She entered the University of Southern California program and was awarded a certificate in occupational therapy in 1945.

Hollis worked in physical disability programs in army hospitals in Temple and San Antonio, Texas, until 1951. She then had a variety of experiences with polio patients at Houston and at Warm Springs, Georgia. From 1957 to 1962 she served as field consultant in physical disabilities for the AOTA. She is perhaps best known for her 15 years as a specialist in hand rehabilitation at Chapel Hill, North Carolina. Hollis frequently lectured at conferences, conducted workshops, and made movies and videotapes of this work.

In 1977 the North Carolina Occupational Therapy Association presented her the Scullin award. She received the Award of Merit from AOTA in 1973 and was named a Fellow.

BIBLIOGRAPHY

Sniderman M, ———: The use of self-curing acrylic in the making of a mouthpiece to aid the upper extremity paralytic patient. *AJOT* 8:3, 115-117, 1954

Splint substitutes. *AJOT* 21:3, 139-146, 1967

Clip for use with prosthesis. *AJOT* 23:2, 152, 1969

———, Harrison E: An improved surface electrode for monitoring myopotentials. *AJOT* 24:1, 28-31, 1970

Skinnerian occupational therapy. *AJOT* 28:4, 208-213, 1974

Innovative splinting ideas. In *Rehabilitation of the Hand*, Hunter JM, Schneider LH, Mackin EJ, Bell JA, Editors. St. Louis: CV Mosby, 1978

Remember? *AJOT* 33:8, 493-499, 1979

Hand rehabilitation. In *Willard and Spackman's Occupational Therapy*, 6th edition, Hopkins HL, Smith HD, Editors. Philadelphia: JB Lippincott, 1983

Carolyn Manville Baum, MA, OTR, FAOTA 1980

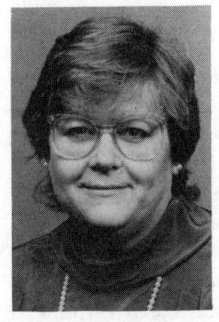

Carolyn Manville Baum is director of Occupational Therapy Services at Irene Walter Johnson Institute of Rehabilitation, and instructor in the Program in Occupational Therapy at Washington University Medical School, St. Louis, Missouri.

Baum holds a bachelor of science degree in occupational therapy from Kansas University and a master of arts degree in health management from Webster University. Formerly she was director of physical medicine and rehabilitation and, before that, director of occupational therapy and staff occupational therapist at Research Medical Center, Kansas City, Missouri.

Her honors include: *Who's Who in the Midwest*, 18th and 19th editions; President, American Occupational Therapy Association, 1982-83; and *Outstanding Young Women of America*, 1976. Baum was named Therapist of the Year, Kansas Occupational Therapy Association in 1973; and Employee of the Year, Research Medical Center in 1972. She was named an AOTA Fellow in 1975. In 1984 she received the AOTA Award of Merit.

BIBLIOGRAPHY

A management tool: The departmental audit. *AJOT* 26:6, 299, 1972

AOTA Continuing Competency Project Contract #1AM-44116, contributing author, 1976

Third Party Reimbursement Manual, Rockville, MD: AOTA, contributing author, 1977

Management and documentation of occupational therapy services. In *Willard and Spackman's Occupational Therapy*, Hopkins H, Smith H, Editors. Philadelphia: JB Lippincott, 1978

Occupational therapists put care in the health system. *AJOT* 34:8, 505-516, 1980

Nationally speaking. Independent living: A critical role for occupational therapy. *AJOT* 34:12, 773-774, 1980

A look into the '80s. *Swiss Journal of Occupational Therapy*, August 1981

Opportunity for occupational therapy: The time is now. *AJOT* 36:6, 363-364, 1982

A perspective of occupational therapy in the U.S. Health System. Proceedings of the 8th International Congress World Federation of Occupational Therapists, 1: 29-36, Hamburg: Federal Republic of Germany, 1982

Letter to the Editor: A study of sensory integration therapies. *Journal of Learning Disabilities* 15:1, January 1982

Nationally speaking. Strategic integrated management system—SIMS. *AJOT* 37:9, 595-600, 1983

A look at our strengths in the '80s: Presidential address. *AJOT* 37:7, 451-455, 1983

———, Devereaux E: A systems perspective: Conceptualizing and implementing occupational therapy in today's complex environment. In *Willard and Spackman's Occupational Therapy*, 6th Edition, Hopkins H, Smith H, Editors. Philadelphia: JB Lippincott, 799-814, 1983

———, Boyle MA, Edwards D: Initiating occupational therapy clinical research. *AJOT* 38:4, 267-269, 1984

Robert K. Bing, EdD, OTR, FAOTA   1981

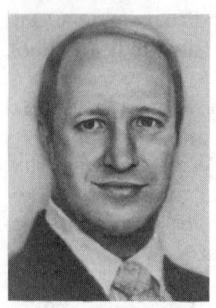

by April McConnell, OTS

Robert K. Bing received his bachelor of science degree in occupational therapy from the University of Illinois and master of arts and doctor of education degrees from the University of Maryland. His major fields of study were human development education and recreation.

He has held clinical occupational therapy appointments in the US Army; Norwich, Connecticut Hospital; Illinois State Psychiatric Institute, Chicago; and The University of Texas Medical Branch Hospitals, Galveston. His faculty appointments have been at Richmond Professional Institute (Virginia Commonwealth University); the Universities of Nebraska, Florida, and Illinois; and The University of Texas Medical Branch. For fourteen years he served as planning director and, subsequently, Dean, The University of Texas School of Allied Health Sciences, Galveston, where he currently is professor of occupational therapy.

Bing has been active in state and national occupational therapy associations, including the presidency of two state organizations. He has chaired several committees. In the AOTA, he has served on the Executive Board; the *AJOT* Editorial Board and numerous committees. In 1982, he was elected President-Elect for one year and for a three-year term as President of the AOTA.

Bing's honors include the Texas Occupational Therapist of the Year award; Honorary Citizen, Hidalgo, Texas; Outstanding Research, The University of Texas School of Allied Health Sciences; and in the AOTA, a Certificate of Appreciation and Fellow. He is cited in *Who's Who in Health Care*; *Who's Who in the South and Southwest*; and *Who's Who in America*.

BIBLIOGRAPHY

Action research—How can we? *Proceedings*, AOTA Annual Conference, Rockville, MD: AOTA, 1961

Adult recreation and the 'Becoming of Youth': A proposal for prevention of deviant behavior. *Illinois Parks*, November-December 1964

Offenkrantz W, ———: A psychoanalytically oriented case conference for occupational therapy students. *AJOT* 21:2, 70, 1967

William Rush Dunton, Jr.: American psychiatrist and occupational therapist 1868-1966, *AJOT* 21:3, 1967

Therapeutic use of self: A formulation. Methods of measurement and evaluation in psychiatric dysfunction. The therapist's responsibility to the patient and the community. In *Expanding Dimensions in Rehabilitation*, Zamir LJ, Editor. Springfield, IL: Charles C Thomas, 1969

Requisites for relevance: Changing concepts in occupational therapy education. *New York Academy of Science Monograph 2559*, 1969

Study guide: Learning theory. In *Reference Handbook for Continuing Education*, Rockville, MD: AOTA, 1970

Occupational therapy revisited: A paraphrastic journey. *AJOT* 35:8, 499-518, 1981
————, et al: Rehabilitation services. In *The Health Professions*, Boylen MV, Morgan MK, McCaulley MH. Philadelphia: WB Saunders, 1982
Nationally speaking. Professional nationalism. *AJOT* 37:5, 301-304, 1983
Beliefs at a new beginning: Inaugural address. *AJOT* 37:6, 375-379, 1983
Nationally speaking. The industry, the art, and the philosophy of history. *AJOT* 37:12, 800-801, 1983
Nationally speaking. Living forward, understanding backwards, Part I. *AJOT* 38:6, 363-366, 1984
Nationally speaking. Living forward, understanding backwards, Part II. *AJOT* 38:7, 435-439, 1984

Joan C. Rogers, PhD, OTR, FAOTA   1983

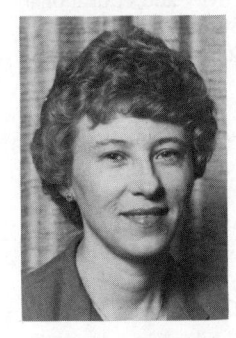

Joan C. Rogers holds a bachelor's degree in biology from Canisius College, Buffalo, New York; a master's degree in occupational therapy from the University of Southern California; and a doctor of philosophy degree, with a major in educational psychology, from the University of Illinois at Urbana.

She has worked clinically at the Edward J. Meyer Memorial Hospital, Buffalo, New York, and in numerous programs as a private practitioner. Rogers has held academic appointments at the State University of New York at Buffalo, the University of Southern California, and the University of North Carolina, Chapel Hill. Currently, she is an associate professor in occupational therapy and an assistant professor in psychiatry at the University of Pittsburgh. She has provided volunteer services to the AOTA and Foundation in a variety of capacities, including membership on the Editorial Board of *The American Journal of Occupational Therapy* and *The Occupational Therapy Journal of Research*, and serving as regional research consultant for the southeast.

Rogers was named a Fellow of the AOTA in 1981 and received service awards for chairing the Gerontology Special Interest Section (SIS) and serving as the SIS liaison to the Commission on Practice in 1983. She was named the Third Brookdale Visiting Scholar by the Brookdale Institute on Aging and Human Development of Columbia University for 1983-84. She was selected as a charter member of the AOTF Academy of Research in 1984.

BIBLIOGRAPHY

————, Figone JJ: The avocational pursuits of rehabilitants with traumatic quadriplegia. *AJOT* 32:9, 571-576, 1978
————, Weinstein JM, Figone JJ: The interest check list: An empirical assessment. *AJOT* 32:10, 628-630, 1978
The design of master's programs in baccalaureate level professions. In *Proceedings of the Conference on the Assessment of Quality Master's Programs*: Commission on Higher Edu-

cation of the Middle States Association of Colleges and Schools, Council of Graduate Schools in the US, College Park, MD: Univ of Maryland, 1979

———, Figone JJ: Psychosocial parameters in treating the person with quadriplegia. *AJOT* 33:7, 432-439, 1979

Advocacy: The key to assessment for the elderly. *The Journal of Gerontological Nursing* 6: 33-36, 1980

Design of the master's degree in occupational therapy, Part 1: A logical approach. *AJOT* 34:2, 113-118, 1980

Design of the master's degree in occupational therapy, Part 2: An empirical approach. *AJOT* 34:3, 176-184, 1980

———, Figone JJ: Traumatic quadriplegia: A follow-up study of self-care skills. *Archives of Physical Medicine and Rehabilitation* 61: 316-321, 1980

———, Mann WC. The relationship between professional productivity and educational level, Part I: Review of literature and methodology. *AJOT* 34:6, 387-392, 1980

———, Mann WC: The relationship between professional productivity and educational level, Part II: Results and discussion. *AJOT* 34:7, 460-468, 1980

———, Hill DJ: Learning style preferences of bachelor's and master's students in occupational therapy. *AJOT* 34:12, 789-793, 1980

Gerontic occupational therapy. *AJOT* 35:10, 663-666, 1981

Order and disorder in medicine and occupational therapy. *AJOT* 36:1, 29-35, 1982

Educating the scholarly practitioner. *Occupational Therapy Journal of Research* 2: 3-11, 1982

Terminology quandary in education. *AJOT* 36:3, 188-192, 1982

Sponsorship: Developing leaders for occupational therapy. *AJOT* 36:5, 309-313, 1982

———, Snow T: An assessment of the feeding behaviors of the institutionalized elderly. *AJOT* 36:6, 375-380, 1982

Teaching clinical reasoning for practice in geriatrics. *Physical and Occupational Therapy in Geriatrics* 1: 29-37, 1982

———, Masagatani G: Clinical reasoning of occupational therapists during the initial assessment of physically disabled patients: A pilot study. *Occupational Therapy Journal of Research* 2: 195-219, 1982

The spirit of independence: The evolution of a philosophy. *AJOT* 36-11, 709-715, 1982

The occupational needs of older persons: A focus of occupational therapy practice. *Physical and Occupational Therapy in Geriatrics* 2: 1-3, 1982

———, Snow TL: Fieldwork in indirect service. In *Service-Learning in Aging: Implications for Occupational Therapy*. Washington, DC: The National Council on the Aging, Inc., 1982

———, Cordes D: Role delineation: Re-employment of older workers. In *Monograph, Service-Learning in Aging: Implications for Occupational Therapy*. Washington, DC: The National Council on the Aging, 1982

Assistive devices—Aids to functional independence. *American Health Care Association Journal*: 31-36, March 1983

Clinical reasoning: The ethics, science, and art. *AJOT* 37:9, 601-616, 1983

Roles and functions of occupational therapy in long-term care: Occupational therapy and activities programs. *AJOT* 37:12, 807-812, 1983

The study of human occupation. In *Occupational Therapy Toward a Definition of Practice for the Future*, Kielhofner G, Editor. Philadelphia: FA Davis, 94-124, 1983

Why study human occupation? *AJOT* 38:1, 47-49, 1984

Occupational therapy for the older disabled adult. *Generations*, Summer 1984

———, Snow T: The model of human occupation applied to aging. Gerontic occupational therapy. In *A Model of Human Occupation: Theory and Application*, Kielhofner G, Editor. Baltimore: Williams and Wilkins, Spring 1985

———, Kielhofner G: Treatment planning. In *A Model of Human Occupation: Theory and Application*, Kielhofner G, Editor. Baltimore: Williams and Wilkins, Spring 1985

Elnora M. Gilfoyle, DSc, OTR, FAOTA   1984

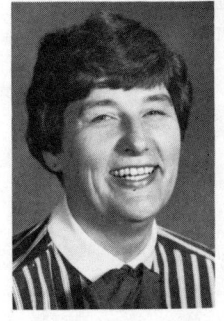

Elnora M. Gilfoyle is an associate professor and head of the Department of Occupational Therapy at Colorado State University in Fort Collins. A graduate of the State University of Iowa with a degree in occupational therapy, she holds an honorary doctor of science degree from Colorado State University.

Gilfoyle served as Project Coordinator for the Training: Occupational Therapy Education Management in Schools (TOTEMS) project funded by the Department of Education; consultant and faculty member for the John F. Kennedy Child Development Center, University of Colorado; director of occupational therapy, The Denver Children's Hospital; and staff therapist at Craig Rehabilitation Center and Denver General Hospital.

She has served as an officer of the AOTA and Occupational Therapy Association of Colorado. Her awards include the Marjorie Ball Lectureship Award from the Occupational Therapy Association of Colorado and listing in *Who's Who in America*. She was named to the AOTA Roster of Fellows in 1973.

BIBLIOGRAPHY

Young J, Gordon G, ———: Functional use of 'nylon' muscle in severe quadriplegia. *Archives of Physical Medicine and Rehabilitation*, April 1961

Functional hand bracing. *Children's Hospital Medical Journal*, Denver, CO, 1962

Functional bracing in the treatment of cerebral palsy. In *Occupational Therapy for the Multiply Handicapped Child*, West W, Editor. Chicago: Univ of Illinois Press, 1965

The three faces of Ev. In *Evaluation and treatment of perceptual-motor dysfunction*, West W, Editor. Madison. Univ of Wisconsin Press, 1966

Martin H, ———: Assessment of perceptual development. *AJOT* 23:1, 1-14, 1969

———, Grady A: cognitive-perceptual-motor development. In *Occupational Therapy*, 4th Edition, Willard, Spackman, Editors. Philadelphia: JB Lippincott, 1970

———, Grady A: A developmental theory of sensory-motor reactions and spontaneous integrative behavior. *Symposium for Somatosensory Perceptual Deficits*. Boston: Boston Univ Press, 1971

Research in sensory-integrative development. *AJOT* 27:4, 189-191, 1973

Yerxa E, ———: Research seminar. *AJOT* 30:8, 509-514, 1976

Henderson A, Llorens L, ———: (Editors) *The Development of Sensory Integrative Theory and Practice*—A collection of the works of A. Jean Ayres. Rockville, MD: AOTA, 1976

Price A, ———, Myers C (Editors): *Research in Sensory-Integrative Development*. Rockville, MD: AOTA, 1976

————, Grady A: Posture and movement development: Minimal brain dysfunction. In *Willard and Spackman's Occupational Therapy*, 5th Edition, Smith, Hopkins, Editors. Philadelphia: Lippincott, 1978

Current occupational therapy roles and functions in the education of handicapped students. *AJOT* 33:9, 1979

Training: Occupational Therapy Educational Management in Schools. (Editor and major author). Rockville, MD: AOTA, 1980

Caring—A philosophy for practice. *AJOT* 34:9, 1980

————, Grady A, Moore J: *Children Adapt*. Thorofare, NJ: Charles B Slack, 1981

————, Grady A: Spatiotemporal adaptation. In *Willard and Spackman's Occupational Therapy*, 6th Edition, Smith, Hopkins, Editors. Philadelphia: JB Lippincott, 1983

Transformation of a profession. *AJOT* 38:9, 575-584, 1984